Thyroid Ultrasound
and Ultrasound-Guided FNA

H. Jack Baskin, Sr. • Daniel S. Duick
Robert A. Levine
Editors

Thyroid Ultrasound and Ultrasound-Guided FNA

Third Edition

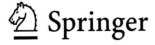 Springer

Editors
H. Jack Baskin, Sr.
University of Central Florida
Orlando, FL, USA

Daniel S. Duick
Endocrinology Associates, PA
Scottsdale, AZ, USA

Robert A. Levine
Thyroid Center of New
    Hampshire
Nashua, NH, USA

ISBN 978-1-4614-4784-9   ISBN 978-1-4614-4785-6 (eBook)
DOI 10.1007/978-1-4614-4785-6
Springer New York Heidelberg Dordrecht London

Library of Congress Control Number: 2012947989

Foreword

This third edition of "Thyroid Ultrasound and Ultrasound-Guided FNA" by Drs. Baskin, Duick, and Levine expands upon the first two editions, including new chapters and authors, and is an essential guide for endocrinologists, endocrine fellows, radiologists, general surgeons with an interest in thyroid and parathyroid surgery, and head and neck surgeons. Over the past decade, the incidence of thyroid cancer in the United States continues to rise (estimated to be 57,000 men and women during 2012), including those patients with more locally invasive and systemic disease.

The use of sophisticated neck ultrasound to detect benign and malignant thyroid nodules, lymph nodes, and cysts, parathyroid adenomas, salivary gland tumors, and other neck lesions has markedly improved our ability to find even smaller thyroid nodules, to help differentiate benign from malignant thyroid nodules and lymph nodes, and to confirm the presence of parathyroid adenomas.

Several new and extremely informative chapters have been added to this third edition: the use of ultrasound in the pediatric population; mapping of neck lymph nodes; surgical trends in the management of thyroid nodules and cancer, and parathyroid disease; evaluation of the salivary glands and nonendocrine tumors; extensive use of thyroid cancer molecular markers in fine needle aspirates; and an up-to-date guideline on preparing ultrasound reports. The chapters on the use of laser and radiofrequency ablation of thyroid nodules and ultrasound elastography to differentiate between benign and malignant thyroid nodules are updated. Although these techniques are innovative, their practical use remains to be determined.

This textbook is extremely informative and should be available to all physicians and trainees with an interest in the diagnostic and operative approach to thyroid and parathyroid disease.

Lewis E. Braverman

Preface to First Edition

Over the past two decades, ultrasound has undergone numerous advances in technology, such as gray-scale imaging, realtime sonography, high resolution 7.5–10 Mtz transducers, and color-flow Doppler that make ultrasound unsurpassed in its ability to provide very accurate images of the thyroid gland quickly, inexpensively, and safely. However, in spite of these advances, ultrasound remains drastically underutilized by endocrinologists. This is due in part to a lack of understanding of the ways in which ultrasound can aid in the diagnosis of various thyroid conditions, and to a lack of experience in ultrasound technique by the clinician.

The purpose of this book is to demonstrate how ultrasound is integrated with the history, physical examination, and other thyroid tests (especially FNA biopsy) to provide valuable information that can be used to improve patient care. Numerous ultrasound examples are used to show the interactions between ultrasound and tissue characteristics and explain their clinical significance. Also presented is the work of several groups of investigators worldwide who have explored new applications of ultrasound that have led to novel techniques that are proving to be clinically useful.

To reach its full potential, it is critical that thyroid ultrasound be performed by the examining physician. This book instructs the physician on how to perform the ultrasound at the bedside so that it becomes part of the physical examination. mong the new developments discussed are the new digital phased-array transducers that allow ultrasound and FNA biopsy to be combined in the technique of ultrasound-guided FNA biopsy. Over the next decade, this technique will become a part of our routine clinical practice and a powerful new tool in the diagnosis of thyroid nodules and in the follow-up of thyroid cancer patients.

H. Jack Baskin, MD
Editor

Preface to Second Edition

In the eight years since the publication of the first edition of this book, ultrasound has become an integral part of the practice of endocrinology. Ultrasound guidance for obtaining accurate diagnostic material by FNA is now accepted normal procedure. As the chief editor of Thyroid wrote in a recent editorial: "I do not know how anyone can see thyroid patients without their own ultrasound by their side." The widespread adoption of this new technology by clinicians in a relatively short span of time is unprecedented.

While most endocrinologists now feel comfortable using ultrasound for the diagnosis of thyroid nodules, many are reluctant to expand its use beyond the thyroid. Its value as a diagnostic tool to look for evidence of thyroid cancer in neck lymph nodes, or to evaluate parathyroid disease is at least as great as it is in evaluating thyroid nodules. In this second edition, we continue to explore these diagnostic techniques that are readily available to all clinicians.

Since the first edition, clinical investigators have continued to discover new techniques and applications for thyroid and neck ultrasound. Power Doppler has replaced color flow Doppler for examining blood flow in the tissues of the neck. Other new advances in diagnosis include ultrasound contrast media, ultrasound elastography, and harmonic imaging.

The only ultrasound-guided therapeutic procedure addressed in the 2000 edition was percutaneous ethanol injection (PEI), which had not been reported from the United States but was commonly practiced elsewhere in the world. Today, other ultrasound-guided therapeutic procedures such as laser, radiofrequency, and high intensity focused ultrasound (HIFU) are being used for ablation of tissue without surgery. These innovative procedures are discussed by the physicians who are developing them.

We hope that this second edition will inspire clinicians to proceed beyond using ultrasound just for the diagnosis of nodular goiter. The benefits to patients will continue as clinicians advance neck ultrasound to its full potential.

H. Jack Baskin, MD
Editor, 2008

Preface to Third Edition

The ninetieth century essayist, Frédéric Bastiat, in speaking of the qualities of a readable and enduring book, said: "It must be short, clear, accurate and as full of feeling as of ideas; *all at the same time*." We have tried to adhere to these qualities in the current volume. As in the previous editions, we have chosen authors who have enthusiastically adapted ultrasound in the diagnosis and treatment of thyroid and ancillary disease of the neck. Each contributor has extensive hands-on experience and contributed to the accumulating knowledge in the field as well as being ardent teachers of this knowledge to others.

Readers will notice some changes from past editions of this book. Some topics given complete chapters in previous editions have been combined into a single chapter. Other chapters have been expanded and new chapters have been added to encompass recent techniques such as employing UGFNA acquired material for molecular and genetic markers and using ultrasound guidance for radiofrequency ablation. A separate chapter on pediatric ultrasound and congenital abnormalities has been added. Other new chapters focus on the effect ultrasound has had on the surgical management of thyroid and parathyroid disease.

Since the first publication of *Thyroid Ultrasound and UGFNA* in 2000, ultrasound has become established as a primary tool for diagnosing and managing thyroid disease. Indeed, over the last 10 years ultrasound has become a catalyst for bringing together endocrinologists, surgeons, radiologists, and pathologists to create a multidisciplinary approach to the management of thyroid disease which is and will continue to benefit our patients.

Salt Lake City, UT, USA   Henry J. Baskin

Contents

Contributors

Robert A. Levine, MD, FACE, ECNU Thyroid Center of New Hampshire, Dartmouth Medical School, Nashua, NH, USA

Dara R. Treadwell, BS, BT, RDMS Tavares, FL, USA

Henry J. Baskin, Jr MD, DACR Department of Radiology, Primary Children's Medical Center, University of Utah School of Medicine, Salt Lake City, UT, USA

Mark A. Lupo, MD, FACE, ECNU Florida State University College of Medicine, Thyroid & Endocrine Center of Florida, Sarasota, FL, USA

Susan J. Mandel, MD, MPH Perelman School of Medicine, University of Pennsylvania, Philadelphia, PA, USA

Jill E. Langer, MD Perelman School of Medicine, University of Pennsylvania, Philadelphia, PA, USA

Gregory Randolph, MD, FACS General and Thyroid Surgical Divisions Mass Eye and Ear Infirmary, Harvard Medical School, Boston, MA, USA

Barry Sacks, MD Beth Israel Deaconess Medical Center, Natick, MA, USA

H. Jack Baskin, Sr MD, MACE University of Central Florida College of Medicine, Orlando, FL, USA

Dev Abraham, MD, MRCP University of Utah, Salt Lake City, UT, USA

Haengrang Ryu, MD MD Anderson Cancer Center, Yonsei University College of Medicine, Seoul, South Korea

Rachel Harris, MD Department of Surgical Oncology, MD Anderson Cancer Center, The University of Texas MD Anderson Cancer Center, Houston, TX, USA

Nancy D. Perrier, MD, FACS Department of Surgical Oncology, Section of Surgical Endocrinology, The University of Texas MD Anderson Cancer Center, Houston, TX, USA

Robert A. Sofferman, MD University Vermont College of Medicine, Burlington, VT, USA

Roberto Valcavi, MD, FACE Endocrinology Unit, Arcispedale Santa Maria Nuova, Reggio Emilia, Italy

Giorgio Stecconi Bortolani, MD Endocrine Unit, Arcispedale Santa Maria Nuova, Reggio Emilia, Italy

Fabrizio Riganti, MD Endocrine Unit, Arcispedale Santa Maria Nuova, Reggio Emilia, Italy

Andrea Frasoldati, MD Endocrine Unit, Arcispedale Santa Maria Nuova, Reggio Emilia, Italy

Daniel S. Duick, MD, FACP, FACE University of Arizona Health Sciences Center, Endocrinology Associates, PA, Scottsdale, AZ, USA

J. Woody Sistrunk, MD, FACE, ECNU Jackson Thyroid and Endocrine Clinic, Jackson, MS, USA

CHAPTER 1
History of Thyroid Ultrasound

Robert A. Levine

INTRODUCTION

The thyroid is well suited to ultrasound study because of its superficial location, vascularity, size, and echogenicity [1]. In addition, the thyroid has a very high incidence of nodular disease, the vast majority benign. Most structural abnormalities of the thyroid need evaluation and monitoring, but not intervention [2]. Thus, the thyroid was among the first organs to be well studied by ultrasound. The first reports of thyroid ultrasound appeared in the late 1960s. Between 1965 and 1970 there were seven articles published specific to thyroid ultrasound. In the last 5 years there have been over 2,200 articles published. Thyroid ultrasound has undergone a dramatic transformation from the cryptic deflections on an oscilloscope produced in A-mode scanning, to barely recognizable B-mode images, followed by initial low resolution gray scale, and now modern high resolution images. Recent advances in technology, including harmonic imaging, spatial compound imaging, contrast studies, and three-dimensional reconstruction, have furthered the field.

In 1880, Pierre and Jacques Curie discovered the piezoelectric effect, determining that an electric current applied across a crystal would result in a vibration that would generate sound waves, and that sound waves striking a crystal would, in turn, produce an electric voltage. Piezoelectric transducers were capable of producing sonic waves in the audible range and ultrasonic waves above the range of human hearing.

SONAR

The first operational sonar system was produced 2 years after the sinking of the Titanic in 1912. This system was capable of detecting an iceberg located 2 miles distant from a ship. A low-frequency

H.J. Baskin et al. (eds.), *Thyroid Ultrasound and Ultrasound-Guided FNA*,
DOI 10.1007/978-1-4614-4785-6_1,
© Springer Science+Business Media, LLC 2013

audible pulse was generated, and a human operator listened for a change in the return echo. This system was able to detect, but not localize, objects within range of the sonar [3].

Over the next 30 years navigational sonar improved, and imaging progressed from passive sonar, with an operator listening for reflected sounds, to display of returned sounds as a one-dimensional oscilloscope pattern, to two-dimensional images capable of showing the shape of the object being detected.

EARLY MEDICAL APPLICATIONS

The first medical application of ultrasound occurred in the 1940s. Following the observation that very high intensity sound waves had the ability to damage tissues, lower intensities were tried for therapeutic uses. Focused sound waves were used to mildly heat tissue for therapy of rheumatoid arthritis, and early attempts were made to destroy the basal ganglia to treat Parkinson's disease [4].

The first diagnostic application of ultrasound occurred in 1942. In a paper entitled "Hyperphonagraphy of the Brain," Karl Theodore Dussic reported localization of the cerebral ventricles using ultrasound. Unlike the current reflective technique, his system relied on the transmission of sound waves, placing a sound source on one side of the head, with a receiver on the other side. A pulse was transmitted, with the detected signal purportedly able to show the location of midline structures. While the results of these studies were later discredited as predominantly artifact, this work played a significant role in stimulating research into the diagnostic capabilities of ultrasound [4].

Early in the 1950s the first imaging by pulse–echo reflection was tried. A-mode imaging showed deflections on an oscilloscope to indicate the distance to reflective surfaces. Providing information limited to a single dimension, A-mode scanning indicated only distance to reflective surfaces (see Fig. 2.7) [5]. A-mode ultrasonography was used for detection of brain tumors, shifts in the midline structures of the brain, localization of foreign bodies in the eye, and detection of detached retinas. In the first presage that ultrasound may assist in the detection of cancer, John Julian Wild reported the observation that gastric malignancies were more echogenic than normal gastric tissue. He later studied 117 breast nodules using a 15 MHz sound source, and reported that he was able to determine their size with an accuracy of 90%.

During the late 1950s the first two-dimensional B-mode scanners were developed. B-mode scanners display a compilation of sequential A-mode images to create a two-dimensional image (see Fig. 2.2). Douglass Howry developed an immersion tank

B-mode ultrasound system, and several models of immersion tank scanners followed. All utilized a mechanically driven transducer that would sweep through an arc, with an image reconstructed to demonstrate the full sweep. Later advances included a hand-held transducer that still required a mechanical connection to the unit to provide data regarding location, and water-bag coupling devices to eliminate the need for immersion [6].

THYROID ULTRASOUND

Application of ultrasound for thyroid imaging began in the late 1960s. In July 1967 Fujimoto et al. reported data on 184 patients studied with a B-mode ultrasound "tomogram" utilizing a water bath [7]. The authors reported that no internal echoes were generated by the thyroid in patients with no known thyroid dysfunction and nonpalpable thyroid glands. They described four basic patterns generated by palpably abnormal thyroid tissue. The type 1 pattern was called "cystic" due to the virtual absence of echoes within the structure, and negligible attenuation of the sound waves passing through the lesion. Type 2 was labeled "sparsely spotted," showing only a few small echoes without significant attenuation. The type 3 pattern was considered "malignant" and was described as generating strong internal echoes. The echoes were moderately bright and were accompanied by marked attenuation of the signal. Type 4 had a lack of internal echoes but strong attenuation. In the patients studied, 65% of the (predominantly follicular) carcinomas had a type 3 pattern. Unfortunately, 25% of benign adenomas were also type 3. Further, 25% of papillary carcinomas were found to have the type 2 pattern. While the first major publication of thyroid ultrasound attempted to establish the ability to determine malignant potential, the results were nonspecific in a large percentage of the cases.

In December 1971 Manfred Blum published a series of A-mode ultrasounds of thyroid nodules (Fig. 2.1) [5]. He demonstrated the ability of ultrasound to distinguish solid from cystic nodules, as well as accuracy in measurement of the dimensions of thyroid nodules. Additional publications in the early 1970s further confirmed the capacity for both A-mode and B-mode ultrasound to differentiate solid from cystic lesions, but consistently demonstrated that ultrasound was unable to distinguish malignant from benign solid lesions with acceptable accuracy [8].

The advent of gray scale display resulted in images that were far easier to view and interpret [9]. In 1974 Ernest Crocker published "The Gray Scale Echographic Appearance of Thyroid Malignancy" [10]. Using an 8 MHz transducer with a 0.5 mm resolution, he described "low amplitude, sparse and disordered echoes" characteristic of thyroid cancer when viewed with a gray scale display. The pattern felt to be characteristic of malignancy was what would now be considered "hypoechoic and heterogeneous." Forty of the eighty patients studied underwent surgery. All six of the thyroid malignancies diagnosed had the described (hypoechoic) pattern. The percentage of benign lesions showing this pattern was not reported in the publication.

With each advancement, in technology, interest was again rekindled in ultrasound's ability to distinguish a benign from a malignant lesion. Initial reports of ultrasonic features typically describe findings as being diagnostically specific. Later, reports follow showing overlap between various disease processes. For example, following an initial report that the "halo sign," a rim of hypoechoic signal surrounding a solid thyroid nodule, was seen only in benign lesions [11], Propper reported that two of ten patients with this finding had carcinoma [12]. As discussed in Chap. 6 the halo sign is still considered to be one of the numerous features that can be used in determining the likelihood of malignancy in a nodule.

In 1977 Wallfish recommended combining fine-needle aspiration biopsy with ultrasound in order to improve the accuracy of biopsy specimens [13]. Recent studies have continued to demonstrate that biopsy accuracy is greatly improved when ultrasound is used to guide placement of the biopsy needle. Most patients with prior "nondiagnostic" biopsies will have an adequate specimen when ultrasound-guided biopsy is performed [14]. Ultrasound-guided fine-needle aspiration results in improved sensitivity and specificity of biopsies as well as a greater than 50% reduction in nondiagnostic and false negative biopsies [15].

In the 1980s the utility of thyroid ultrasound became evident. Within 4 years after the Chernobyl nuclear accident, the incidence of papillary thyroid cancer increased 100-fold among young children in areas of high radiation exposure. Ultrasound screening of these children detected thousands of patients with early thyroid cancer and allowed surgical cure. Screening continues to be performed on this population, and the death rate from thyroid cancer among these individuals remains nil. Ultrasound screening has also been demonstrated to be of value in patients with relatives having familial papillary or medullary thyroid cancer.

Ultrasound also has a useful role in population screening for iodine deficiency. Ultrasound provides a simple and accurate way to measure thyroid gland volume. It has been shown that thyroid volume in children correlates well with both dietary iodine content and urinary iodine excretion. Thus ultrasound provides an efficient method of identifying iodine deficient areas of the world. Ultrasound screening has proven easier to accomplish and as accurate as 24 h urine collection, and has expedited the treatment of endemic goiter.

Current resolution allows demonstration of thyroid nodules smaller than 1 mm; thus ultrasound has clear advantages over palpation in detecting and characterizing thyroid nodular disease. Nearly 50% of patients found to have a solitary thyroid nodule by palpation will be shown to have additional nodules by ultrasound, and more than 25% of the additional nodules are larger than 1 cm [16]. With a prevalence estimated between 19 and 67%, the management of incidentally detected, nonpalpable thyroid nodules remains controversial [17]. Several guidelines have been developed to assist in deciding which nodules warrant biopsy and which may be monitored without tissue sampling. These guidelines are discussed in Chap. 7.

Over the past several years the value of ultrasound in screening for suspicious lymph nodes prior to surgery in patients with biopsy proven cancer has been established. Current guidelines for the management of thyroid cancer indicate a pivotal role for ultrasound in monitoring for loco-regional recurrence [17].

During the 1980s Doppler ultrasound was developed, allowing detection of flow in blood vessels. As discussed in Chap. 3 the Doppler pattern of blood flow within the thyroid nodules may play a role in assessing the likelihood of malignancy. Doppler imaging may also demonstrate the increased blood flow characteristic of Graves' disease [18], and may be useful in distinguishing between Graves' disease and thyroiditis, especially in pregnant patients or patients with amiodarone-induced hyperthyroidism [19].

Recent technological advancements include intravenous sonographic contrast agents, three-dimensional ultrasound imaging, and elastography. Intravenous sonographic contrast agents are available in Europe, but remain experimental in the United States. All ultrasound contrast agents consist of microspheres, which function both by reflecting ultrasonic waves and, at higher signal power, by reverberating and generating harmonics of the incident wave. Ultrasound contrast agents have been predominantly used to visualize large blood vessels, with less utility in enhancing parenchymal tissues. They have shown promise in imaging peripheral vasculature as well as liver tumors and metastases [20], but no studies have been published demonstrating an advantage of contrast agents in routine thyroid imaging. The use of contrast agents may be helpful in the early assessment of successful laser or radiofrequency ablation of thyroid nodules [21].

Three-dimensional display of reconstructed images has been available for CT scan and MRI for many years and has demonstrated practical application. While three-dimensional ultrasound has gained popularity for fetal imaging, its role in diagnostic ultrasound remains unclear. While obstetrical ultrasound has the great advantage of the target being surrounded by a natural fluid interface, greatly improving surface rendering, three-dimensional thyroid ultrasound is limited by the lack of a similar interface distinguishing the thyroid from adjacent neck tissues. It has been predicted that breast biopsies may eventually be guided in a more precise fashion by real time three-dimensional imaging [22], and it is possible that, in time, thyroid biopsy will similarly benefit. At the present time, however, three-dimensional ultrasound technology does not provide a demonstrable advantage in thyroid imaging.

Elastography is a promising technique in which the compressibility of a nodule is assessed by ultrasound while external pressure is applied. With studies showing a good predictive value for prediction of malignancy in breast nodules, recent investigations of its role in thyroid imaging have been promising. Additional prospective trials are ongoing to assess the role of elastography in predicting the likelihood of thyroid malignancy. The role of elastography in the selection of nodules for biopsy or surgery is discussed in Chap. 15.

With the growing recognition that real time ultrasound performed by an endocrinologist provides far more useful information than that obtained from a radiology report, office ultrasound by endocrinologists has gained acceptance. The first educational course specific to thyroid ultrasound was offered by the American Association of Clinical Endocrinologists (AACE) in 1998. Under the direction of Dr. H. Jack Baskin, 53 endocrinologists were taught to perform diagnostic ultrasound and ultrasound-guided fine-needle aspiration biopsy. By the turn of the century 300 endocrinologists had been trained. Endocrine University, established in 2002 by AACE, began providing instruction in thyroid ultrasound and biopsy to all graduating endocrine fellows. By the end of 2011 over 4,000 endocrinologists had completed an AACE ultrasound course. In 2007 a collaborative effort between the American Institute of Ultrasound in Medicine and the AACE established a certification program for endocrinologists trained in neck ultrasound. By the end of 2011 the ECNU (Endocrine Certification in Neck Ultrasound) program had certified over 200 endocrinologists as having the training, experience, and expertise needed to perform thyroid and parathyroid ultrasound and fine needle aspiration biopsy. In 2011 the American Institute of Ultrasound in

Medicine began accrediting qualified endocrine practices as centers of excellence in thyroid and parathyroid imaging.

In the 40 years since ultrasound was first used for thyroid imaging, there has been a profound improvement in the technology and quality of images. The transition from A-mode to B-mode to gray scale images was accompanied by dramatic improvements in clarity and interpretability of images. Current high resolution images are able to identify virtually all lesions of clinical significance. Ultrasound characteristics cannot predict benign lesions, but features including irregular margins, microcalcifications, and central vascularity may deem a nodule suspicious [3]. Ultrasound plays a clear fundamental role in thyroid nodule evaluation and the selection of which nodules should undergo biopsy. [17] Ultrasound has proven utility in the detection of recurrent thyroid cancer in patients with negative whole body iodine scan or undetectable thyroglobulin [17, 23]. Recent advances including the use of contrast agents, tissue harmonic imaging, elastography, and multiplanar reconstruction of images will likely further enhance the diagnostic value of ultrasound images. The use of Doppler flow analysis and elastography may improve the predictive value for determining the risk of malignancy, but no current ultrasound technique is capable of determining benignity with an acceptable degree of accuracy. Ultrasound guidance of fine-needle aspiration biopsy has been demonstrated to improve both diagnostic yield and accuracy, and is becoming the standard of care. Routine clinical use of ultrasound is often considered an extension of the physical examination by endocrinologists. High quality ultrasound systems are now available at prices that make this technology accessible to virtually all providers of endocrine care [3].

References

1. Solbiati L, Osti V, Cova L, Tonolini M. Ultrasound of the thyroid, parathyroid glands and neck lymph nodes. Eur Radiol. 2001;11(12):2411–24.
2. Tessler FN, Tublin ME. Thyroid sonography: current applications and future directions. AJR Am J Roentgenol. 1999;173:437–43.
3. Levine RA. Something old and something new: a brief history of thyroid ultrasound technology. Endocr Pract. 2004;10(3):227–33.
4. Woo JSK. A short history of the development of ultrasound in obstetrics and gynecology. 2011. http://www.ob-ultrasound.net/history1. html. Accessed 16 Dec 2011.
5. Blum M, Weiss B, Hernberg J. Evaluation of thyroid nodules by A-mode echography. Radiology. 1971;101:651–6.
6. Skolnick ML, Royal DR. A simple and inexpensive water bath adapting a contact scanner for thyroid and testicular imaging. J Clin Ultrasound. 1975;3(3):225–7.

7. Fujimoto F, Oka A, Omoto R, Hirsoe M. Ultrasound scanning of the thyroid gland as a new diagnostic approach. Ultrasonics. 1967;5:177–80.

8. Thijs LG. Diagnostic ultrasound in clinical thyroid investigation. J Clin Endocrinol Metab. 1971;32(6):709–16.

9. Scheible W, Leopold GR, Woo VL, Gosink BB. High resolution real-time ultrasonography of thyroid nodules. Radiology. 1979;133:413–7.

10. Crocker EF, McLaughlin AF, Kossoff G, Jellins J. The gray scale echographic appearance of thyroid malignancy. J Clin Ultrasound. 1974;2(4):305–6.

11. Hassani SN, Bard RL. Evaluation of solid thyroid neoplasms by gray scale and real time ultrasonography: the "halo" sign. Ultrasound Med. 1977;4:323.

12. Propper RA, Skolnick ML, Weinstein BJ, Dekker A. The nonspecificity of the thyroid halo sign. J Clin Ultrasound. 1980;8:129–32.

13. Walfish PG, Hazani E, Strawbridge HTG, Miskin M, Rosen IB. Combined ultrasound and needle aspiration cytology in the assessment and management of hypofunctioning thyroid nodule. Ann Intern Med. 1977;87(3):270–4.

14. Gharib H. Fine-needle aspiration biopsy of thyroid nodules: advantages, limitations, and effect. Mayo Clin Proc. 1994;69:44–9.

15. Danese D, Sciacchitano S, Farsetti A, Andreoli M, Pontecorvi A. Diagnostic accuracy of conventional versus sonography guided fine-needle aspiration biopsy in the management of nonpalpable and palpable thyroid nodules. Thyroid. 1998;8:511–5.

16. Tan GH, Gharib H, Reading CC. Solitary thyroid nodule: comparison between palpation and ultrasonography. Arch Intern Med. 1995;155:2418–23.

17. Cooper DS, Doherty GM, Haugen BR, et al. The American Thyroid Association Guidelines Task Force. Revised management guidelines for patients with thyroid nodules and differentiated thyroid cancer. Thyroid. 2009;19:1167–214.

18. Ralls PW, Mayekowa DS, Lee KP, et al. Color-flow Doppler sonography in Graves' disease: "thyroid inferno". AJR Am J Roentgenol. 1988;150:781–4.

19. Bogazzi F, Bartelena L, Brogioni S, et al. Color flow Doppler sonography rapidly differentiates type I and type II amiodaroneinduced thyrotoxicosis. Thyroid. 1997;7(4):541–5.

20. Grant EG. Sonographic contrast agents in vascular imaging. Semin Ultrasound CT MR. 2001;22(1):25–41.

21. Valcavi R. Personal communication. (2012)

22. Lees W. Ultrasound imaging in three and four dimensions. Semin Ultrasound CT MR. 2001;22(1):85–105.

23. Antonelli A, Miccoli P, Ferdeghini M. Role of neck ultrasonography in the follow-up of patients operated on for thyroid cancer. Thyroid. 1995;5(1):25–8.

CHAPTER 2
Thyroid Ultrasound Physics

Robert A. Levine

SOUND AND SOUND WAVES

Some animal species such as the dolphins, whales, and bats are capable of creating a "visual" image based on receiving reflected sound waves. Man's unassisted vision is limited to electromagnetic waves in the spectrum of visible light. Humans require technology and an understanding of physics to use sound to create a picture. This chapter will explore how man has developed a technique for creating a visual image from sound waves [1].

Sound is transmitted as mechanical energy, in contrast to light, which is transmitted as electromagnetic energy. Unlike electromagnetic waves, sound waves require a propagating medium. Light is capable of traveling through a vacuum, but sound will not transmit through a vacuum. The qualities of the transmitting medium directly affect how sound is propagated. Materials have different speed of sound transmission. Speed of sound is constant for a specific material, and does not vary with sound frequency (Fig. 2.1). *Acoustic impedance* is the inverse of the capacity of a material to transmit sound. When sound travels through a material and encounters a change in acoustic impedance a portion of the sound energy will be reflected and the remainder will be transmitted. The amount reflected is proportionate to the degree of mismatch of acoustic impedance. Acoustic impedance of a material depends on its density, stiffness, and speed of sound [2].

Sound waves propagate by compression and rarefaction of molecules in space (Fig. 2.2). Molecules of the transmitting medium vibrate around their resting position, and transfer their energy to neighboring molecules. Sound waves carry energy rather than matter through space.

H.J. Baskin et al. (eds.), *Thyroid Ultrasound and Ultrasound-Guided FNA*, **9**
DOI 10.1007/978-1-4614-4785-6_2,
© Springer Science+Business Media, LLC 2013

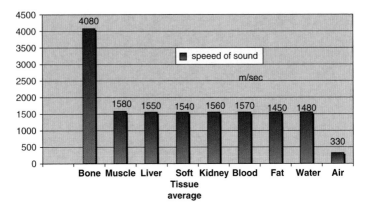

FIG. 2.1. Speed of sound. The speed of sound is constant for a specific material and does not vary with frequency. Speed of sound for various biological tissues is illustrated.

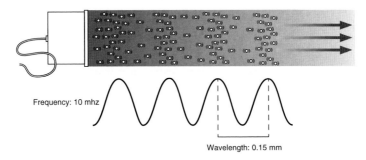

FIG. 2.2. Sound waves propagate in a longitudinal direction, but are typically represented by a sine wave where the peak corresponds to the maximum compression of molecules in space, and the trough corresponds to the maximum rarefaction.

As shown in Fig. 2.2, sound waves propagate in a longitudinal direction, but are typically represented by a sine wave where the peak corresponds to the maximum compression of molecules in space, and the trough corresponds to the maximum rarefaction. Frequency is defined as the number of cycles per time of the vibration of the sound waves. A Hertz (Hz) is defined as one cycle per second. The audible spectrum is between 30 and 20,000 Hz. Ultrasound is defined as sound waves at a higher frequency than the audible spectrum. Typical frequencies used in diagnostic ultrasound vary between 5 and 15 million cycles per second (5 and 15 MHz) [1, 3].

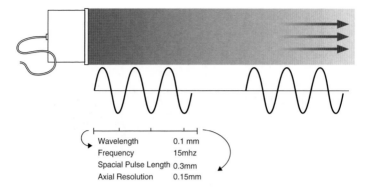

FIG. 2.3. Diagnostic ultrasound uses pulsed waves, allowing for an interval of sound transmission, followed by an interval during which reflected sounds are received and analyzed. Typically three cycles of sound are transmitted as a pulse.

Diagnostic ultrasound uses pulsed waves, allowing for an interval of sound transmission, followed by an interval during which reflected sounds are received and analyzed. Typically three cycles of sound are transmitted as a pulse. The spatial pulse length is the length in space filled by three cycles (Fig. 2.3). Spatial pulse length is one of the determinants of resolution. Since higher frequencies have a smaller pulse length, higher frequencies are associated with improved resolution. As illustrated in Fig. 2.3, at a frequency of 15 MHz the wavelength in biological tissues is approximately 0.1 mm, allowing an axial resolution of 0.15 mm. Although resolution improves with increased frequency, the depth of penetration of the ultrasound waves decreases, limiting the visualization of deeper structures.

As mentioned above, the *speed of sound* is constant for a given material or biological tissue. It is not affected by frequency or wavelength. It increases with stiffness and decreases with density of the material. As seen in Fig. 2.1, common biological tissues have different propagation velocities. Bone, as a very dense and stiff tissue has a high propagation velocity of 4,080 m/s. Fat tissue, with low stiffness and low density, has a relatively low speed of sound of 1,450 m/s. Most soft tissues have a speed of sound near 1,540 m/s. Muscle, liver, and thyroid have a slightly faster speed of sound. By convention, all ultrasound equipment uses an average speed of 1,540 m/s. The distance to an object displayed on an ultrasound image is calculated by multiplying the speed of sound by the time interval for a sound signal to return to the transducer

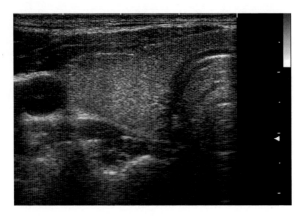

FIG. 2.4. The echotexture of normal thyroid tissue. It has a ground glass appearance and is brighter than muscle tissue.

[2, 3]. By using the accepted 1,540 m/s as the assumed speed of sound, all ultrasound equipment will provide identical distance or size measurements.

Reflection is the redirection of a portion of a sound wave from the interface of tissues with unequal acoustic impedance. Larger differences in impedance will result in greater amounts of reflection. A material that is homogeneous in acoustic impedance does not generate any internal echoes. A pure cyst is a typical example of an anechoic (echoless) structure. Most biological tissues have varying degrees of inhomogeneity both on a cellular and macroscopic level. Connective tissue, blood vessels, and cellular structure all provide mismatches of acoustic impedance, which lead to the generation of characteristic ultrasonographic patterns (Figs. 2.4, 2.5, and 2.6). Reflection is categorized as specular, when reflecting off of smooth surfaces such as a mirror. In contrast, diffuse reflection occurs when a surface is irregular, with variations at or smaller than the wavelength of the incident sound. Diffuse reflection results in scattering of sound waves and production of noise.

CREATION OF AN ULTRASOUND IMAGE

The earliest ultrasound imaging consisted of a sound transmitted into the body, with the reflected sound waves displayed on an oscilloscope. Referred to as A-mode ultrasound, these images in the 1960s and 1970s were capable of providing measurements of internal structures such as thyroid lobes, nodules, and cysts. Figure 2.7a shows an A-mode ultrasound image of a solid thyroid

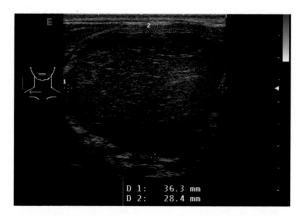

FIG. 2.5. The thyroid from a patient with the acutely swollen inflammatory phase of Hashimoto's thyroiditis. Massive infiltration by lymphocytes has decreased the echogenicity of the tissue resulting in a more homogeneous hypoechoic pattern.

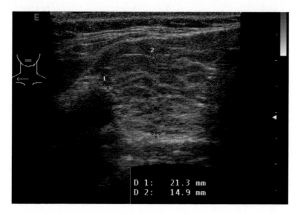

FIG. 2.6 A typical heterogeneous pattern from Hashimoto's thyroiditis with hypoechoic inflammatory regions separated by hyperechoic fibrous tissue.

nodule. Scattered echoes are present from throughout the nodule. Figure 2.7b shows the image from a cystic nodule. The initial reflection is from the proximal wall of the cyst, with no significant signal reflected by the cyst fluid. The second reflection originates from the posterior wall. Figure 2.7c shows the A-mode image from a complex nodule with solid and cystic components. A-mode ultrasound was capable of providing size measurements in one dimension, but did not provide a visual image of the structure [1].

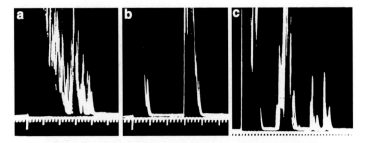

FIG. 2.7. A-mode ultrasound images. (**a**) An A-mode ultrasound image of a solid thyroid nodule. Scattered echoes are present from throughout the nodule. (**b**) The image from a cystic nodule. The initial reflection is from the proximal wall of the cyst, with no significant signal reflected by the cyst fluid. The second reflection originates from the posterior wall. (**c**) The A-mode image from a complex nodule with solid and cystic components.

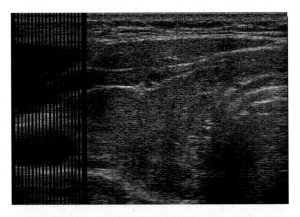

FIG. 2.8. A B-mode ultrasound image is composed of a series of A-mode images aligned to provide a two-dimensional image.

In order to provide a visual two-dimensional image, a series of one-dimensional A-mode images are aligned as a transducer is swept across the structure being imaged. Early thyroid ultrasound images were created by slowly moving a transducer across the neck. By scanning over a structure and aligning the A-mode images, a two-dimensional image is formed. The two-dimensional image formed in this manner is referred to as a B-mode scan (Fig. 2.8). Current ultrasound transducers use a series of piezo-electric crystals in a linear array to electronically simulate a sweep of the transducer. Firing sequentially, each crystal sends a pulse of sound wave into the tissue, and receives subsequent reflections.

The final ultrasound image reflects a cross-sectional image through the tissue defined by the thin flat beam of sound emitted from the transducer. Resolution is the ability to distinguish between two separate, adjacent objects. For example, with a resolution of 0.2 mm, two adjacent objects measuring <0.2 mm would be shown as a single object. Objects smaller than the resolution will not be realistically imaged. Lateral resolution refers to the ability to discriminate in a transverse, or side to side, direction. Azimuthal resolution refers to the image perpendicular to the axis of the ultrasound beam. Axial resolution is the ability to discriminate objects along the path of the ultrasound beam. Axial resolution is determined by the spatial pulse length and therefore frequency. Lateral and azimuthal resolution are dependent on the focusing of the ultrasound beam.

THE USEFULNESS OF ARTIFACTS IN ULTRASOUND IMAGING

A number of artifacts commonly occur in ultrasound images. Unlike most other imaging techniques, artifacts are very helpful in interpreting ultrasound images. Artifacts such as shadows behind objects or unexpected areas of brightness can provide additional understanding of the properties of the materials being imaged.

When sound waves impact on an area of extreme mismatch of acoustic impedance, such as a tissue–air interface or a calcification, the vast majority of the sound waves are reflected, providing a very bright signal from the object's surface and an absence of imaging beyond the structure. Figure 2.9 demonstrates *acoustic shadowing* behind a calcified nodule. Figure 2.10 illustrates a coarse calcification within the thyroid parenchyma with acoustic shadowing behind the calcification. Figure 2.11 shows the typical appearance of the trachea on an ultrasound image. Because there is no transmission of sound through the air–tissue interface of the anterior wall of the trachea, no imaging of structures posterior to the trachea occurs.

Conversely, a cystic structure transmits sound with very little attenuation, resulting in a greater intensity of sound waves behind it, compared to adjacent structures. This results in acoustic *enhancement* with a brighter signal behind a cystic or anechoic structure. This enhancement can be used to distinguish between a cystic and solid nodule within the thyroid. Figure 2.12 illustrates enhancement behind a cystic nodule. Enhancement is not limited to cystic nodules, however. Any structure that causes minimal attenuation of the ultrasound signal will have enhancement posterior to it. Figure 2.13 illustrates enhancement behind a solid

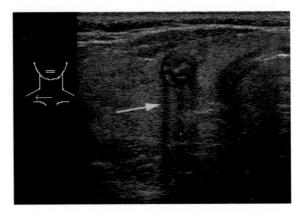

FIG. 2.9. Acoustic shadowing. When sound waves impact on an area of extreme mismatch of acoustic impedance, such as a calcification, the vast majority of the sound waves are reflected, resulting in a shadow beyond the structure. This calcified nodule is from a patient with familial papillary carcinoma.

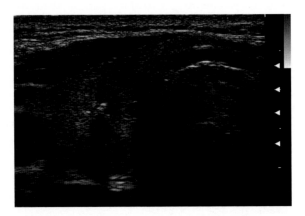

FIG. 2.10. Acoustic shadowing. A shadow is observed behind a coarse calcification within the thyroid parenchyma. Unlike calcification within a nodule, amorphic calcification within the parenchyma is not typically associated with malignancy.

parathyroid adenoma. Figure 2.14 illustrates enhancement behind a benign colloid nodule. Due to the high content of fluid and colloid within the nodule, and resultant decrease in cellularity, there is less attenuation of signal within the nodule than within the surrounding thyroid tissue.

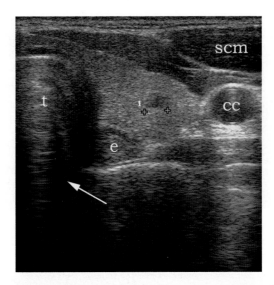

FIG. 2.11. Acoustic shadowing. Due to the extreme reflection from the tissue–air interface of the trachea, no image is seen behind the trachea on an anterior ultrasound.

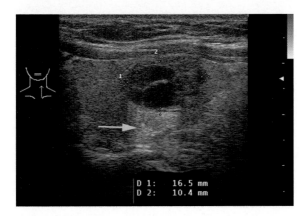

FIG. 2.12. Enhancement. A cystic structure transmits sound with very little attenuation, resulting in a greater intensity of sound waves behind it. Enhancement is typical behind a cystic nodule.

Figure 2.15 shows a nodule exhibiting "eggshell" calcification. A layer of calcium surrounding the nodule results in an absence of reflected signal behind the nodule. As can be seen in the figure, reflection is greatest from the surfaces perpendicular to the sound

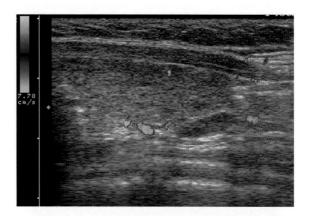

FIG. 2.13. Enhancement. Parathyroid adenomas have relatively homogeneous tissue and, like a parathyroid cyst, may demonstrate enhancement behind them.

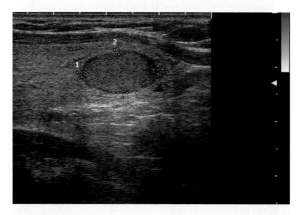

FIG. 2.14. Enhancement. This benign colloid nodule has a high content of fluid and colloid with a result in decrease in cellularity. The decreased attenuation of signal within the nodule results in enhancement despite it being a solid nodule.

waves: the front and back walls. Because the angle of incidence approaches 180° along the side walls, most of the reflected waves are reflected away from the transducer, resulting in a decreased signal corresponding to the sides of the structure.

Edge artifacts are extremely useful in identifying nodules in the thyroid. Figure 2.16 shows dark lines extending posteriorly from the sides of a nodule, aligned with the ultrasound beam. This is another example of a reflection artifact. As described above, the sound waves

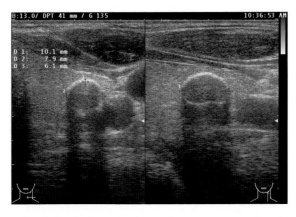

FIG. 2.15. Eggshell calcification. A layer of calcium surrounding the nodule results in reflection from the surface, along with marked posterior acoustic shadowing.

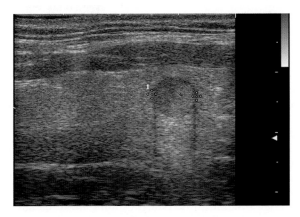

FIG. 2.16. Edge artifact. *Dark lines* are seen extending posteriorly from the sides of a nodule. This artifact can be used to help identify a nodule or other structure.

striking the object along the side are reflected away, rather than back towards the transducer. When two parallel dark lines are seen aligned vertically in an image, they can be followed "up" on the display to help identify a nodule or other structure.

Several artifacts arise due to reverberation. When sound waves reflect off of a very reflective surface, some may be re-reflected from the skin surface producing multiple phantom images beyond the actual image. Figure 2.17 illustrates the very common *reverberation*

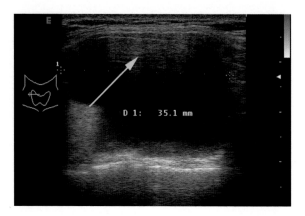

FIG. 2.17. Reverberation artifact. It is very common to see this artifact in the anterior aspect of cysts. This arises due to reverberation of signal between the skin surface and the anterior wall of the cyst, resulting in the late signals being received, and giving the appearance of solid tissue in the anterior aspect of the cyst.

artifact which occurs due to this reverberation of sound waves between the skin surface and deeper tissue interfaces. Since some of the reflected sound waves will bounce back from the skin surface into the tissue multiple times, phantom images are produced. As shown, it is very common to see this artifact in the anterior aspect of cysts, raising doubt as to whether the lesion is a true cyst, or partly solid. Changing the angle at which the sound strikes the lesion will usually clarify the situation. Figure 2.18 shows this common artifact behind the anterior wall of the trachea.

The "comet tail" artifact is another extremely common finding arising due to reverberation [4] (Figs. 2.19 and 2.20). Colloid nodules may contain tiny crystals resulting from the desiccation of the gelatinous colloid material. Reflection of the sound waves off of the crystal results in a bright spot. However, in contrast to a soft tissue calcification, the crystals begin to vibrate under the influence of the ultrasound energy. The vibration generates sound waves, which return to the transducer after the initial reflected signal. Also referred to as a *ringdown artifact*, a *cat's eye* (Fig. 2.21), or *stepladder artifact*, these "comet tails" help differentiate between the typically benign densities found in a colloid nodule and highly suspicious microcalcifications. While comet tail artifacts most commonly arise within a benign colloid nodule, they may also be seen in resolving hematomas, and have rarely been described within papillary carcinoma.

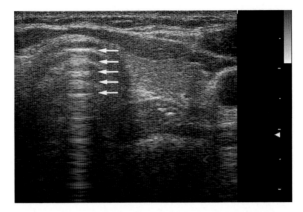

FIG. 2.18. Reverberation artifact. Numerous *parallel lines* are seen posterior to the anterior wall of the trachea. These are commonly misconstrued as the tracheal rings, but are actually reverberation artifact.

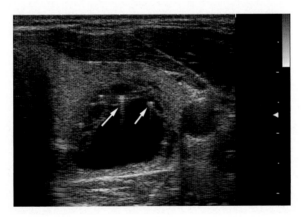

FIG. 2.19. "Comet tails." Colloid nodules may contain tiny crystals resulting from the desiccation of the gelatinous colloid material. Reflection of the sound waves off of the crystal results in a bright spot. However, in contrast to a soft tissue calcification, the crystals begin to vibrate under the influence of the ultrasound energy. The vibration generates sound waves, which return to the transducer after the initial reflected signal.

Refraction is the alteration of direction of the transmitted sound at an acoustic interface when the angle of incidence is not 90°. A sound wave striking an interface at 90° is reflected straight back. When waves strike at an angle other than 90° the transmitted wave is bent as it propagates through the interface. A greater

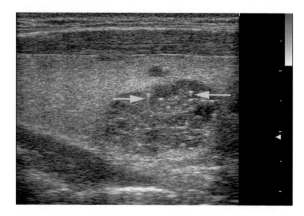

FIG. 2.20. "Comet tails." Another example of comet tail artifacts within a benign colloid nodule.

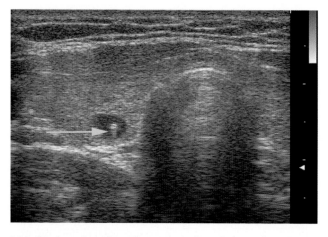

FIG. 2.21. "Cat's-eye" artifact. The comet tail artifacts is also referred to as a ringdown artifact, a stepladder artifact, or, when a single lesion is seen within a small cyst, a cat's-eye.

degree of mismatch of acoustic impedance between tissues results in a greater degree of refraction. While not typically seen in near field ultrasound used in thyroid and other small parts imaging, refraction artifacts can result in a second "ghost" image when a refracting object exists in the path of an ultrasound beam.

As sound waves propagate through any tissue, the intensity of the wave is *attenuated*. Attenuation of acoustic energy results

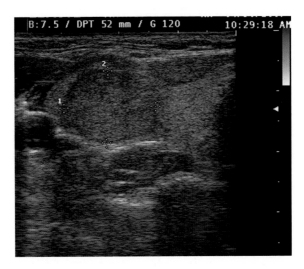

FIG. 2.22. Comparison of images produced with frequencies of 7.5 and 13 MHz. In this image utilizing 7.5 MHz the nodule is less well defined, but the posterior structures are better visualized. Compare to figure 2.23.

from a combination of reflection, scattering, and absorption, with conversion of sound energy to heat. Attenuation is frequency dependent, with higher frequencies having greater attenuation. As a result, while higher frequencies provide improved resolution, the depth of imaging decreases with increasing frequency. Current ultrasound technology utilizes sound waves as high as 16 MHz for thyroid imaging. However, imaging is limited to less than 5 cm of depth at this frequency. Visualization of deeper structures, as with abdominal or pelvic ultrasound, requires lower frequencies. In obese patients, or when imaging very deep structures, frequencies of 5–7.5 MHz may be needed for adequate penetration and visualization of the deep neck structures. Figures 2.22 and 2.23 compare images made at 7.5 and 15 MHz. Loss of detail of proximal structures is evident with the lower frequency.

Shadowing and enhancement, as described above, are examples of attenuation artifacts. Shadowing occurs behind structures with extreme acoustic mismatch due to the attenuation of transmission of sound waves caused by nearly complete reflection. Enhancement occurs behind structures with little to no attenuation, with higher intensity sound waves present behind the structure in comparison to the adjacent tissues.

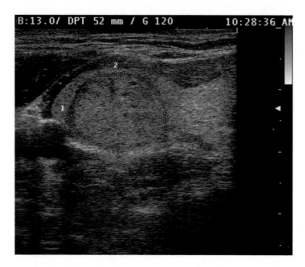

FIG. 2.23. Comparison of images produced with frequencies of 7.5 and 13 MHz. In this image utilizing 13 MHz the nodule shows much better definition. Compare to figure 2.22.

ADVANCES IN ULTRASOUND IMAGING

Ultrasound transducers consist of an array of crystals capable of transmitting and receiving ultrasound energy. Piezo-electric crystals vibrate when exposed to an electrical current. Conversely, when energy strikes the crystal, it results in an electrical signal, with a frequency corresponding to the frequency of the incident sound wave. Thyroid ultrasound typically uses a linear array of several hundred crystals within a transducer. The transverse width of the image produced is equal to the length of the array of crystals in the transducer. Curved array transducers are less often used in thyroid ultrasound (but are commonly used in abdominal, pelvic, and cardiac imaging). By producing a divergent beam of ultrasound they allow visualization of structures larger than the transducer. They are occasionally used as an aid in fine needle aspiration biopsy, but the image produced has spatial distortion due to the lack of a linear relationship between the transverse and longitudinal planes (see Chap. 12).

Once received, the ultrasound signal undergoes image reconstruction, followed by image enhancement. Noise reduction and edge sharpening algorithms are used to clarify the image. Most ultrasound equipment allows the user to select the degree of noise reduction, dynamic range, and edge sharpening, to optimize image quality. Ultrasound equipment allows for user adjustment of the gain of the received signal. Overall gain can be adjusted, and separate channels corresponding to individual depths may be adjusted (time gain compensation) to provide the best image quality at the region of interest. Most ultrasound equipment also allows for user adjustment of the focal zone, the depth at which the ultrasound beam is ideally focused. Multiple focal zones may also be selected on most ultrasound equipment. While providing a slight increase in image sharpness, the use of multiple focal zones typically slows the refresh rate of the image, resulting in a more jumpy image when visualized during real time scanning.

While standard ultrasound receives only the frequency identical to that transmitted for imaging, tissue harmonic imaging capitalizes on the tendency of tissues to reverberate when exposed to higher power ultrasound energy. Different tissues have a different degree of reverberation, and produce unique signatures of tissue harmonics (multiples of the original frequency). Selective detection of the harmonic signal produces an alternative image. Because higher frequencies are being detected, the resolution may be improved, but the original transmitted frequency is typically lower when using tissue harmonic imaging. Since the distance traveled by a harmonic signal is one half that of the transmitted and received signal there is less noise. The increased resolution and decreased noise may result in increased conspicuity of some objects [5], but tissue harmonic imaging has not had widespread application in thyroid imaging.

Recently ultrasound image quality has benefitted by transition to complete digital processing. In conventional ultrasound a linear transducer transmits and receives parallel ultrasonographic waves in a single direction. With compound spatial imaging the ultrasound beam is electronically or mechanically steered into multiple angles. Compound spatial imaging combines multiple images obtained from different angles and reconstructs them into a single image [6]. This results in much less speckle and noise, and a much more realistic appearing image (Figs. 2.24 and 2.25). Artifacts are reduced, but careful selection of the degree of noise reduction applied allows useful artifacts such a shadowing, enhancement and edge artifacts to remain, aiding in interpretation of the image (Figs. 2.26 and 2.27) [7].

In summary, sound transmission is dependent on the conducting medium. Sound is reflected at interfaces of mismatch of acoustic impedance. The resolution of an ultrasound image is dependent on the frequency, the focused beam width, and the quality of the electronic processing. Resolution improves with higher

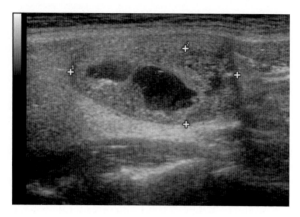

FIG. 2.24. A conventional ultrasound image without spatial compound imaging shows speckle artifact and more noise than the processed image shown in figure 2.25.

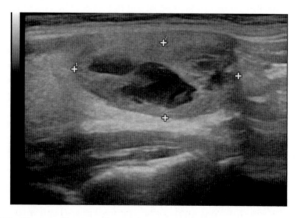

FIG. 2.25. After application of spatial compound imaging there is a reduction of speckle artifact, less noise, and overall improved image quality.

frequencies, but the depth of imaging suffers. Image artifacts such as shadowing and enhancement provide useful information, rather than just interfering with creation of a clear image. The current image quality, affordable cost, and ease of performance make real time ultrasound an integral part of the clinical evaluation of the thyroid patient.

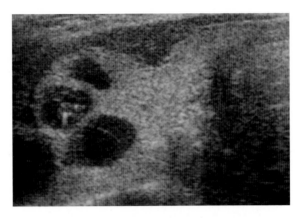

Fɪɢ. 2.26. A comet tail artifact and posterior acoustic enhancement are present prior to application of spatial compound imaging.

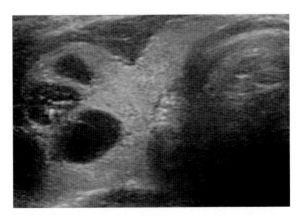

Fɪɢ. 2.27. The comet tail artifact and posterior enhancement remain visible with compound spatial imaging despite the reduction of speckle and noise artifact.

References

1. Meritt CRB. Physics of ultrasound. In: Rumack CM, Wilson SR, Charboneau JW, Levine D, editors. Diagnostic ultrasound. 4th ed. St. Louis: Mosby; 2011. p. 2–33.
2. Levine RA. Something old and something new: a brief history of thyroid ultrasound technology. Endocr Pract. 2004;10(3):227–33.
3. Coltrera MD. Ultrasound physics in a nutshell. Otolaryngol Clin North Am. 2010;43(6):1149–59.

4. Ahuja A, Chick W, King W, Metreweli C. Clinical significance of the comet-tail artifact in thyroid ultrasound. J Clin Ultrasound. 1996;24(3):129–33.

5. Szopinski KT, Wysocki M, Pajk AM, et al. Tissue harmonic imaging of thyroid nodules: initial experience. J Ultrasound Med. 2003;22(1):5–12.

6. Lin DC, Nazarian L, O'Kane PL, et al. Advantages of real-time spatial compound sonography of the musculoskeletal system versus conventional sonography. AJR Am J Roentgenol. 2002;179(6):1629–31.

7. Shapiro RS, Simpson WL, Rauch DL, Yeh HC. Compound spatial sonography of the thyroid gland: evaluation of freedom from artifacts and of nodule conspicuity. AJR Am J Roentgenol. 2001;177:1195–8.

CHAPTER 3
Doppler Ultrasound of the Neck

Robert A. Levine

DOPPLER PHYSICS

The Doppler shift is a change in frequency that occurs when sound (or light) is emitted from, or bounced off of, a moving object. When a moving target reflects a sound, the frequency of the reflected sound wave is altered. The frequency is shifted up by an approaching target and shifted down by a receding target. This is illustrated in Fig. 3.1. The amount the frequency is shifted is proportional to the velocity of the moving object. Because the Doppler shift was originally described for energy in the visible light spectrum, an upward Doppler shift is referred to as a blue shift (a shift to a higher visible light frequency) and a downward Doppler shift is referred to as a red shift.

Ultrasound utilization of the Doppler shift falls into three main categories. Analysis of the Doppler frequency spectrum allows for calculation of velocity, and is used in vascular studies. Color-flow Doppler and power Doppler superimpose a color image representing motion onto a B-mode image to illustrate location of motion (blood flow).

In thyroid ultrasound, Doppler imaging is used predominantly to assess the vascularity of tissues. The leading use is to help determine the likelihood of a thyroid nodule being malignant. However, other applications of Doppler imaging include assessing the etiology or subtype of amiodarone thyrotoxicosis, clarifying images, and helping to assess the etiology of hyperthyroidism.

Analysis of the Doppler spectrum allows for the determination of flow velocity and calculation of resistance to flow. By analyzing the waveform, the peak systolic velocity and diastolic velocity can be calculated. Resistive index and pulsatility index can be derived

H.J. Baskin et al. (eds.), *Thyroid Ultrasound and Ultrasound-Guided FNA*, **29**
DOI 10.1007/978-1-4614-4785-6_3,
© Springer Science+Business Media, LLC 2013

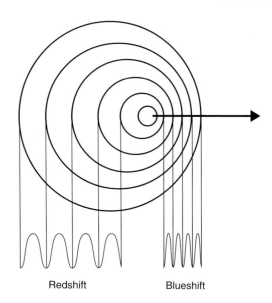

Redshift   Blueshift

Fig. 3.1. Illustration of the Doppler shift. When a moving target reflects a sound, the frequency of the reflected sound wave is altered. The frequency is shifted up by an approaching target and shifted down by a receding target. The amount the frequency is shifted is proportional to the velocity of the moving object.

from these measurements. While these values are typically used in studies of peripheral vascular disease, the peak flow velocity and resistive index are occasionally used in reporting the degree of vascularity of thyroid tissue.

For most imaging of the thyroid color-flow Doppler and power Doppler are utilized. In color-flow Doppler, a unique color (or brightness) is assigned to an individual frequency. Typically a greater frequency shift (corresponding to a higher velocity) is assigned a brighter color. Analysis of the color-flow image gives a graphic illustration of the direction and speed of blood flow within soft tissue. In contrast, power Doppler considers all frequency shifts to be equivalent, integrating the total amount of motion detected. The assigned color represents the total amount of flow present, independent of the velocity. The color image, therefore, is indicative of the total amount of flow present, without information regarding velocity (Figs. 3.2 and 3.3).

Color-flow Doppler provides information regarding both direction and velocity, and is more useful in vascular studies. In contrast, power Doppler does not provide information regarding

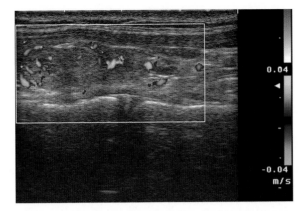

Fig. 3.2. Color Doppler. In color-flow Doppler, a unique color (or brightness) is assigned to an individual frequency. Typically, a greater frequency shift (corresponding to a higher velocity) is assigned a brighter color. Analysis of the color-flow image gives a graphic illustration of the direction and speed of blood flow within soft tissue.

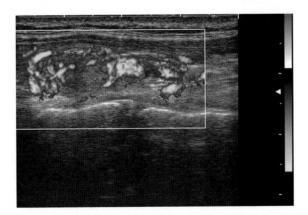

Fig. 3.3. Power Doppler. In contrast, power Doppler considers all frequency shifts to be equivalent, integrating the total amount of motion detected. The assigned color represents the total amount of flow present, independent of the velocity. Power Doppler has increased sensitivity for the detection of low degrees of flow, has less noise interference, and is less dependent on the angle of incidence between the ultrasound waves and the moving object.

velocity. However, it has increased sensitivity for the detection of low degrees of flow, has less noise interference, and is less dependent on the angle of incidence between the ultrasound waves and the moving object. Power Doppler is generally the preferred imaging technique for assessing the vascularity of thyroid tissue [1].

DOPPLER ANALYSIS OF THYROID NODULES

Figure 3.4 shows a follicular carcinoma in the inferior pole of the thyroid, with a very high degree of blood flow. The inferior thyroid artery can be seen feeding the nodule. In contrast, Fig. 3.5 shows a nodule with no significant intranodular vascularity, with only scattered blood vessels around the periphery. This nodule was a benign follicular adenoma.

Color and power Doppler imaging has been considered to have predictive value for the determination of the probability of malignancy in thyroid nodules. A number of studies have shown that most benign nodules have absent intranodular blood flow on power Doppler analysis, and most malignancies have demonstrable central flow [2–4]. However, a large series has recently challenged that concept [5].

Papini et al. [2] studied 494 consecutive patients with nonpalpable nodules measuring 8–15 mm. All patients had a Doppler ultrasound study performed prior to fine needle aspiration biopsy. An intranodular vascular pattern was observed in 74% of all nodules with thyroid cancer. Eighty-seven percent of the cancers were solid and hypoechoic, and 77% of the cancers had irregular or blurred margins. Only 29% of the cancers had microcalcifications. Independent risk factors for malignancy included irregular margins (RR = 16.8%), intranodular Doppler blood flow (RR = 14.3), and microcalcifications (RR = 5).

Berni et al. [3] analyzed 108 patients with thyroid nodules demonstrated to be hypofunctioning on nuclear medicine study. All of the patients had subsequent surgical excision of the nodule. Half of the patients were found to have malignancy, so this clearly was not a random population. Of the 108 patients, 92 would have been correctly diagnosed based on their color Doppler pattern. There were six false negative cancers with no blood flow, and 10 false positive benign lesions with significant intranodular flow. The calculated sensitivity was 88.8%, and the specificity was 81.5%. The positive predictive value of blood flow was 83%, and the negative predictive value was 88%.

Recently, Moon retrospectively reviewed ultrasounds of 1,083 nodules (with 269 malignancies) in 1,024 patients and found that vascularity was not associated with malignancy [5]. Vascularity

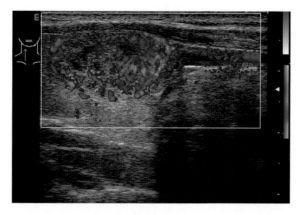

FIG. 3.4. Vascular nodule. A follicular carcinoma is present in the inferior pole of the thyroid, with a very high degree of blood flow. The inferior thyroid artery can be seen feeding the nodule.

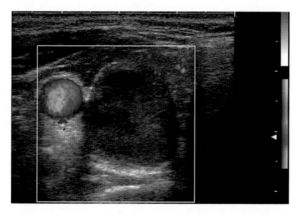

FIG. 3.5. Avascular nodule. This benign follicular adenoma has no intranodular blood flow.

was classified as none, peripheral, and intranodular. Vascularity was present in 31% of the benign nodules and only 17% of papillary cancers. Absent vascularity was more common in malignant nodules (60%) than in benign nodules (43%). It is not clear why such disparate results were seen. It is possible that it relates to a very high number of (small) papillary cancers in the Moon series (>97% papillary cancers). Moon suggests that prior studies may have suffered from selection bias, analyzing only hypoechoic, cold nodules, or nodules only >1 cm. In contrast, Moon included nodules regardless of size, echogenicity, or results of radioisotope scan [5]. It has been suggested that a pattern of central versus peripheral vascularity may be more predictive of malignancy, and this was not considered in the Moon series [6, 7].

The current ATA and AACE/AME guidelines for the management of thyroid nodules consider intranodular vascularity to be a risk factor [8, 9]. However, recently revised guidelines published by the Korean Society of Radiology have eliminated vascularity as a risk factor [10]. Additional studies, including a large multicenter study, are currently in progress and will hopefully help clarify the relationship between vascularity and likelihood of malignancy.

In summary, color and power Doppler imaging may provide useful information regarding the likelihood of malignancy in thyroid nodules. However, absence of vascularity on a Doppler study should not obviate the need for fine needle aspiration biopsy. The power Doppler flow pattern should be interpreted along with other ultrasonographic characteristics including echogenicity, edge definition, and calcifications, as well as clinical features such as nodule size and sex of the patient to help in the decision regarding the need for biopsy.

DOPPLER ANALYSIS OF NODULES WITH FOLLICULAR CYTOLOGY

Fukunari et al. [11] studied 310 patients with a solitary thyroid nodule in which a prior fine needle aspiration biopsy had demonstrated a follicular lesion. All patients underwent a color Doppler flow mapping study prior to surgery. The amount of flow in the nodule was classified on a four-point scale. Grade 1 nodules had no flow detectable. Grade 2 nodules had only peripheral flow, without intranodular flow. Grade 3 nodules had low velocity central flow, and grade 4 nodules had high-intensity central flow (Figs. 3.6–3.10). For purposes of statistical analysis, the absence of intranodular flow (grades 1 and 2) was considered a negative result, and the presence of central flow (grades 3 and 4) was considered a positive result. Of 177 benign adenomatous nodules, 95% were grade 1 or 2, and only 5% were grade 3. No benign adenomatous nodules had grade 4 blood flow. Of 89 benign follicular adenomas, 66% showed grade 1 or 2 Doppler flow, and 34% showed grade 3 or 4 flow. Of the 44 follicular carcinomas, none showed grade 1 Doppler flow, 13.6% showed grade 2 flow, and 86.4% showed either grade 3 or 4 flow.

Using the data of Fukunari, the sensitivity of intranodular blood flow in predicting malignancy was 86%. The specificity was

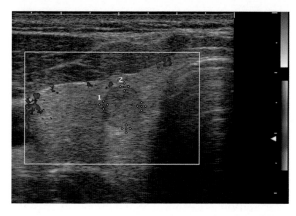

FIG. 3.6. Grade 1 Doppler flow. Grade 1 lesions have no intranodular flow and no flow to the periphery.

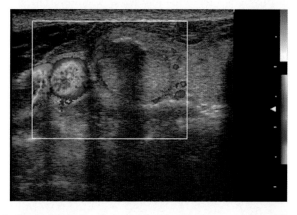

FIG. 3.7. Grade 2 Doppler flow. Grade 2 lesions have peripheral flow only, without intranodular flow.

85%, and the diagnostic accuracy was 81%. The prevalence of cancer in this group of follicular nodules was 14%.

In a similar analysis, De Nicola et al. [12] studied 86 patients in whom nodules had prior follicular biopsies. The flow pattern was characterized on a scale from 0 to 4, with 0 defined as no visible flow, 1 as peripheral flow only, 2 as peripheral flow with a small amount of central flow, 3 as peripheral flow plus extensive intranodular flow, and 4 as central flow only. Patterns 0–2 were grouped as negative results, and nodules with pattern 3 and 4

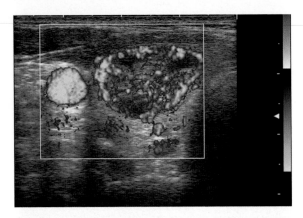

FIG. 3.8. Grade 3 Doppler flow. Grade 3 lesions have low to moderate velocity central flow.

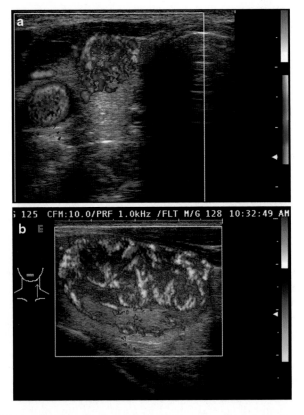

FIG. 3.9. Grade 4 Doppler flow. Grade 4 lesions have high-intensity central blood flow. 3.9a illustrates color Doppler imaging and 3.9b shows power Doppler imaging.

were considered positive. Of 59 non-neoplastic nodules, 93% were grade 0–2, and only 7% were grade 3. No non-neoplastic nodules had grade 4 blood flow. Of 14 benign follicular adenomas, 71% showed grade 0–2 Doppler flow, and 29% showed grade 3 or 4 flow. Of the ten carcinomas, 20% showed grade 0–2 Doppler flow, and 80% showed grade 3 or 4 flow. Based on this analysis, sensitivity was 80% and the specificity was 89%.

Applying Bayes' theorem to the data of Fukinari and De Nicola suggests that follicular nodules with no intranodular flow have only a 3% probability of malignancy rather than the generally accepted 15–20% likelihood in unselected follicular nodules. Conversely, vascular follicular nodules have a probability of malignancy approaching 50% [13, 14].

In summary, absence of flow in a nodule with a prior follicular biopsy makes malignancy much less likely. The power Doppler flow pattern should be interpreted along with other ultrasonographic features, as well as clinical features such as size of the nodule and age and sex of the patient, to help in the decision regarding the need for, and extent of, surgery.

DOPPLER ULTRASOUND OF AMIODARONE-INDUCED THYROTOXICOSIS

Amiodarone may cause thyroid dysfunction in 15–20% of treated patients [15]. Doppler ultrasound has been shown to help in the differentiation of the etiology of Amiodarone-induced thyrotoxicosis [16, 17]. Type 1 Amiodarone thyrotoxicosis resembles Graves' disease. It typically occurs in patients with preexisting thyroid autoimmunity. The gland is hyperthyroid, overproducing thyroid hormone. It may respond to treatment with Thionomides and Perchlorate. Typically, type 1 Amiodarone-induced thyrotoxicosis is associated with normal or increased vascularity on Doppler ultrasound. Type 2 Amiodarone-induced thyrotoxicosis more closely resembles painless thyroiditis. In this entity, inflammation and destruction of thyroid tissue results in the release of preformed thyroid hormone. It may respond to glucocorticoid therapy, and typically does not respond to Thionomides or Perchlorate. An elevated interleukin-6 level has been suggested as indicative of type 2 Amiodarone thyrotoxicosis, but its predictive value is poor. Typically, type 2 Amiodarone thyrotoxicosis is associated with absent or a very low degree of vascularity on power Doppler analysis [16, 17].

Eaton et al. demonstrated color-flow Doppler to be useful in the differentiation between the subtypes, but did report 20% falling into an "indeterminate" subtype [18]. Bogazzi demonstrated a

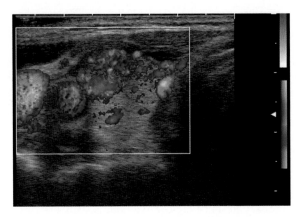

FIG. 3.10. Grade 4 Doppler flow in a benign nodule. While high-intensity blood flow within a nodule raises the likelihood of malignancy, benign hyperplastic colloid nodules may also show very intense intranodular blood flow. Note the similarity of this image of a benign nodule to the malignant nodule shown in Fig. 3.9a.

58% response to steroid therapy when flow was absent on color Doppler imaging, and only a 14% steroid response rate when flow was present [17]. A suggested treatment algorithm, using power Doppler analysis, suggests the use of steroid therapy when no flow is present. If flow is present, and especially if extremely vascular, Thionomides with or without Perchlorate are recommended. Combined therapy or surgery should be considered for any patient who does not respond to the initial treatment protocol, or who presents with the indeterminate Doppler pattern of mild flow [15].

DOPPLER ULTRASOUND OF GRAVES' DISEASE AND THYROIDITIS

With the recognition that the Doppler pattern was useful in Amiodarone-induced thyrotoxicosis, it seemed likely that Doppler would be useful for distinguishing hyperthyroidism of Graves' disease from thyrotoxicosis due to destructive (subacute, painless, or postpartum) thyroiditis. Graves' disease has been described as the "thyroid inferno" [19], with intense blood flow and peak systolic velocity up to 20 cm/s (Fig. 3.11). On the other hand, the vascular pattern observed in destructive thyroiditis is variable, ranging from totally absent to extremely hypervascular. During the acute inflammatory phase, vascularity is typically extremely low or absent. However, normal, increased, or intense vascularity may

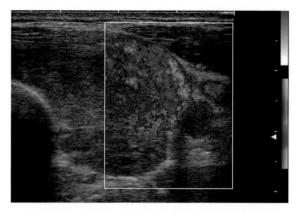

FIG. 3.11. Graves' disease. Graves' disease has been described as the "thyroid inferno" typically showing very intense blood flow.

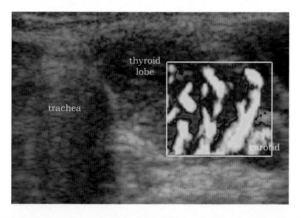

FIG. 3.12. Postpartum thyroiditis. Thyroiditis may be associated with any level of vascular flow, ranging from totally absent to intense, as is seen in this patient with postpartum thyroiditis.

be seen during the recovery phase. Similarly, while Graves' disease may exhibit intense vascularity, in mild cases the blood flow may be normal or only mildly increased. Figure 3.11 illustrates hypervascularity associated with Graves' disease. Figure 3.12 shows the thyroid from a patient with postpartum thyroiditis, in this case demonstrating extreme hypervascularity. Figure 3.13 shows intense blood flow in a patient with Hashitoxicosis, and Fig. 3.14 shows low vascularity in subacute thyroiditis.

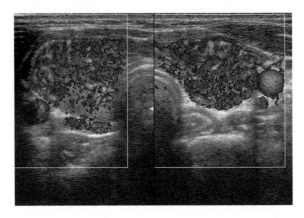

FIG. 3.13. Hashitoxicosis. Hashimoto's thyroiditis may also be associated with any degree of vascular flow. This patient with the hyperthyroid phase of early Hashimoto's thyroiditis (hashitoxicosis) has intense blood flow and could be easily confused with Graves' disease.

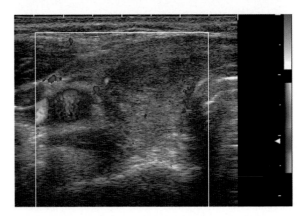

FIG. 3.14. Subacute thyroiditis. Subacute thyroiditis may also be associated with any degree of vascular flow. This image shows decreased flow associated with subacute thyroiditis.

The recent guidelines for the management of hyperthyroidism and other causes of thyrotoxicosis issued by the American Thyroid Association and the American Association of Clinical Endocrinologists recommended against the routine use of ultrasound in the evaluation of the thyrotoxic patient, stating, "Ultrasonography does not generally contribute to the differential diagnosis of thyrotoxicosis." The authors did concede that in situations in which radioactive iodine scanning was contraindicated or not useful (e.g., pregnancy, breast feeding, or recent iodine exposure) that "increased color Doppler flow may be useful in confirming a diagnosis of thyroid hyperactivity" [20]. In an editorial discussing these guidelines, Kahaly, Bartelena, and Hegedus argued that, "Thyroid US is a highly sensitive, convenient, inexpensive and noninvasive technique to aid in determining the underlying pathophysiology of thyrotoxicosis." They further stated that, "Addition of color-flow Doppler US improves the diagnostic spectrum and accuracy through its ability to quantify thyroid vascularity. This method accurately distinguishes GD from destructive thyroiditis" [21].

Because there is an overlap in color Doppler imaging between Graves' disease and destructive thyroiditis, attempts have been made to apply quantitative techniques to differentiate the two. Kurita et al. [22] calculated the "thyroid blood flow area" (TBFA) by measuring the percentage of thyroid area exhibiting Doppler flow. While they demonstrated a statistically significant difference between 22 patients with untreated Graves' disease and 10 patients with destructive thyroiditis, there was considerable overlap. Using a TBFA cutoff of 8%, 14% of patients with Graves' disease had low blood flow area and would have been misdiagnosed, and 10% of thyroiditis patients had high flow and would have been erroneously classified as Graves' disease.

Uchida et al. [23] attempted to differentiate Graves' from destructive thyroiditis, using measurement of the superior thyroid artery mean peak systolic velocity. While also demonstrating a statistical difference between 44 patients with untreated Graves' disease and 13 with destructive thyroiditis, there again was a significant overlap, with over 15% of the Graves' disease patients having a peak systolic velocity low enough to be misdiagnosed as destructive thyroiditis.

Hari Kumar et al. [24] reported ability to distinguish GD from destructive thyroiditis using color-flow Doppler imaging and peak systolic velocity of the inferior thyroid artery. They reported a small overlap between the groups using both modalities. Ota et al. [25] reported results of a novel technique, with dedicated software calculating the TBFA. Comparing 56 patients with GD to 58 patients with DT they observed no overlap with a cutoff of 4% TBFA.

Since Graves' disease typically has very intense flow, the absence of flow in a thyrotoxic patient is suggestive of thyroiditis, and the presence of the "thyroid inferno" is highly suggestive of Graves' disease. However, the presence of normal or mildly increased vascularity may reflect either Graves' disease or destructive thyroiditis in a thyrotoxic patient. Significant overlap exists, even in most reports of quantitative techniques, and caution should be used in assignment of diagnosis solely based on color or power Doppler images. Both ultrasound and Doppler ultrasound are extremely operator dependent. As stated by Professor Fausto Bogazzi in a commentary to the Ota study: "Thyroidal RAIU still maintains full validity in helping to distinguish between hyperthyroid, thyrotoxic and euthyroid individuals. Color Doppler can be considered a supplemental technique that might overtake RAIU only if further technical improvement and standardization can be achieved" [26]. When evaluating a thyrotoxic patient the clinician should consider the clinical history, physical examination, and laboratory studies. Ultrasonography and Doppler analysis may provide supportive evidence for the clinical impression. If doubt remains, RAI uptake may provide additional diagnostic information.

OTHER USES OF DOPPLER IMAGING

Doppler imaging may be useful to clarify images. For example, the margins of an isoechoic nodule may be difficult to discern, but Doppler imaging often shows peripheral vascularity, helping to identify the boundaries of the nodule (Figs. 3.15 and 3.16). What appear to be small hypoechoic nodules may in fact be small intrathyroidal blood vessels, apparent only when Doppler imaging is used. Doppler imaging is also useful prior to biopsy, to avoid laceration of large feeding vessels (Fig. 3.17).

Doppler imaging may help distinguish benign from malignant lymph nodes. As discussed in Chap. 8, in a normal lymph node the vascular supply enters centrally at the hilum, and spreads along the long axis, within the hilar line. In malignant lymph nodes, aberrant vessels enter peripherally through the lymph node capsule. Increased and disordered vascularity may be seen both peripherally and centrally. Figures 3.18 and 3.19 demonstrate the vascular pattern in benign and malignant lymph nodes. Doppler flow study may indicate compression of the jugular vein by a malignant lymph node, as seen in Fig. 3.20.

When examining lymph nodes for possible metastatic disease, it is important to set the ultrasound equipment to be able to detect very small amounts of flow in the hilum and cortex of the lymph node. Maximum sensitivity can be achieved by setting the Doppler pulse repetition frequency to less than 800 cycles per second and the wall filter to the lowest setting. This is in contrast to standard thyroid imaging, in which a PRF of 1,000 and a medium wall

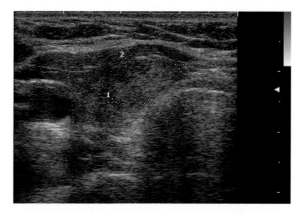

FIG. 3.15. The margins of the nodule are not entirely clear in this figure. With application of power Doppler ultrasound the boundaries of the nodule become evident.

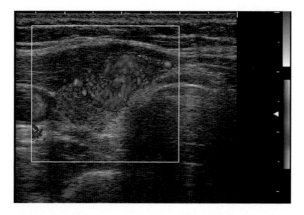

FIG. 3.16. The margins of the nodule are not entirely clear in Fig. 3.15. With application of power Doppler ultrasound the boundaries of the nodule become evident.

filter will provide acceptable detection of parenchymal or nodular vascularity.

As discussed in Chap. 9, parathyroid adenomas frequently have a pulsatile polar artery, and Doppler imaging may be useful in establishing that a nodule posterior to the thyroid represents a parathyroid rather than a central compartment lymph node (Fig. 3.21).

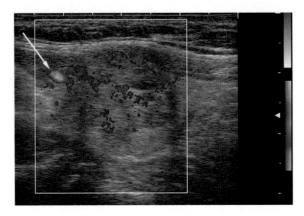

FIG. 3.17. Doppler imaging is useful prior to biopsy. The high-intensity signal associated with a thyroidal artery is noted in the projected path of the biopsy needle in this image. Repositioning prior to biopsy can help avoid the rare complication of lacerating the artery.

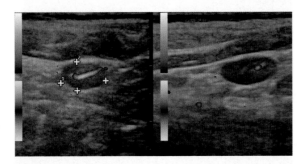

FIG. 3.18. Normal lymph node. In a normal lymph node, the vascular supply enters centrally at the hilum, and spreads along the long axis, within the hilar line.

CONCLUSIONS

In summary, Doppler ultrasound plays an important role in thyroid imaging. Power Doppler imaging may play an important role in the prediction of the likelihood of malignancy in a thyroid nodule and most of the current guidelines recommend documentation of

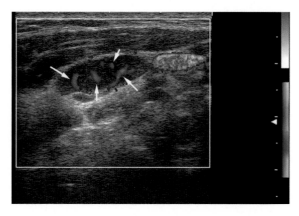

FIG. 3.19. Lymph node with metastatic papillary carcinoma. In contrast to the preceding figure, this malignant lymph node has disordered and chaotic blood flow.

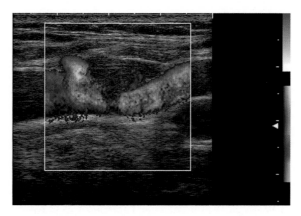

FIG. 3.20. A malignant lymph node in a patient with papillary carcinoma is seen compressing the jugular vein in this Doppler image. Benign lymph nodes may cause deviation of the major vessels but typically do not indent the vessel or cause abnormality in the blood flow.

vascularity in all significant thyroid nodules [8, 9]. However, an absent flow pattern does not have sufficient predictive value to eliminate the need to biopsy an avascular nodule. Doppler imaging is useful in the evaluation of goiter, thyroid nodules, lymph nodes, and parathyroid glands.

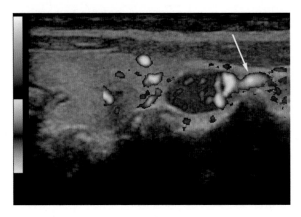

FIG. 3.21. Parathyroid adenomas frequently have a pulsatile polar artery, and Doppler imaging may be useful in establishing that a nodule posterior to the thyroid represents a parathyroid rather than a central compartment lymph node.

References

1. Cerbone G, Spiezia S, Colao A, Sarno D, et al. Power Doppler improves the diagnostic accuracy of color Doppler ultrasonography in cold thyroid nodules: follow-up results. Horm Res. 1999;52(1):19–24.
2. Papini E, Guglielmi R, Bianchini A, Crescenzi A, et al. Risk of malignancy in nonpalpable thyroid nodules: predictive value of ultrasound and color Doppler features. J Clin Endocrinol Metab. 2002;87(5):1941–6.
3. Berni A, Tromba L, Falvo L, Marchesi M, et al. Malignant thyroid nodules: comparison between color Doppler diagnosis and histological examination of surgical samples. Chir Ital. 2002;54(5):643–7.
4. Frates MC, Benson CB, Doubilet PM, Cibs ES, Marqusee E. Can color Doppler sonography aid in the prediction of malignancy of thyroid nodules? J Ultrasound Med. 2003;22:127–31.
5. Moon HJ, Kwak JY, Kim MJ, et al. Can vascularity at power Doppler US help predict thyroid malignancy? Radiology. 2010;255(1):260–9.
6. Chammas MC, Gerhard R, de Oliveira IR, et al. Thyroid nodules: evaluation with power Doppler and duplex Doppler ultrasound. Otolaryngol Head Neck Surg. 2005;132(6):874–82.
7. Chammas MC. Why do we have so many controversies in thyroid nodule Doppler US? Radiology. 2011;259(1):304.
8. Cooper DS, Doherty GM, Haugen BR, et al. The American Thyroid Association Guidelines Task Force. Revised management guidelines for patients with thyroid nodules and differentiated thyroid cancer. Thyroid. 2009;19:1167–214.
9. Gharib H, Papini E, Paschke R, Duick DS, et al. American Association of Clinical Endocrinologists, Associazione Medici Endocrinologi, and European Thyroid Association medical guidelines for clinical practice

for the diagnosis and management of thyroid nodules. Endocr Pract. 2010;16 Suppl 1:1–43.

10. Moon WJ, Baek JH, Jung SLK, et al. Ultrasonography and the ultra-sound-based management of thyroid nodules: consensus statement and recommendations. Korean J Radiol. 2011;12(1):1–14.

11. Fukunari N, Nagahama M, Sugino K, et al. Clinical evaluation of color Doppler imaging for the differential diagnosis of thyroid follicular lesions. World J Surg. 2004;28(12):1261–5.

12. De Nicola H, Szejnfeld J, Logullo AF, et al. Flow pattern and vascular resistance index as predictors of malignancy risk in thyroid follicular neoplasms. J Ultrasound Med. 2005;24:897–904.

13. Levine RA. Value of Doppler ultrasonography in management of patients with follicular thyroid biopsies. Endocr Pract. 2006;12(3):270–4.

14. Iared W, Shigueoka DC, Cristófoli JC, et al. Use of color Doppler ultrasonography for the prediction of malignancy in follicular thyroid neoplasms: systematic review and meta-analysis. J Ultrasound Med. 2010;29(3):419–25.

15. Bogazzi F, Bartelena L, Martino E. Approach to the patient with amiodarone-induced thyrotoxicosis. J Clin Endocrinol Metab. 2010;95(6):2529–35.

16. Macedo TA, Chammas MC, Jorge PT, et al. Differentiation between the two types of amiodarone-associated thyrotoxicosis using duplex and amplitude Doppler sonography. Acta Radiol. 2007;48(4):412–21.

17. Bogazzi F, Bartelena L, Brogioni S, et al. Color flow Doppler sonog-raphy rapidly differentiates type I and type II amiodarone-induced thyrotoxicosis. Thyroid. 1997;7(4):541–5.

18. Eaton SE, Euinton HA, Newman CM, et al. Clinical experience of amiodarone-induced thyrotoxicosis over a 3-year period: role of colour-flow Doppler sonography. Clin Endocrinol (Oxf). 2002;56(1):33–8.

19. Ralls PW, Mayekowa DS, Lee KP, et al. Color-flow Doppler sonog-raphy in Graves disease: "Thyroid Inferno". AJR Am J Roentgenol. 1988;150:781–4.

20. Bahn RS, Burch HB, Cooper DS, et al. Hyperthyroidism and other causes of thyrotoxicosis: Management Guidelines of the American Thyroid Association and American Association of Clinical Endocrinologists. Thyroid. 2011;21(6):593–646.

21. Kahaly GJ, Bartalena L, Hegedus L. The American Thyroid Association/American Association of Clinical Endocrinologists Guidelines for hyperthyroidism and other causes of thyrotoxicosis: a European perspective. Thyroid. 2011;21(6):585–91.

22. Kurita S, Sakurai M, Kita Y, et al. Measurement of thyroid blood flow area is useful for diagnosing the cause of thyrotoxicosis. Thyroid. 2005;15(11):1249–52.

23. Uchida T, Takeno K, Goto M, Kanno R, et al. Superior thyroid artery mean peak systolic velocity for the diagnosis of thyrotoxicosis in Japanese patients. Endocr J. 2010;57(5):439–43.

24. Hari Kumar KVS, Pasupuleti V, Jayaraman M, et al. Role of thyroid Doppler in differential diagnosis of thyrotoxicosis. Endocr Pract. 2009;15(1):6–9.

25. Ota H, Amino N, Morita S, et al. Quantitative measurement of thyroid blood flow for differentiation of painless thyroiditis from Graves' disease. Clin Endocrinol. 2007;67:41–5.
26. Bogazzi F, Vitti P. Could improved ultrasound and power Doppler replace thyroidal radioiodine uptake to assess thyroid disease? Nat Clin Pract Endocrinol Metab. 2008;4(2):70–1.

CHAPTER 4
Normal Neck Anatomy and Method of Performing Ultrasound Examination

Dara R. Treadwell

INTRODUCTION

Successful performance of an ultrasound examination of the neck requires knowledge of the anatomy of the normal neck. It also requires suitable ultrasound equipment, an understanding of the equipment's operation, application of principles of ultrasound physics, and the appropriate setup for performing the procedure.

ANATOMY OF THE NECK

The thyroid gland is a butterfly-shaped gland draped over the trachea. The right and left lobes lie on each side of the trachea, connected by the isthmus lying anterior to the trachea. Each lobe is approximately 4.5–5.5 cm in length, 1–2 cm wide, and 1–2 cm thick. The isthmus is typically 0.2–0.3 cm in thickness, with the normal isthmus less than 0.5 cm in thickness. Anterior to the thyroid are the strap muscles. These include the sternohyoid, the sternothyroid, and more laterally, the omohyoid. Anterior and lateral to the strap muscles is the much larger sternocleidomastoid (SCM) muscle which divides the neck into the anterior and posterior triangles. Posterior to each thyroid lobe is the longus colli muscle which abuts the posterior capsule of the thyroid gland (Fig. 4.1).

Adjacent to the lateral borders of the thyroid gland are the common carotid artery (CCA) and the internal jugular vein (IJV). The artery usually defines the lateral border of the thyroid lobe, and the IJV is typically located lateral to the CCA. However, because

H.J. Baskin et al. (eds.), *Thyroid Ultrasound and Ultrasound-Guided FNA*, **49**
DOI 10.1007/978-1-4614-4785-6_4,
© Springer Science+Business Media, LLC 2013

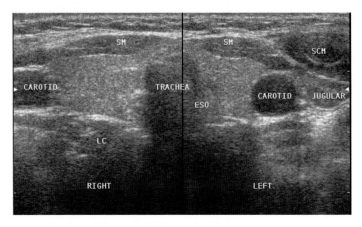

Fɪɢ. 4.1. Sonographic cross-sectional anatomy.

its soft walls allow it to conform to the surrounding tissue, the IJV sometimes shifts anteriorly to the CCA, a factor to consider in determining angle of approach in fine needle aspiration biopsy.

Behind the centrally located trachea and coursing in the same direction is the esophagus. Ultrasound does not allow visualization behind the trachea; however, a portion of the esophagus is often seen protruding out behind the trachea against the left lobe of the thyroid. Infrequently, the esophagus is seen on the right. It may resemble a donut ring with a hypoechoic center. It is sometimes difficult to distinguish the boundary between the esophagus and the thyroid lobe in the longitudinal plane. Identification of the esophagus can be facilitated by observing esophageal contraction and peristalsis, in real time, while the patient swallows.

EQUIPMENT

The basic components of an ultrasound system include the ultrasound unit itself, the transducer, and the monitor. The unit has a keyboard for inputting patient data and control functions such as depth of view, location, and number of focal zones, overall gain adjustment, time gain compensation, frequency selection, zoom mode, freeze frame, and Doppler imaging. The standard transducer for neck imaging is a multi-frequency, linear array probe in the 10–15 MHz range which is ideal for examining the superficial structures of the neck (Fig. 4.2). The length (or footprint) of the probe is generally 3.5–4 cm, which allows sufficient movement of the probe from the chin to the clavicles in the longitudinal plane.

FIG. 4.2. High frequency
linear array transducer.

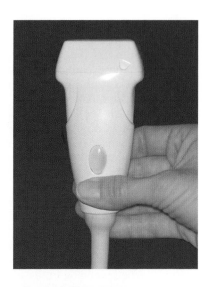

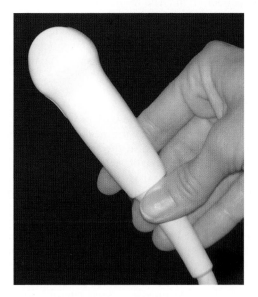

FIG. 4.3. Microconvex curvilinear transducer.

An optional (microconvex curvilinear) transducer has a tightly
curved convex footprint with a frequency range of 5–8 MHz
(Fig. 4.3). Although this probe was originally designed for viewing

the neonatal brain through the fontanel, it can be used to visualize the inferior aspect of the thyroid lobe from the sternal notch. This is especially useful for evaluating goiter in patients with severe kyphosis or those patients who have difficulty in hyperextending the neck. It is also useful for imaging substernal parathyroid glands and lymph nodes, and can be used in the performance of routine biopsies (See Chap. 12).

The monitor can be of any size but must be clearly visible to the examiner while conducting an ultrasound study or ultrasound-guided procedure. The monitor only shows a two-dimensional image. Therefore, images of the thyroid must be obtained in both the transverse and longitudinal planes to complete three-dimensional imaging. In either probe orientation, the top of the monitor display will indicate the surface area directly in contact with the probe and the bottom of the screen will display structures that are deep within the neck. For proper orientation, one end of the probe will be marked with a light, a raised dot, an indentation, or some other identifiable marking. When scanning in the transverse plane, the mark will be toward the patient's right. The resulting image will depict the right side of the neck on the left side of the screen and the left side on the right (Fig. 4.1). Correspondingly, in the longitudinal plane, the identification mark is positioned toward the patient's head, demonstrating the superior aspect on the left side of the monitor and the inferior aspect on the right.

PROCEDURE

For routine imaging, position the patient lying supine with a pillow under their shoulders and the neck extended. The anterior aspect of the neck is scanned in the transverse and longitudinal planes with the use of acoustic gel as a couplant. The central trachea with its reverberation artifact and the CCA and IJV serve as landmarks. The IJV can be made to distend and appear more prominent by having the patient perform a Valsalva maneuver. The normal thyroid gland is relatively homogeneous with a "ground glass" appearance on ultrasound (See Chap. 2). Connective tissue in the neck has a higher echodensity (hyperechoic) than thyroid tissue, and muscles have lower echodensity (hypoechoic). The sternothyroid and sternohyoid muscles are seen anterior to the thyroid gland, the SCM muscle is seen laterally, and the longus colli muscle lies posteriorly.

Transverse planes of the lobes above and below the level of the isthmus demonstrate the upper and lower poles of the thyroid. It is customary to start with the right thyroid lobe in the transverse plane. Scan through the entire lobe from superior to inferior poles

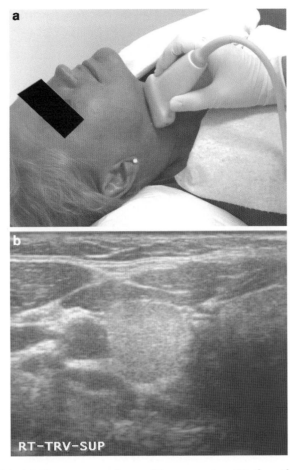

F$_{IG}$. 4.4. (**a**) Transverse probe position, superior RT thyroid gland. (**b**) Transverse image, superior RT thyroid gland.

first to determine the anatomical relationships and echotexture of the gland. To comply with the AIUM protocol for practice accreditation and to satisfy ECNU requirements, still images should be obtained through the superior segment (Fig. 4.4a, b), the mid portion (Fig. 4.5a, b) and the inferior segment of the lobe (Fig. 4.6a, b). Each image should include at least a part of the CCA in cross section and if possible, the IJV. Images should be labeled to provide information regarding location and orientation. At the mid portion, measure the transverse dimension of the gland. The lateral cursor

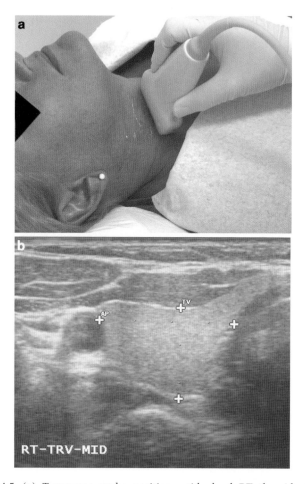

FIG. 4.5. (a) Transverse probe position, mid gland RT thyroid gland. (b) Transverse image, mid gland RT thyroid gland.

should include thyroid tissue that might extend beyond the carotid artery and the medial cursor should be placed at the lateral edge of the trachea. The depth (anterior–posterior dimension) of the thyroid lobe may be measured in either the transverse or longitudinal plane. In the transverse plane, place a cursor on the anterior border of the thyroid and extend a line from there to the deepest point of the thyroid lobe. The line should be at right angles to the lateral-medial line.

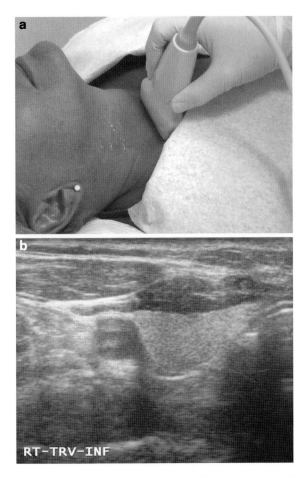

FIG. 4.6. (**a**) Transverse probe position, inferior RT thyroid gland. (**b**) Transverse image, inferior RT thyroid gland.

Rotating the transducer 90 ° shows the longitudinal plane of each lobe. Turn the patient's head approximately 10 ° toward the opposite side and align the probe with carotid artery (Fig. 4.7a, b). With the probe directly over the CCA, move the probe slowly imaging the lateral (Fig. 4.8a, b), mid (Fig. 4.9a, b), and medial (Fig. 4.10a, b) sections of each lobe. In most cases, the length of the thyroid lobe will be greater than the footprint of the probe.

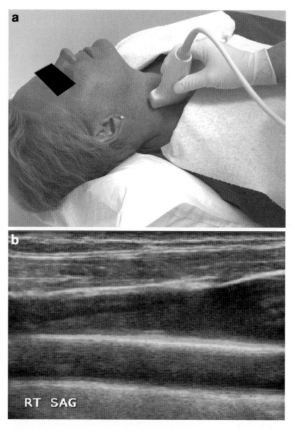

FIG. 4.7. (**a**) Longitudinal probe position, RT neck. (**b**) Longitudinal image demonstrating the RT IJV and CCA relationship.

To obtain the image of the entire thyroid lobe in one frame, utilize either the split screen function (Fig. 4.11), the extended, panoramic view (Fig. 4.12), or the trapezoidal display (Fig. 4.13). Measure the length of the lobe from the superior tip to the inferior pole. Measure the anterior to posterior dimension at the widest point. The anterior to posterior measurement in the longitudinal plane is the most accurate, but because the posterior border is sometimes difficult to visualize, it is acceptable to measure this dimension in the transverse plane. Figure 4.14a, b demonstrate imaging of the isthmus.

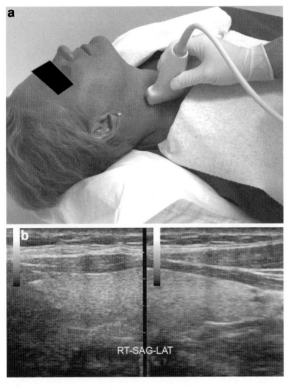

FIG. 4.8. (**a**) Longitudinal probe position, lateral RT thyroid lobe. (**b**) Longitudinal image, lateral RT thyroid lobe.

There are some variations to scanning that prove helpful. If the patient is unable to sufficiently hyperextend the neck or if the patient has a large goiter such that the inferior aspect of the thyroid lobe is not clearly visualized in the longitudinal plane, have the patient swallow. This may elevate the lobe sufficiently to view the inferior aspect of the lobe. By capturing this action in a digital clip, one can scroll through, frame by frame, until the desired image is observed and documented (Fig. 4.15). An alternative to this is to utilize the tightly curved microconvex curvilinear probe. Place the probe in the sternal notch; rotate down and to the side of interest to capture the inferior margin of the thyroid lobe (Fig. 4.16a, b).

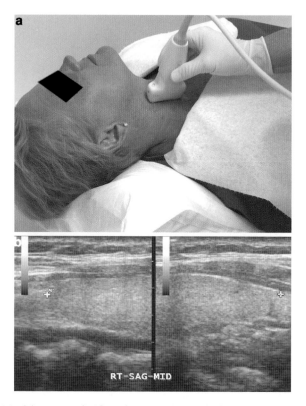

Fig. 4.9. (**a**) Longitudinal probe position, mid gland RT thyroid lobe. (**b**) Longitudinal image, mid gland RT thyroid lobe.

This chapter has focused on the normal ultrasound anatomy of the thyroid. It is essential that ultrasound of the thyroid always includes the entire neck, looking for abnormal lymph nodes, enlarged parathyroid glands, and abnormal masses. These, along with other conditions of the neck, will be discussed in the following chapters.

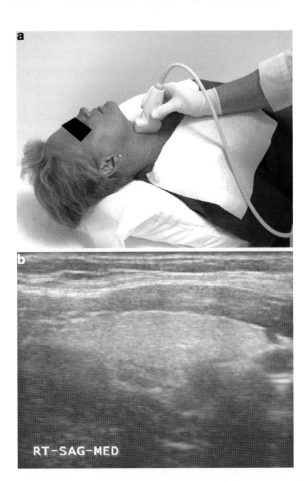

FIG. 4.10. (**a**) Longitudinal probe position, medial RT thyroid lobe. (**b**) Longitudinal image, medial RT thyroid lobe.

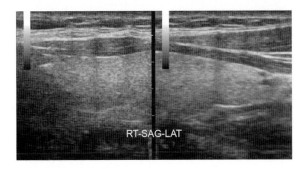

FIG. 4.11. Split screen longitudinal thyroid image.

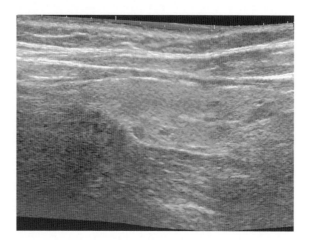

FIG. 4.12. Panoramic view longitudinal thyroid image.

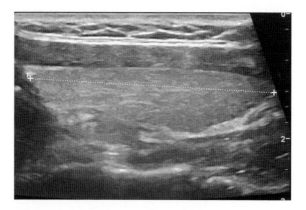

FIG. 4.13. Trapezoidal longitudinal thyroid image.

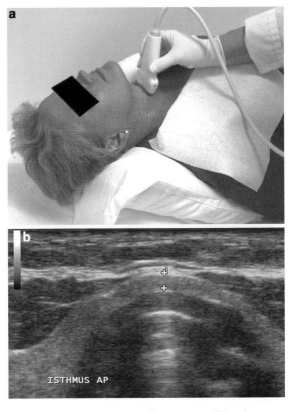

FIG. 4.14. (**a**) Isthmus transverse probe position. (**b**) Isthmus transverse image.

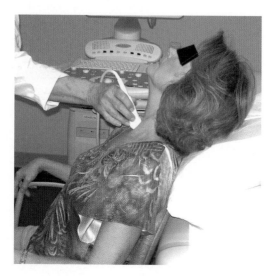

FIG. 4.15. Positioning a patient with neck or back physical limitations.

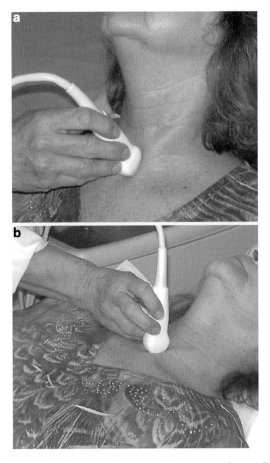

FIG. 4.16. (**a**) Using the microconvex curvilinear transducer. (**b**) Sternal notch application of the microconvex curvilinear transducer.

References

1. Ahuja AT, Evans RM, editors. Practical head and neck ultrasound. London: Greenwich medical limited; 2000.
2. Blum M, Yee J. Method of performing ultrasonography of the neck. In: Jack Baskin MD H, editor. Thyroid ultrasound and ultrasound-guided FNA biopsy. Massachusetts: Kluwer; 2000. p. 35–58.
3. AIUM. Standards for performance of the thyroid and parathyroid ultrasound examination (AIUM Standard, approved 1998). Laurel, MD: American Institute of Ultrasound in Medicine; 1999.

CHAPTER 5
Pediatric Ultrasound of the Neck

Henry J. Baskin, Jr

INTRODUCTION

The spectrum of imaging abnormalities encountered during pediatric neck ultrasound extends well beyond the thyroid gland—both anatomically and conceptually—to include normal anatomic variants and embryologically derived pathologies that are less commonly seen in older patients. This chapter will briefly discuss an approach to scanning children's necks and then focus on the spectrum of abnormalities that may be encountered during pediatric neck ultrasound, first addressing embryologically derived pathology, normal variants, and non-thyroidal cervical abnormalities, before focusing on the appearance of specific diseases that involve the thyroid itself.

PATIENT PREPARATION

The key to successful pediatric neck ultrasound lies in appropriate patient preparation. For a very young child, the procedure can be frightening: A trip to the doctor in and of itself is scary, but then you are forced to lie on your back while a stranger in a white coat smears cold goo all over your neck and someone else holds you down, forcing you to stay still while your parents sit nervously on the side. Without proper planning, such an endeavor is difficult at best and an utter failure at worst. Understanding the child's perspective helps one prepare better for this examination and thus allows better diagnostic imaging.

Ideally, as with all pediatric medical care, an ultrasound should be performed in an environment that is welcoming and nonthreatening to children. Age-appropriate toys and, if available, Child Life

H.J. Baskin et al. (eds.), *Thyroid Ultrasound and Ultrasound-Guided FNA*, **65**
DOI 10.1007/978-1-4614-4785-6_5,
© Springer Science+Business Media, LLC 2013

Specialists, should be at hand to comfort the child. Newborns are especially soothed by ceiling projectors and warming pads on the scanning bed. Transducer gel warmers should be used to make the gel a comfortable temperature and, if appropriate, the child should be offered a chance to feel the gel and transducer prior to the examination. If not actually performing the study, the interpreting physician should be closely involved in image acquisition so as to decrease the time that the child needs to stay still.

Ultrasound performed by the physician is also helpful because many pediatric neck abnormalities extend into the lateral neck, where children's small size and the complex regional anatomy can become quite confusing and real-time scanning helps to better conceptualize any complex transspatial lesions. In addition to being skilled and experienced with imaging pediatric neck lesions, the interpreting physician should be knowledgeable as to when computed tomography, magnetic resonance imaging, or scintigraphy would better elucidate a given abnormality; they should also be facile in correlating any ultrasound abnormalities with findings made visible by other modalities. For these reasons, at our institution, all pediatric ultrasound is performed or directly supervised by subspecialty-trained pediatric radiologists.

Finally, it is crucial to use a high-resolution, high-frequency (at least 15 MHz), linear-array transducer to best visualized the pediatric thyroid gland and cervical soft tissues. Unfortunately, traditional high-resolution transducers offered with most ultrasound packages are often too large to comfortably use on the very short necks of neonates and young infants. Likewise, infants and toddlers often have quite chubby chins and necks and, because the thyroid lies relatively higher in the neck at this age, the transducer may not be able to obtain close contact with the skin. In these young children, the thyroid gland may be best imaged by a specialized small footprint probe, such as those used in neonatal echoencephalography; of course, the sonographer should be familiar with and experienced at using such probes.

EMBRYOLOGICALLY DERIVED PATHOLOGY

Embryology of the Thyroid Gland

The thyroid gland originates at the base of the tongue in an embryological structure known as the foramen cecum and then descends into the lower neck by way of the thyroglossal duct. As the developing gland descends into the lower neck, it divides into separate lobes connected to each other by an isthmus.

After the thyroid gland reaches its final location—inferior to the hyoid bone and anterior to the trachea—the thyroglossal duct involutes. Aberrations of this normal development result in various forms of thyroid dysgenesis or thyroglossal duct remnants that one may encounter during pediatric neck ultrasound.

Congenital Hypothyroidism

Congenital hypothyroidism (CH) is relatively common, occurring in approximately 1 per 3,000 births. It is classified as either transient or permanent; the transient form accounts for 20% of newborns with CH and occurs as a result of maternal iodine deficiency or secondary to in utero exposure to antithyroid drugs, maternal TSH-receptor antibodies, or very high levels of iodine. Permanent CH results from dyshormonogenesis, autoimmune disease in the newborn, or from thyroid dysgenesis (aplasia, hypoplasia, or ectopy).

CH is the most easily treated form of developmental delay and ultrasound is clinically useful to help differentiate its many causes. In patients with transient CH or with CH due to dyshormonogenesis or autoimmune thyroiditis, ultrasound will demonstrate an orthotopic thyroid gland; the gland may be normal sized in transient CH or enlarged in cases of dyshormonogenesis (Fig. 5.1) or autoimmune disease. If CH is secondary to thyroid dysgenesis then ultrasound will demonstrate an absent or small thyroid gland.

Thyroid Aplasia

Thyroid aplasia presents with CH and an absence of any thyroidal tissue. The defect is usually sporadic, but there are some familial forms and both autosomal dominant and autosomal recessive inheritance patterns have been reported. Neck ultrasound fails to reveal any thyroid tissue in the thyroid bed and no uptake is seen with I-123 scintigraphy.

Thyroid Hypoplasia

Ultrasound in children with CH may sometimes demonstrate a small, but otherwise normal-appearing thyroid gland (Fig. 5.2). This is particularly common in those children who have CH and trisomy 21 (children with trisomy 21 are also more likely to have small benign thyroid cyst) (Fig. 5.3). There are published charts of normal thyroid volumes for different populations and these should be used to evaluate the size of the thyroid in children with hypothyroidism, congenital or otherwise.

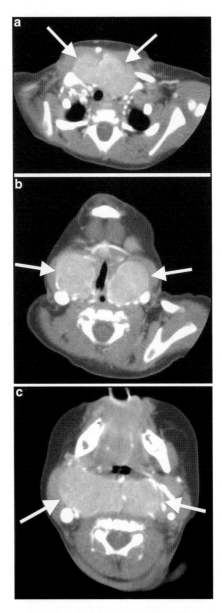

Fig. 5.1. Goitrous thyroid in congenital hypothyroidism. Axial CT images (**a**, **b**, **c**) show a massively enlarged thyroid (*arrows*) in a 5-month-old with a TSH over 300. Full ultrasonic visualization of the thyroid gland is difficult in young children because of the overall short length of their necks

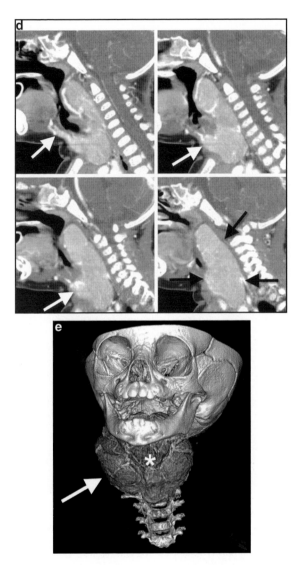

FIG. 5.1. (continued) compared to the size of most high-frequency transducers and because of the relatively high positioning of the thyroid gland in the neck compared to adults. This is best appreciated on sagittal CT images from the same patient, which well demonstrates the patient's short neck and how the path of least resistance for the thyroid to enlarge is posterior (*arrows*, **d**). On a 3D CT reconstruction (**e**), note how the thyroid gland (*arrow*) wraps around the airway (*asterisk*).

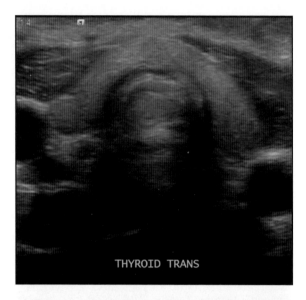

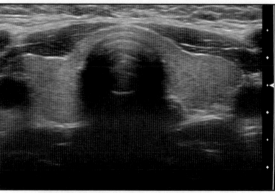

FIG. 5.2. Thyroid hypoplasia. In thyroid hypoplasia, the gland is small and difficult to visualize; the right and left lobes may both be small and the isthmus may be relatively normal thickness, as shown in a patient with congenital hypothyroidism and trisomy 21 (**a**). Compare this to the thyroid of a normal child (**b**), which is well-defined, normal volume, and well-proportioned.

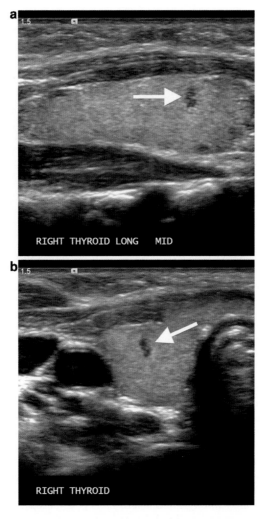

FIG. 5.3. Benign thyroid cyst in trisomy 21. Longitudinal (**a**) and transverse (**b**) ultrasound images in a 26-month-old boy with trisomy 21 shows the typical appearance of a very small hypoechoic cyst (*arrows*) seen in patients with Down syndrome. Note lack of significant posterior acoustic enhancement because these cysts are so small.

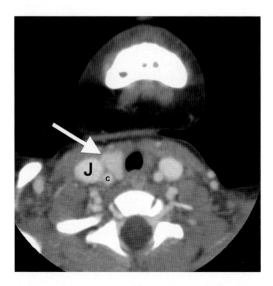

FIG. 5.4. Left thyroid hemiagenesis. Axial CT image in a 26-month-old with a retropharyngeal abscess shows absence of the left lobe of the thyroid gland. The right lobe is shown with an arrow, and the right jugular vein (*J*) and carotid artery (*c*) are also annotated. Although not present in this child, patients with an absent left thyroid lobe usually have a small, but blunted isthmus.

Thyroid Hemiagenesis

Thyroid hemiagenesis is a rare congenital anomaly in which one lobe of the thyroid fails to form. It is the most innocuous form of thyroid dysgenesis and is much more common in girls. In hemiagenesis it is almost always the left lobe that is absent; the right lobe has a normal size and appearance and, although blunted, the isthmus is usually present (Fig. 5.4). For unknown reasons, the isthmus will be absent in rare cases of right hemiagenesis (Fig. 5.5). Although hemiagenesis is considered an incidental finding, numerous studies have shown that these patients have a slightly increased rate of all forms of thyroid pathology, from hyperthyroidism to carcinoma. The diagnosis of thyroid hemiagenesis should be clearly communicated to the surgeon in patients who are to undergo any type of neck surgery.

Ectopic Thyroid

Ectopic, or aberrant, thyroid tissue can be found anywhere along the normal path of thyroid descent, but is most commonly found at the base of the tongue, in which case it may be referred

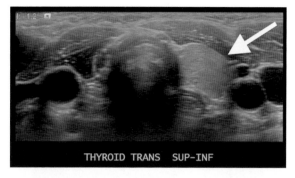

FIG. 5.5. Right thyroid hemiagenesis. A transverse image of the thyroid reveals a normal left lobe (arrow), but no right lobe or isthmus. Right thyroid hemiagenesis is quite rare.

to as a lingual thyroid (Fig. 5.6). Ultrasound of the thyroid bed may reveal a hypoplastic thyroid or no thyroid tissue at all. Further imaging workup varies according to local preferences and practice; although I-123 scintigraphy is very sensitive for the presence of ectopic thyroid tissue, it fails to localize exactly where along the path from the base of the tongue to the inferior neck any potential aberrant thyroid tissue exists. Contrast-enhanced CT is especially helpful for the evaluation of thyroid ectopia because of its excellent spatial resolution and ability to provide multiplanar images, which best identify smaller rests of ectopic thyroid tissue (Fig. 5.7) or any potential thyroglossal duct remnants.

Thyroglossal Duct Cysts
The thyroglossal duct is a normally transient structure that involutes during fetal life; if it fails to do so, any remnants may slowly collect fluid and eventually manifest as a cystic neck mass. Ninety percent of thyroglossal duct cysts (TGCs) present before age 10, and the typical history is a young child with a painless and compressible midline or paramidline mass. There is often a history of waxing and waning size, which occurs when there is irritation from recurrent upper respiratory tract infection or minor trauma. Sometimes TGCs become secondarily infected and present as an acutely painful, inflamed mass. If a TGC has not been complicated by prior infection or bleeding, then it appears as an anechoic cystic mass with increased through transmission and sharp,

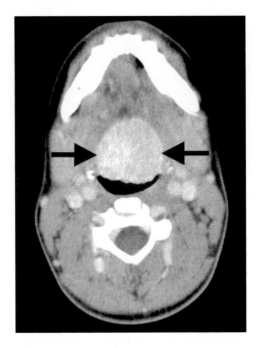

FIG. 5.6. Lingual thyroid. An axial enhanced CT scan through the neck in a young child with hypothyroidism, a long-standing sensation of neck fullness, and tongue mass on radiographs shows a clump of high attenuation thyroid tissue in the base of the tongue, known as a lingual thyroid.

well-defined margins. They are usually spherical but may have tubular configuration (Fig. 5.8). About half are found at the level of the hyoid bone, a quarter above it, and another quarter below it; they should never be found below the level of the thyroid. If complicated by prior hemorrhage or infection, TGCs may have more echogenic contents, small septations, and a thickened, irregular margin; they occasionally appear solid (although should still cause increased through transmission) (Fig. 5.9). Complete surgical resection is needed or TGCs will recur.

Fourth Branchial Apparatus Anomalies
Another embryologic anlage that may cause pediatric thyroid abnormalities is the fourth branchial apparatus. Fourth branchial apparatus anomalies (BAAs) include a spectrum of epithelial lined remnants that only involve the left lobe of the thyroid. Fourth

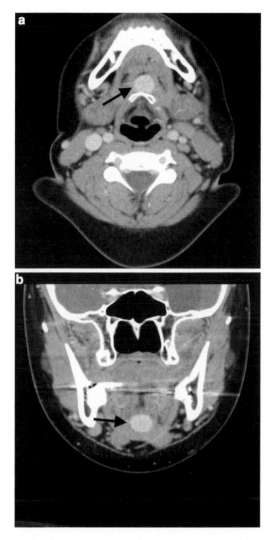

FIG. 5.7. Ectopic thyroid. Aberrant thyroid tissue may be found anywhere along the course of the thyroglossal duct, from the base of the tongue to the thyroid bed. Although scintigraphy is often espoused as the study of choice to identify ectopic thyroid tissue, it provides little spatial resolution. CT has the advantage of significantly better spatial resolution and the ability to provide multiplanar reconstructions, which can often better demonstrate rest of aberrant tissue, as shown in this patient with hypothyroidism, no thyroid tissue in the thyroid bed, and a small rest of aberrant thyroid (*arrows*) anterior to the hyoid bone.

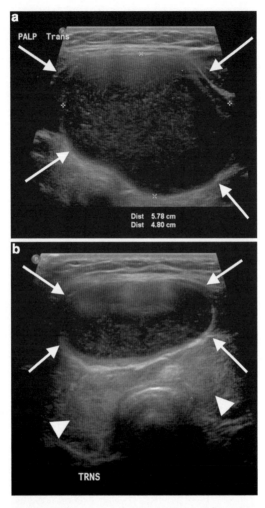

FIG. 5.8. Thyroglossal duct cyst. An US was obtained on this teenager to evaluate a long-standing palpable thyroid mass. The mass turned out to be a thyroglossal duct cyst. Transverse US images show a predominantly anechoic cyst with scattered low-level echos (*arrows*, **a** and **b**). This minimally complex thyroglossal duct cyst sits just above the level of the thyroid gland (*arrowheads*, **b**).

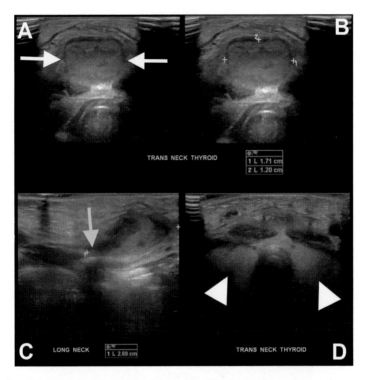

TRANS NECK THYROID

1 L 1.71 cm
2 L 1.20 cm

LONG NECK

1 L 2.69 cm

TRANS NECK THYROID

FIG. 5.9. Complex thyroglossal duct cyst. US was performed to evaluate a new painful thyroid mass in a 2-year-old boy. The images demonstrate that the mass is actually a heterogeneous, isoechoic cystic collection (*calipers and white arrows*) separate from the thyroid gland (*arrowheads*). This was an infected thyroglossal duct cyst; note its "tail" (*yellow arrow*) extending cephalad towards the tongue, reflecting this TDG's embryologic origins.

BAAs may become infected and cause suppurative thyroiditis, abscess, cystic mass, or sinus tract to the pyriform sinus; imaging depends on the specific patient's complication. Suppurative thyroiditis—which can be caused by a BAA or occur primarily—begins as a focal area of abnormally decreased echogenicity within the thyroid (Fig. 5.10). With worsening infection and abscess

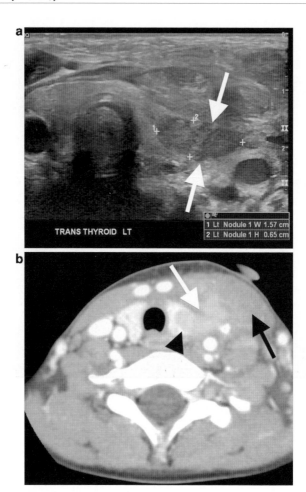

Fig. 5.10. Fourth branchial apparatus anomalies. Suppurative thyroiditis in a 6-year-old boy with fever and neck pain. Embryologic remnants from the fourth branchial apparatus are almost always left-sided and may lead to any one of several abnormalities, from suppurative thyroiditis to a sinus track to infected cysts or abscesses. In this child, transverse US shows a well-defined, focal, heterogeneously hypoechoic nodule (*calipers*, **a**) extending through the thyroid capsule (*arrows*, **a**). Axial CT in the same patient also shows the focal area of suppuration in the upper pole of the left lobe (*arrowhead*, **b**) as well as more detail of the extracapsular extension (*white arrow*, **b**) and inflammation of the overlying strap musculature (*black arrow*, **b**).

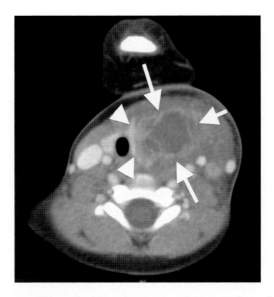

FIG. 5.11. Fourth branchial apparatus anomalies. An enhanced CT in a 13-year-old with fever, neck pain, and new thyroid mass shows a "claw" of thyroid tissue (*arrowheads*) around a large, complex, peripherally enhancing fluid collection emanating from the superior pole of the left thyroid lobe, typical for an infected fourth BAA cyst.

formation, a complex focal fluid collection may develop, usually with heterogeneous but hypoechoic internal contents; if caused by a BAA, a sinus tract may extend up into the deep neck towards the pyriform sinus. Such complications are best visualized by contrast-enhanced CT imaging (Fig. 5.11).

Inclusion Cysts

Small epidermal inclusion cysts are another common cause of palpable neck or "thyroid" masses in children. These cysts are characterized pathologically as either dermoids or epidermoids, both of which are benign congenital cysts derived from inclusion of ectodermic elements. On ultrasound, they appear as well-defined, avascular masses with internal echogenicity similar to the thyroid gland. The ultrasound findings of inclusion cysts are nonspecific (Fig. 5.12), but, because they contain dermal appendages, dermoids may have imaging characteristics identical to fat and therefore have a pathognomonic appearance on MRI and CT.

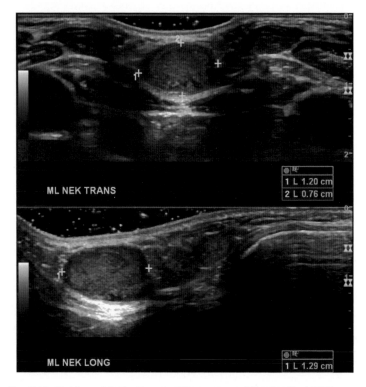

Fig. 5.12. Epidermal inclusion cyst. Transverse and longitudinal US images show a well-defined isoechoic nodule (*calipers*) in the subcutaneous soft tissues of the infrahyoid midline neck, just above the thyroid gland. Images are characteristic, but not diagnostic, of an epidermal inclusion cyst; tissue diagnosis is needed and in this case confirmed the diagnosis of dermoid.

Vascular Malformations

Vascular malformations are a common cause of pediatric neck masses. Broadly speaking, these lesions are a group of nonneoplastic congenital malformations caused by disordered development of vascular channels. They are categorized by the predominant channel involved and are therefore termed either lymphatic, venous, venolymphatic, or arteriovenous malformations. They may range from predominately solid to mostly cystic masses. Although they often infiltrate the thyroid gland, vascular malformations usually extend into the lateral neck.

Lymphatic malformations are usually transspatial, multicystic masses with numerous fluid–fluid levels (as a result of prior hemorrhage or infection) (Fig. 5.13). If predominately microcystic, lymphatic malformations may appear solid on ultrasound.

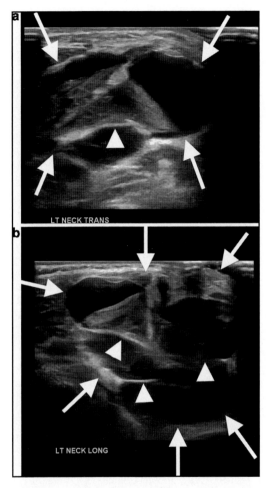

FIG. 5.13. Lymphatic malformation. Transverse (**a**) and longitudinal
(**b**) neck ultrasound in a 3-year-old boy with new swelling near the thyroid
gland reveals a very complex, transspatial, multiloculated fluid collection
(*white arrows*, **a** and **b**) extending from the region of the thyroid (not
shown) into the left lateral neck. Note the presence of thin septations
(*arrowheads*, **a** and **b**), typical of macrocystic lymphatic malformations.
Two axial fluid-sensitive sequence MR images (**c**) better show the internal
characteristics of this complex cystic lesion (*yellow arrows*) as well as its
relationship regional structures, including the thyroid gland (*small white
arrows*, upper image). Again, note numerous thin septations (*arrowheads*)
and fluid–fluid levels (*large white arrows*) from prior internal hemorrhage. Two contrast-enhanced MR images (**d**) show that the lesion (*yellow arrows*) does not enhance, supporting the diagnosis of lymphatic

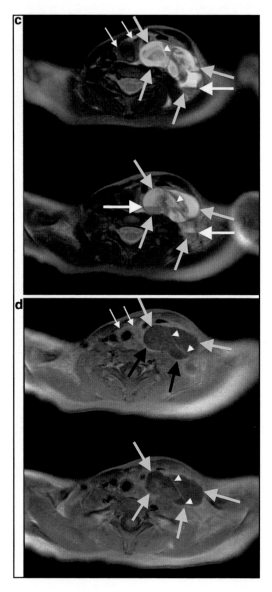

FIG. 5.13. (continued) malformation. The thin septations (*arrowheads*) are again well seen, as are regional soft tissues, including the thyroid gland (*small white arrows*, upper image).

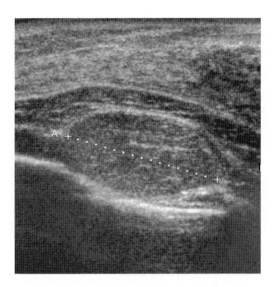

FIG. 5.14. Venous malformation. A longitudinal US image shows a well-defined, hypoechoic neck mass (*calipers*) in a 14-year-old girl. This appearance is nonspecific and excisional biopsy is mandatory to exclude a soft tissue sarcoma; biopsy in this case revealed a venous malformation.

Venous malformations generally appear as a lobulated, hyperechoic soft tissue mass that may contain phleboliths (which cause posterior acoustic shadowing) (Fig. 5.14). CT and MRI are very useful to demonstrate enhancement of the solid components of these lesions and are much better than ultrasound for delineating the entire extent of disease; these modalities usually help provide a confident diagnosis without biopsy.

Infantile Hemangioma

Unfortunately, the adult medical literature is littered with reports of masses related to the thyroid (and elsewhere in the body) that are inaccurately classified as a "hemangioma." These masses are in fact venous malformations and should be referred to as such. True infantile hemangiomas are benign neoplasms seen exclusively in young children. They also follow a very predictable natural history: they develop in early infancy, proliferate during the first year of life, and involute shortly thereafter. They may be seen near the thyroid gland but, unlike the aforementioned malformations,

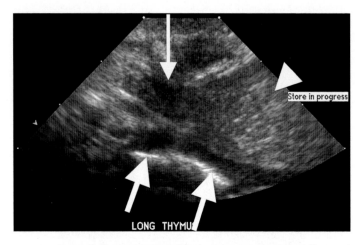

Store in progress

LONG THYMU

Fig. 5.15. Normal thymus tissue. The thymus may extend well into the neck in younger children and may be confounding when unexpectedly seen on ultrasound. Here a longitudinal US image shows a finger of thymic tissue extending in the neck (*small arrow*), just lateral to the thyroid gland and next to the carotid artery (*large arrows*). Note the normal appearance of the remainder of the thymus (*arrowhead*), which has a similar echotexture as the liver.

infantile hemangiomas are never seen in older children and adults. Infantile hemangiomas should not be confused with other lesions and are treated conservatively.

Thymic Tissue

The thymus is also derived from the branchial apparatus and, like the thyroid, descends into the neck early during fetal life. The two lobes of the thymus course behind the thyroid and sterno-cleidomastoid muscles and fuse at the level of the aortic arch, but occasionally a portion of the thymus will extend into the upper neck and may be visible on thyroid ultrasound. Knowledge of its normal appearance helps avoid any diagnostic dilemma. In younger children, the thymus is hypoechoic with an echotexture similar to that of the liver (Fig. 5.15). As children grow, the thymus becomes infiltrated with fat, which accentuates its internal septations and gives it a pattern sometimes referred to as a "starry sky" appearance. The thymus gland should never cause mass effect or displacement of vessels or other structures. On real-time imaging, the thymus gently pulsates with cardiac motion.

DIFFUSE THYROID DISEASES

Hashimoto thyroiditis is by far the most common diffuse thyroid abnormality seen in children. Early changes almost always involve the posterior portion of the gland, first manifesting as subtle coarsening of the normally smooth, homogeneous echotexture in the deeper part of the gland. As thyroiditis progresses, the posterior portion of the gland will develop very small (1–2 mm) round or oval areas of hypoechogencity. Eventually these subtle sonographic abnormalities progress to involve the entire gland and over several years (or with particularly pernicious disease, even sooner), the entire thyroid becomes increasingly heterogeneous (Fig. 5.16). Although these abnormalities are almost always present in children with Hashimoto thyroiditis, these sonographic features may at first be quite subtle and therefore it is important to use a high-resolution transducer to achieve adequate image resolution.

With chronic Hashimoto disease, the thyroid develops course, thickened septa that appear on ultrasound as branching, echogenic reticulations that form conspicuous rounded or oval foci of relatively hypoechoic thyroid tissue, small lesions known as pseudonodules (Fig. 5.17). It is this pattern of coarse reticular echoes and pseudonodules that becomes the dominant ultrasound feature in children with severe or chronic thyroiditis (Fig. 5.18).

Severe thyroiditis—especially early on—may cause diffuse enlargement of the gland, sometimes accompanied by marked hyperemia visible with power Doppler (Fig. 5.19). These changes are generally not, but may be, encountered in chronic disease. Also, unlike the early grayscale findings described earlier, increased Doppler flow seen in Hashimoto thyroiditis is often inhomogeneous and has no predictable pattern, sometimes sparing large swaths of the gland (Fig. 5.20).

One should not expect thyroid ultrasound to offer specificity with regard to other diffuse thyroid diseases; there are no imaging features that accurately suggest alternative diagnoses such as Graves' disease or nodular hyperplasia (both of which are far less common than Hashimoto thyroiditis in children) (Fig. 5.21). The clinical usefulness of ultrasound in the evaluation of children with Hashimoto thyroiditis lies in the identification of the very early grayscale abnormalities described earlier. In children, these subtle findings can suggest the diagnosis well before thyroid antibodies become positive.

Other important ultrasonic findings to be cognizant of in children with thyroiditis are the potential of associated lymphoma (which may cause regional lymphadenopathy) or the presence of a dominant nodule (which may represent a superimposed adenoma or thyroid malignancy).

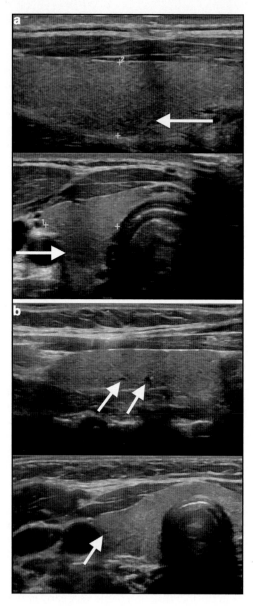

FIG. 5.16. Ultrasound findings in five children with thyroiditis of increasing severity. (a) 17-year-old boy: There is subtle coarsening of the thyroid echotexture in the posterior portion of the gland (*arrows*). (b) 13-year-old boy: In addition to mild coarsening, there are a few oval hypoechoic foci (*arrows*) in the posterior portion of the gland. (c) 12-year-old boy: The posterior gland has become progressively more heterogeneous (*arrows*), losing the smooth echotexture that characterizes the normal thyroid. (d) 7-year-old girl: Numerous thin, echogenic septations (*arrowheads*) have become visible

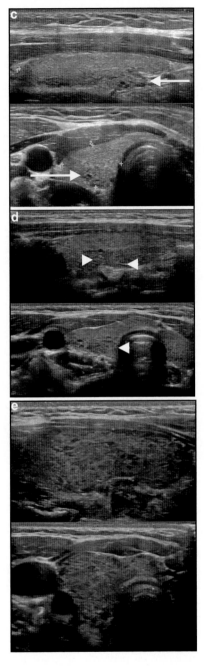

FIG. 5.16. (continued) within the area of coarse echogenicity. (**e**) 13-year-old girl: The whole gland now has a coarse, heterogeneous echotexture with thin septations and innumerable small hypoechoic foci visible throughout.

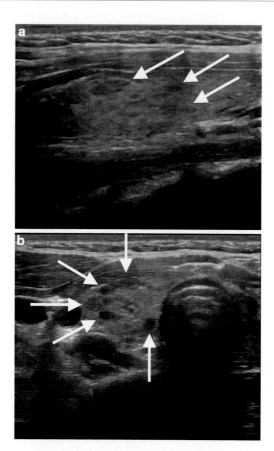

FIG. 5.17. Pseudonodules. Longitudinal (**a**) and transverse (**b**) US in a 14-year-old girl with chronic Hashimoto disease show innumerable rounded and oval hypoechoic foci known as pseudonodules (*arrows*).

FOCAL THYROID LESIONS

Focal thyroid nodules and masses are rare in children, accounting for less than 2% of pediatric thyroid diseases. Thyroid cancer in this age group is rarer still, occurring in less than 2 per 100,000 children. There are no specific imaging features unique to pediatric thyroid nodules and any dominant lesion should be biopsied as discussed in other chapters of this book.

The vast majority of pediatric thyroid nodules are benign, the most common diagnosis being benign follicular adenoma. Adenomas may have variable echogenicity, ranging from mostly

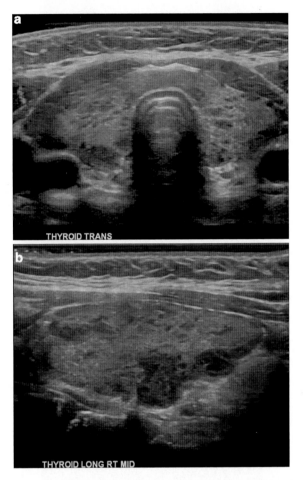

FIG. 5.18. Chronic Hashimoto disease. Transverse (**a**) and longitudinal (**b**) US in a 12-year-old boy show the typical appearance of chronic Hashimoto disease: a diffuse pattern of coarse reticular echoes and pseudonodules throughout the gland.

solid (Fig. 5.22) to mostly cystic (Fig. 5.23) masses. Other common benign thyroid lesions seen in children include colloid cysts and cystic degenerating or hemorrhagic nodules (Fig 5.24).

Like in adults, papillary carcinoma is the most common thyroid neoplasm in the pediatric age group. Unfortunately, it tends to behave more aggressively than in adults, with higher

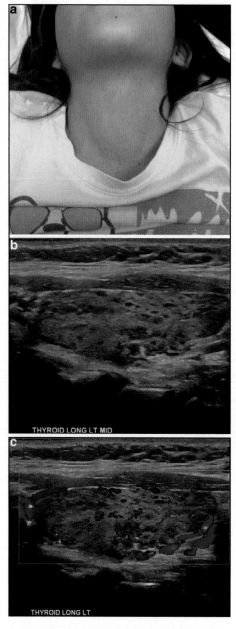

FIG. 5.19. Thyromegaly. Photograph (**a**) of a 9-year-old girl with severe thyroiditis shows marked enlargement of the thyroid gland. Grayscale (**b**) and color Doppler (**c**) images show the typical pattern of severe thyroiditis with innumerable pseudonodules. The gland is hyperemic and enlarged, with a volume over twice the upper limits of normal for her age.

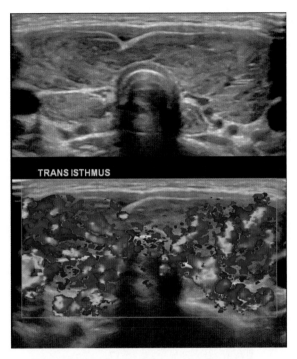

FIG. 5.20. Thyromegaly and hyperemia. Grayscale and color Doppler US images demonstrate diffuse thyroid enlargement and typical findings of severe thyroiditis. Note the diffuse, but inhomogeneous, pattern of hyperemia.

rates of multifocality, neck lymph node disease, and extracapsular extension (Fig 5.25). Other malignancies that may be seen include follicular carcinoma, medullary carcinoma, papillary oncocytic neoplasm, and metastatic disease, none of which have any specific imaging features.

SUMMARY

The most important concepts to remember about pediatric thyroid ultrasound can be distilled into two points. The first is that one must keep an open mind about what ultrasound of a "thyroid mass" may actually reveal in a child. The complex embryologic development of neck can result in disparate but predictable abnormalities that are, in fact, separate from the thyroid gland itself and

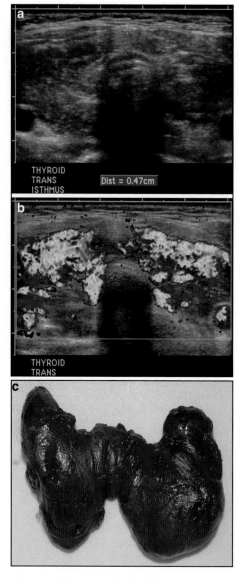

FIG. 5.21. Graves' disease. US cannot reliably differentiate between Hashimoto thyroiditis and Graves' disease in children. Grayscale (**a**) and color Doppler (**b**) US images in a 16-year-old girl with Graves' disease show sonographic features similar to those seen in Hashimoto thyroiditis, including diffuse enlargement, coarsening of the echotexture and echogenic septations. (**c**) A gross pathologic photograph of the thyroid from the same patient.

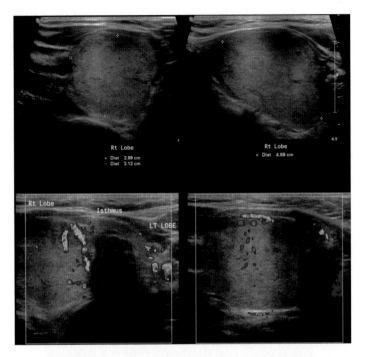

Fig. 5.22. Follicular adenoma. Imaging features of thyroid neoplasms are not specific. The most common thyroid neoplasm in children is benign follicular adenoma, which may range from completely solid to mostly cystic. Here, grayscale and color Doppler US images show a large, well-defined mass (*calipers*) in the right lobe of the thyroid of a 12-year-old boy with follicular adenoma.

the interpreting physician must be familiar with how to best diagnose these abnormalities, especially when further workup involves the use of other imaging techniques.

The second important concept to remember when performing pediatric thyroid ultrasound is that early thyroiditis may be quite subtle and often precedes the clinical detection of antithyroid antibodies in children. When imaging children with thyroiditis, one should be highly sensitive to subtle abnormalities seen in early disease. In children with chronic thyroiditis, the focus should be on the identification of any dominant nodule or regional lymphadenopathy. The sonographic approach and features of focal thyroid nodules in children is not unique and the other chapters of this text cover these topics in excellent detail.

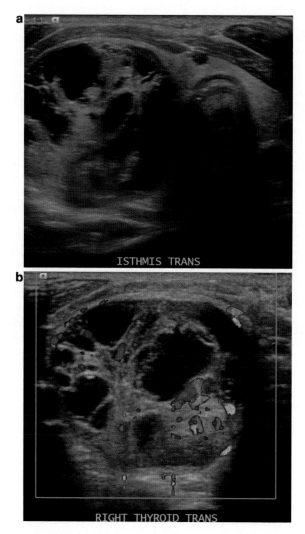

FIG. 5.23. Follicular adenoma. Transverse grayscale (**a**) and color Doppler (**b**) US images in a 17-year-old boy show an example of a mostly cystic follicular adenoma.

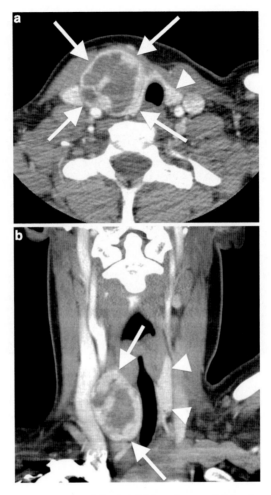

FIG. 5.24. Degenerating nodule. Axial (**a**) and coronal (**b**) enhanced CT in a 11-year-old boy with a long-standing thyroid mass show a nonspecific, partially enhancing cystic mass (*arrows*) found to be a degenerating nodule on pathology. Note the normal left thyroid lobe (*arrowheads*).

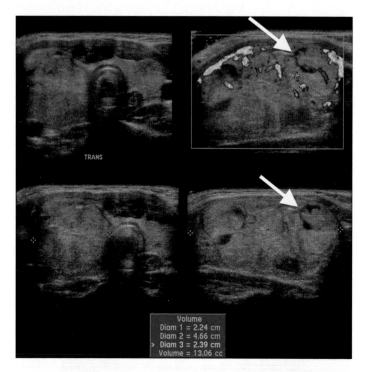

FIG. 5.25. Papillary carcinoma. Transverse (*top left & bottom left*) and longitudinal color Doppler (*top right*) and grayscale (*bottom right*) US images show a large, heterogeneous, multilobulated mass (*calipers*) almost replacing the entire right lobe of the thyroid in a 12-year-old boy. There is focal extracapsular extension (*arrows*) of this papillary carcinoma.

Bibliography

1. Chang Y-W, Hong HS, Choi DL. Sonography of the pediatric thyroid: a pictorial essay. J Clin Ultrasound. 2009;37(3):149–57. doi:10.1002/jcu.20555.
2. Frates MC, Benson CB, Charboneau JW, Cibas ES, Clark OH, Coleman BG, et al. Management of thyroid nodules detected at US: society of radiologists in ultrasound consensus conference statement. Radiology. 2005;237(3):794–800. doi:10.1148/radiol.2373050220.
3. Hoang JK, Lee WK, Lee M, Johnson D, Farrell S. US features of thyroid malignancy: pearls and pitfalls. Radiographics. 2007;27(3):847–60. doi:10.1148/rg.273065038.
4. Marwaha RK, Tandon N, Kanwar R, Ganie MA, Bhattacharya V, Reddy DHK, et al. Evaluation of the role of ultrasonography in

diagnosis of autoimmune thyroiditis in goitrous children. Indian Pediatr. 2008;45(4):279–84.

5. Nasseri F, Eftekhari F. Clinical and radiologic review of the normal and abnormal thymus: pearls and pitfalls. Radiographics. 2010;30(2): 413–28. doi:10.1148/rg.302095131.

6. Ruchala M, Szczepanek E, Szaflarski W, Moczko J, Czarnywojtek A, Pietz L, et al. Increased risk of thyroid pathology in patients with thyroid hemiagenesis: results of a large cohort case–control study. Eur J Endocrinol. 2009;162(1):153–60. doi:10.1530/EJE-09-0590.

7. Takashima S, Nomura N, Tanaka H, Itoh Y, Miki K, Harada T. Congenital hypothyroidism: assessment with ultrasound. AJNR Am J Neuroradiol. 1995;16(5):1117–23.

CHAPTER 6
Ultrasound of Diffuse Thyroid Enlargement: Thyroiditis

Mark A. Lupo and Robert A. Levine

INTRODUCTION

Diffuse enlargement of the thyroid gland is a common finding during both physical examination and ultrasound evaluation. While iodine deficiency is still the most common cause of goiter worldwide, chronic lymphocytic thyroiditis (CLT), also referred to as Hashimoto's thyroiditis, is the most common cause of goiter and hypothyroidism in the USA, most of Europe, and other countries with adequate dietary iodine. Table 6.1 lists the common causes of diffuse thyroid enlargement. Thyroiditis describes a diverse group of conditions characterized by thyroid inflammation. While there is significant overlap in the sonographic findings of these various entities, ultrasound provides insight into the etiology and clinical course of the disease process, and may identify nodules that may require fine needle aspiration (FNA) biopsy.

CHRONIC LYMPHOCYTIC (HASHIMOTO'S) THYROIDITIS (CLT)

CLT is the most common form of thyroiditis. Approximately 10% of the US population overall and an estimated 25% of women over the age of 65 years exhibit antibodies to thyroperoxidase [1]. The presence of thyroid autoantibodies predicts future thyroid dysfunction in patients who are euthyroid. The pathologic hallmark of Hashimoto's thyroiditis is lymphocytic infiltration of the gland by B cells and cytotoxic T cells. A decrease in echogenicity is seen on ultrasound, as the lymphocytic infiltrate allows greater through transmission of sound than intact thyroid follicles.

H.J. Baskin et al. (eds.), *Thyroid Ultrasound and Ultrasound-Guided FNA*, **99**
DOI 10.1007/978-1-4614-4785-6_6,
© Springer Science+Business Media, LLC 2013

Table 6.1 Causes of diffuse thyroid enlargement

Hashimoto's thyroiditis
Graves' disease
Silent thyroiditis/postpartum thyroiditis
Subacute thyroiditis
Suppurative thyroiditis
Drug-induced thyroiditis
Riedel's thyroiditis
Iodine deficiency
Organification defect

This hypoechogenicity has been used to predict the presence of autoimmune thyroid disease and the risk of subsequent hypothyroidism. Pederson studied 485 patients with diffuse thyroid hypoechogenicity and 100 normal patients and found that hypoechogenicity had a positive predictive value of autoimmune thyroid disease of 88% and a negative predictive value of 95% [2]. Hypoechogenicity on ultrasound has been shown to have a greater predictive value for development of hypothyroidism than the presence of thyroid autoantibodies [3, 4]. This finding is less robust in morbidly obese subjects, as the thyroid may be more hypoechoic than normal [5].

The degree of change in echogenicity seen in Hashimoto's thyroiditis is very variable. Normal thyroid (Figs. 2.4, 2.5, and 2.6) has a ground glass, homogeneous appearance that is comparatively brighter (more hyperechoic) than the surrounding strap muscles. As lymphocytic infiltration progresses, the thyroid echogenicity decreases, approaching that of the surrounding strap muscles and in some cases even exceeding that of the strap muscles. The progression and degree of hypoechogenicity generally predicts the severity of hypothyroidism [6].

Heterogeneity is another common ultrasonographic feature of autoimmune thyroid disease. A variety of patterns is seen in CLT, reflecting the histopathologic features and the dynamic nature of chronic inflammatory disease. Hallmark pathologic findings include lymphoplasmacytic aggregates with germinal centers, atrophic thyroid follicles, oxyphilic change of the epithelial cells (Hürthle cells), and variable fibrosis [7]. These histopathologic changes parallel the spectrum of changes seen on ultrasound.

We have categorized seven patterns of heterogeneity in CLT (Table 6.2). It should not be construed that there is a sequential progression through the patterns described. While fibrosis and goiter regression is typically a later event in the progression of the

Table 6.2 Sonographic patterns of Hashimoto's thyroiditis

Hypoechoic and heterogeneous
Pseudomicronodular
  Swiss cheese pattern
  Honeycomb pattern
Pseudomacronodular
Profoundly hypoechoic
Developing fibrosis
Hyperechoic
Speckled

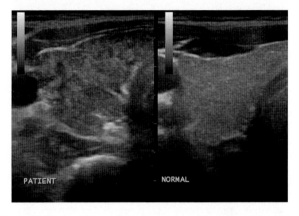

FIG. 6.1. (**a, b**) Hypoechoic and heterogeneous. The normal thyroid, shown in the *right frame*, has a bright, ground glass appearance. In contrast, the Hashimoto's gland in the *left frame* is hypoechoic, with the anterior portion almost as dark as the adjoining SCM muscle. It is mildly heterogeneous, without nodularity.

disease, any of the other patterns can be seen early in the disorder, as inflammation may be diffuse or patchy, and does not typically progress through the various patterns.

Patterns of Heterogeneity Seen in Chronic Lymphocytic Thyroiditis

Pattern 1: Hypoechoic and Heterogeneous
Normal thyroid tissue is hyperechoic compared to muscle tissue and is relatively homogeneous, with a ground glass appearance (Fig. 6.1: right panel). Areas of lymphocytic infiltration of the thyroid appear hypoechoic compared to normal thyroid parenchyma. When lymphocytic infiltration is mild and diffuse, the ultrasonographic

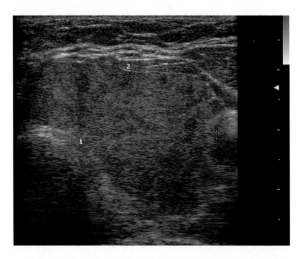

Fɪɢ. 6.2. Hypoechoic and Heterogeneous. The lobe and isthmus are enlarged, with a hypoechoic, mildly heterogeneous echotexture commonly seen in, and characteristic of, Hashimoto's thyroiditis.

pattern is mildly hypoechoic and mildly heterogeneous (Fig. 6.1: left panel, Fig. 6.2).

Pattern 2: Pseudomicronodular
When the areas of inflammation are more discrete, the hypoechoic pattern appears more focal, forming localized hypoechoic regions or pseudonodules (Fig. 6.3). The corresponding histopathology includes numerous germinal centers, areas of inflammation scattered throughout the gland. Pseudonodules are occasionally difficult to distinguish from true nodules. In contrast to true nodules, pseudonodules often have less well-defined borders on all views, gradually blending into the surrounding parenchyma. They typically do not have scalloped or infiltrative borders. As the location, number, and size of areas of inflammation are dynamic, the appearance may vary from study to study.

The common variants of pseudomicronodules are described as Swiss cheese and honeycomb. In the former, areas of inflammation are more discrete and well-defined, giving an appearance of numerous hypoechoic areas (pseudonodules) similar to the holes in Swiss cheese (Fig. 6.4). The hypoechoic regions are often misinterpreted as nodules, and ultrasound reports may refer to "a heterogeneous background with numerous subcentimeter hypoechoic nodules." This is a very common pattern, and should

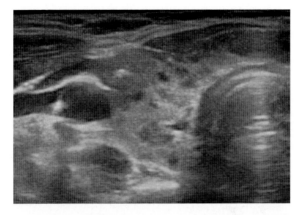

FIG. 6.3. Pseudomicronodular. Numerous ill-defined, subcentimeter hypoechoic areas are present, corresponding to small localized areas of inflammation. None appear different from the rest, and none have "suspicious features." The remaining thyroid parenchyma has an isoechoic echotexture.

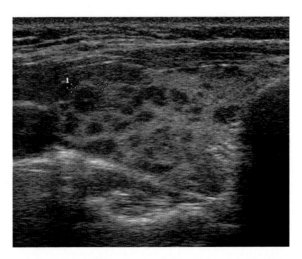

FIG. 6.4. Pseudomicronodular Swiss cheese. In this pattern the pseudonodules are better defined and slightly larger. This is commonly misinterpreted as a multinodular goiter.

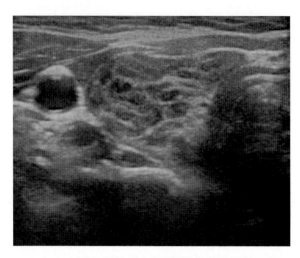

FIG. 6.5. Pseudomicronodular honeycomb. The areas of hypoechogenicity (pseudonodules) are more confluent, separated by thin bands of "normal" thyroid parenchyma. In contrast to the preceding image, more than 50% of the lobe is composed of the pseudonodules.

suggest Hashimoto's thyroiditis, rather than multinodular goiter. The pseudonodules are usually subcentimeter in size, and all have a similar appearance. If an individual pseudonodule appears different, especially with calcifications or infiltrative margins, the possibility of malignancy should be entertained.

In contrast to the Swiss cheese variant of pseudomicronodular, in which the thyroid parenchyma predominates with multiple discrete small pseudonodules, the honeycomb variant is composed of almost confluent small pseudonodules with very little parenchyma or fibrotic tissue separating the hypoechoic tissue (Fig. 6.5). Often ultrasound reports will erroneously indicate "a multinodular goiter with too numerous to count small nodules."

Pattern 3: Pseudomacronodular
When the areas of inflammation are larger, pseudonodules also appear larger, and are often mistaken for true large nodules (Figs. 6.6a, b and 6.7a, b). The pseudonodules may appear confluent, with little or no normal intervening thyroid parenchyma. Once again, the possibility of coexisting malignancy should be considered if an individual region has suspicious features.

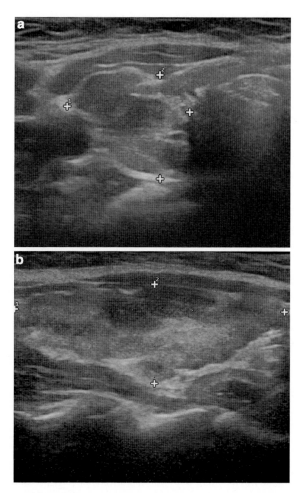

FIG. 6.6. (**a**, **b**) Pseudomacronodular. The hypoechoic areas of inflammation are larger, but again are without suspicious features. The edges are ill-defined but not infiltrative. This pattern is also frequently misinterpreted as multinodular goiter.

Pattern 4: Profoundly Hypoechoic

This pattern is typically seen in a large, inflamed goiter. The thyroid parenchyma is almost entirely replaced by lymphocytes, as opposed to discrete germinal centers. The ultrasonographic appearance is homogeneous and profoundly hypoechoic, equal to or darker than adjacent muscle tissue (Fig. 6.8a, b). As discussed

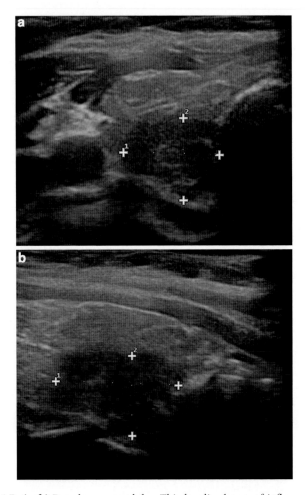

Fig. 6.7. (**a**, **b**) Pseudomacronodular. This localized area of inflammation appears as a suspicious nodule, with a deep hypoechoic echotexture and ill-defined edges. Biopsy of this nodule was benign, with characteristics of chronic lymphocytic thyroiditis (CLT). Pseudomacronodules such as this may require biopsy.

subsequently, thyroid lymphoma may have a very similar appearance, and should be considered in the differential diagnosis, especially if there has been rapid growth.

Pattern 5: Developing Fibrosis
Later in the progression of thyroid inflammation, fibrosis develops. Hyperechoic bands are seen separating the typical hypoechoic

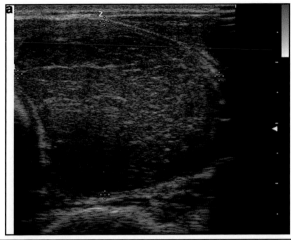

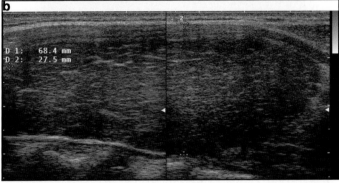

FIG. 6.8. (**a**, **b**) Profoundly hypoechoic. With an echotexture very similar to the neck muscles, this pattern is often seen in inflamed and swollen glands. As discussed in the text, rapid growth with this appearance should prompt evaluation for thyroidal lymphoma.

tissue (Fig. 6.9). Occasionally pseudonodules will be separated by fibrous bands. The hyperechoic bands may be suggestive of peripheral (rim) calcification, but do not produce the characteristic profound posterior shadowing seen in peripheral calcification (Fig. 6.10).

Pattern 6: Hyperechoic and Heterogeneous
When fibrosis is more diffuse, a goiter may appear hyperechoic (Fig. 6.11). This pattern has been observed less frequently,

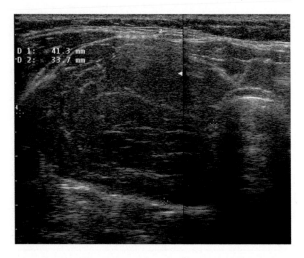

FIG. 6.9. Developing fibrosis. Developing fibrosis results in hyperechoic bands and echogenic foci without posterior acoustic shadowing. As fibrous bands separate the inflamed areas, the appearance may be "pseudomacronodular." However, true thyroid nodules rarely have a hyperechoic halo.

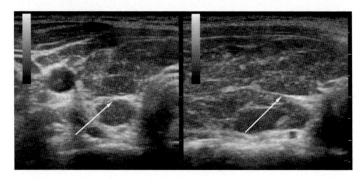

FIG. 6.10. Cleft sign. A thick fibrotic band separates the anterior and posterior portions of the right lobe. This finding may occur in a normal thyroid, but is often very prominent in Hashimoto's thyroiditis. (*Right Frame*) right lobe transverse, (*Left Frame*) right lobe longitudinal.

but may be more common later in the course of autoimmune hypothyroidism, associated with regression of the goiter.

Pattern 7: Speckled
In this very uncommon pattern, numerous punctate densities are scattered throughout a goiter (Fig. 6.12a, b). With an appearance suggestive of microcalcifications, biopsy is usually required to

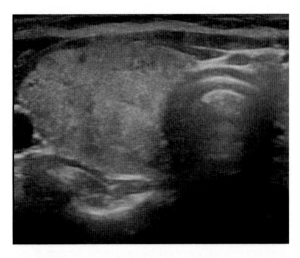

FIG. 6.11. Hyperechoic and heterogeneous. While the typical pattern in Hashimoto's thyroiditis is hypoechoic, later in the course of the disease diffuse scarring may predominate over follicles and inflammation. The result is a less commonly seen pattern of diffuse hyperechogenicity. Note the paratracheal lymph node, a frequent finding in autoimmune thyroiditis.

exclude diffuse infiltration by papillary carcinoma. The pattern is very similar to that described for diffuse sclerosing papillary carcinoma [8]. The punctate densities do not cast an acoustic shadow, and may be similar in origin to the bright linear densities commonly seen in benign colloid nodules [9].

Thyroid Nodules in Chronic Lymphocytic Thyroiditis

It has been suggested that there is a higher prevalence of papillary thyroid cancer in patients with Hashimoto's thyroiditis [10–14]. Due to the heterogeneous echotexture in CLT it may be challenging to detect true nodules and to identify potentially suspicious neoplasms. Real-time imaging in two planes along with Doppler interrogation is necessary to differentiate areas of concern that should undergo ultrasound-guided FNA.

The sonographic appearance of papillary thyroid cancer (PTC) in CLT does not differ from PTC found in an otherwise normal thyroid [10, 13, 14]. Therefore, the same criteria discussed in the nodule chapter should be applied to the evaluation of nodules detected in CLT. There may be a tendency toward denser calcification and less psammomatous calcification in PTC found in Hashimoto's thyroiditis, but any calcification within a nodule should be a cause for concern [15] (Figs. 6.13 and 6.14).

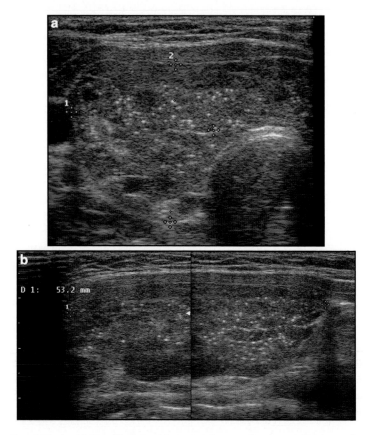

FIG. 6.12. (**a**, **b**) Speckled. In this very infrequently observed pattern the gland is enlarged and hypoechoic. Numerous punctate, nonshadowing echogenic foci are present, some with the appearance of "comet tail" artifacts. Biopsy was performed due to the concern that these might represent microcalcifications, but cytology confirmed benign lymphocytic thyroiditis.

A recently described specific nodular pattern in Hashimoto's is suggestive of a benign process. A hyperechoic nodule with a background of heterogeneous hypoechogenicity has been termed a "white knight" by Bonavita et al. [16] and is thought to represent a benign regenerative nodule (Fig. 6.15). A variant of this is the "giraffe pattern," also described by Bonavita et al. [16], characterized by multiple hyperechoic nodules surrounded by linear thin areas of hypoechogenicity (Fig. 6.16).

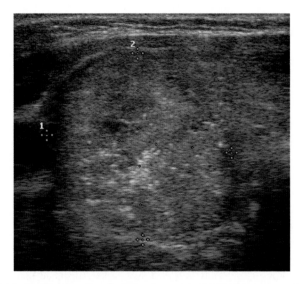

FIG. 6.13. Papillary carcinoma in background of CLT. This patient also had clearly pathological regional lymph nodes, with microcalcifications. Note the similarity to Fig. 6.12a, b. However, in this case the punctate echogenic foci were localized to one region of the gland.

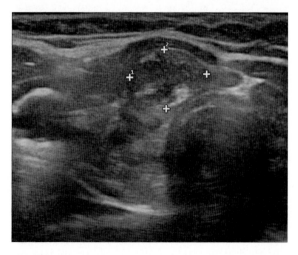

FIG. 6.14. Papillary carcinoma in background of CLT. This nodule was easily palpable and very firm. The appearance is not profoundly different from the remaining parenchyma, but subtle microcalcifications are present.

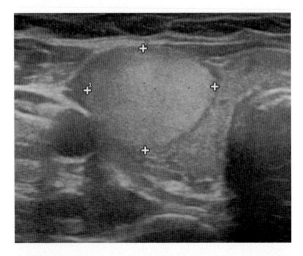

FIG. 6.15. "The White Knight" hyperechoic nodules in a background of CLT are almost uniformly benign. Bonavita has suggested that nodules with this appearance do not require biopsy.

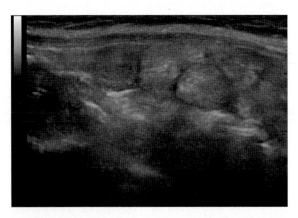

FIG. 6.16. "Giraffe" pattern. Also described by Bonavita as a benign pattern, multiple hyperechoic nodules are separated by hypoechoic bands. This pattern is actually a photographic negative of a giraffe hide.

Lymph Nodes in CLT

Lymph node reactivity and enlargement is almost invariably present in Hashimoto's thyroiditis. These prominent nodes are commonly found in the paratracheal and pretracheal space surrounding the thyroid, particularly at the inferior aspect of

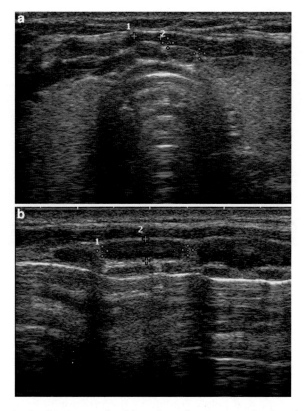

FIG. 6.17 (**a**, **b**) Paratracheal lymph nodes. Paratracheal nodes are extremely common in CLT, and are rarely seen without CLT. They are occasionally misinterpreted as isthmus nodules. Transverse image is shown in (**a**) and sagittal in (**b**). Note the tracheal rings posterior to the lymph nodes.

the isthmus, as well as in surgical levels III and IV of the lateral neck. These lymph nodes may be confluent and tend to appear somewhat rounded. The presence of an echogenic hilum is variable (Fig. 6.17a, b). The prominence and atypical appearance may cause concern in the evaluation for lymph node involvement in patients with both Hashimoto's and thyroid cancer. Any suspicious findings such as calcification, cystic necrosis, or disordered vascularity should prompt FNA evaluation of a lymph node. In addition, a lymph node at the inferior pole of the thyroid may resemble a parathyroid adenoma, making the sonographic evaluation of primary hyperparathyroidism more challenging in patients with CLT.

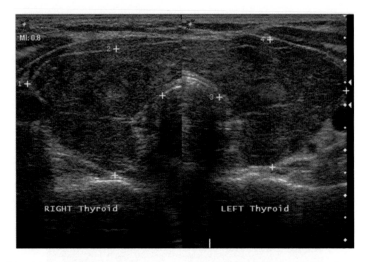

FIG. 6.18. Diffuse lymphoma. The appearance is very similar to that shown in Fig. 6.8—profoundly hypoechoic. Rapid growth of a diffusely hypoechoic goiter should prompt evaluation for lymphoma.

Lymphoma in CLT

Primary thyroid lymphoma is rare. The thyroid contains no native lymphoid tissue, so the infiltration of lymphocytes in autoimmune thyroid disease is a prerequisite to the development of thyroid lymphoma [17]. There are two typical patterns: (1) a diffuse enlargement and goiter similar to the profoundly hypoechoic pattern described above, and (2) nodular lymphoma with distinct borders between the tumor and the surrounding thyroid parenchyma. In both cases, a pseudocystic appearance is often seen owing to the through transmission of sound and subsequent posterior acoustic enhancement [18, 19] (Figs. 6.18 and 6.19). These changes may be indistinguishable from the heterogeneous hypoechogenicity commonly seen in Hashimoto's thyroiditis. Therefore, if a hypoechoic nodule or goiter exhibits rapid growth, biopsy with flow cytometry should be performed.

Atrophic Thyroiditis

CLT may ultimately result in atrophy of the gland with heterogeneous hypoechogenicity and fibrosis (Fig. 6.20).

Graves' Disease

The grayscale ultrasound appearance of Graves' disease is in many ways similar to that of Hashimoto's thyroiditis. Histopathologically,

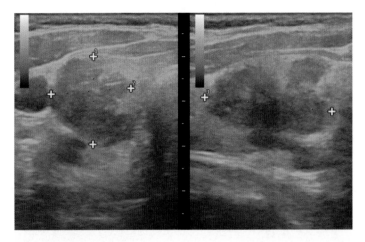

FIG. 6.19. Nodular lymphoma. This irregular hypoechoic nodule, with lobulated and infiltrative margins, appears suspicious and would require fine needle biopsy. When rapid growth is present flow cytometry should be performed in addition to cytology.

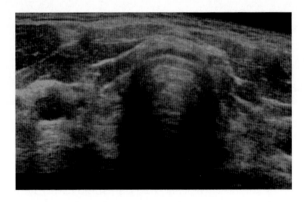

FIG. 6.20. Atrophic thyroiditis. Long-standing CLT may result in atrophy, with a shrunken, hypoechoic, fibrotic gland.

Graves' disease exhibits lymphoid infiltration, sometimes with germinal center formation. However, the lymphoid cells are strewn in the interfollicular stroma and do not encroach on the follicles themselves. The follicles often show marked epithelial hyperplasia. Fibrosis is unusual unless the disease is long-standing [7]. Accordingly, on ultrasound there is less heterogeneity than seen in Hashimoto's thyroiditis. In Graves' disease the hypoechogenicity

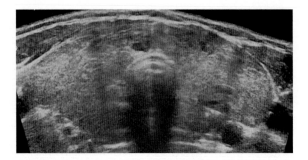

FIG. 6.21. Graves' disease. The goiter of Graves' disease typically appears less hypoechoic and less heterogeneous than that of Hashimoto's thyroiditis, but considerable overlap in appearance exists.

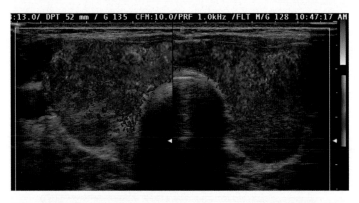

FIG. 6.22. Graves' disease. Color-flow or power Doppler may show the "Thyroid Inferno" in Graves' disease. Also see Fig. 3.11.

is not as pronounced because the intact and enlarged follicles are reflective of sound waves (Fig. 6.21). In some cases the gland is even hyperechoic.

The classic sonographic feature of Graves' disease is intense Doppler flow in the gland referred to as the "thyroid inferno" [20] (Fig. 6.22). Some authors have suggested that Doppler flow can distinguish Graves' disease from thyrotoxicosis due to thyroiditis, with the latter showing decreased flow [21, 22]. In this setting, total blood flow correlates strongly with radioiodine uptake, suggesting it may be a useful technique for patients in whom nuclear studies are contraindicated (pregnancy and breast-feeding) or not readily available [23]. It must be noted, however, that there is overlap in the amount of blood flow between Graves' and thyroiditis, so Doppler characteristics alone may not be sufficient to distinguish between these two entities [24]. Radioiodine uptake remains the gold standard in differentiating Graves' hyperthyroidism from thyrotoxicosis due to thyroiditis [24, 25], although when used along with clinical history and laboratory assays, ultrasound with Doppler flow may be more convenient, as sensitive, and more cost-effective than the routine use of nuclear imaging [26, 27]. Chapter 3 (Doppler Ultrasound) contains additional discussion of this topic.

Several authors have suggested that the incidence of thyroid cancer is greater in patients with Graves' disease. Cancers occurring in patients with Graves' disease may be more aggressive owing to the stimulating effect of thyrotropin receptor antibodies [28, 29]. A recent series from Japan [30] did not report an increased aggressiveness of thyroid cancer in Graves' disease; however, this might be explained by geographic differences in iodine intake. While the recent American Thyroid Association and American Association of Clinical Endocrinologists guidelines did not recommend routine use of ultrasound in the evaluation of thyrotoxicosis [25], it has been suggested that screening all Graves' disease patients with ultrasound to identify otherwise occult thyroid nodules is clinically appropriate and cost-effective [26, 27].

Painless Thyroiditis

Painless thyroiditis includes both silent and postpartum thyroiditis. Silent thyroiditis is considered to be an autoimmune process and has been referred to subacute lymphocytic thyroiditis, as it may be a form of transient Hashimoto's thyroiditis [1]. It occurs primarily in women aged 30–50 years and levels of thyroid autoantibodies tend to be lower than those seen in Hashimoto's thyroiditis. When it presents within 1 year of parturition it is termed postpartum thyroiditis. Postpartum thyroiditis is seen in up to 10% of all pregnancies and up to 30% of type 1 diabetics [1]. The recurrence rate is up to 70% in subsequent pregnancies. Patients with painless thyroiditis may present either in the thyrotoxic phase (which is usually mild and lasts 1–2 months) or the hypothyroid phase (which is typically transient and lasts up to 4–6 months). The probability of full recovery can be predicted by antibody titers and serial sonographic assessment of echogenicity [31]. Ultrasound evaluation shows hypoechogenicity similar to other forms of autoimmune thyroid disease. The histopathology is similar to Hashimoto's but with relative lack of oncocytic metaplasia, minimal to absent follicular atrophy, and mild to no fibrosis [7]. These differences are reflected in the ultrasound appearance in that hyperechoic fibrotic

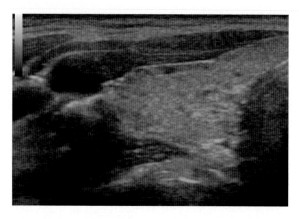

FIG. 6.23. Painless thyroiditis. Destructive thyroiditis, including postpartum and silent thyroiditis, has a nonspecific appearance with a mild goiter and a hypoechoic, mildly heterogeneous echotexture. Vascularity is typically low, but may be normal or increased, especially in the recovery phase.

changes are not seen and the degree of parenchymal hypoechogenicity is not typically profound (Fig. 6.23). During the thyrotoxic phase, there tends to be little to no blood flow on Doppler imaging; however, significant flow may be seen especially in the recovery phase. As discussed further in Chap. 3, there is significant overlap in the color Doppler patterns seen in destructive thyroiditis and Graves' disease. When evaluating a thyrotoxic patient, the clinician should consider the clinical history, physical examination, and laboratory data. Ultrasonography and Doppler interrogation often provide supportive evidence for the clinical impression. If doubt remains, radioactive iodine uptake can offer additional diagnostic information.

Subacute Thyroiditis

Patients with subacute thyroiditis present with marked neck tenderness and thyrotoxicosis, with elevated markers of inflammation (ESR). Patients may have fever, weakness, and other systemic symptoms. Three classic phases occur: thyrotoxic, hypothyroid, and recovery. Various terms have been used to describe this type of thyroiditis including: De Quervain's thyroiditis, subacute granulomatous thyroiditis, and nonsuppurative thyroiditis. Most commonly, subacute thyroiditis occurs following a viral upper respiratory infection. It is the most common cause of thyroid pain, which is caused by stretching of the thyroid capsule from inflammation and edema. Thyrotoxicosis occurs due to the

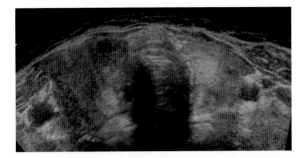

FIG. 6.24. Subacute thyroiditis. Subacute thyroiditis typically appears as ill-defined patchy areas of hypoechogenicity, corresponding to the areas of tenderness on exam. They may be unilateral, bilateral, or migratory.

disruption of thyroid follicles and release of stored thyroid hormone. Ultrasound is useful in evaluating the cause of the neck pain and swelling, and to differentiate thyroiditis from a hemorrhagic cyst or other neck mass. The typical sonographic findings are focal patchy areas of marked hypoechogenicity, which may elongate along the long-axis of the gland. Calcification is not typically seen in subacute thyroiditis [32] (Fig. 6.24). These ill-defined hypoechoic areas typically correspond to the areas of tenderness and may be unilateral, bilateral, or migrate over time to the contralateral side. Adjacent reactive lymph node enlargement is common. Blood flow is usually absent in focal painful thyroiditis [33]. Due to the lobulated irregular borders, the areas of inflammation often are difficult to differentiate from thyroid nodules, but in most cases sequential ultrasounds show resolution (Figs. 6.25a, b and 6.26a, b). If FNA is not performed on initial evaluation, repeat ultrasound should be performed in 4–6 months to confirm improvement.

Suppurative Thyroiditis

The thyroid is generally resistant to acute infection due to its high blood flow, iodine content, excellent lymphatic drainage, and protective capsule. Bacterial infection may occur in patients with preexisting thyroid disease, particularly in children with a congenital fourth branchial pouch sinus tract [1] (Fig. 5.10). Patients with suppurative thyroiditis typically present with rapid onset of fever, pain, and compressive symptoms. Infections usually start in the perithyroidal soft tissue. Early in suppurative thyroiditis, a sonographic finding may be a thin, hypoechoic border surrounding the thyroid lobe. Later, intrathyroidal and extrathyroidal abscesses are seen as ill-defined hypoechoic, heterogeneous masses with internal

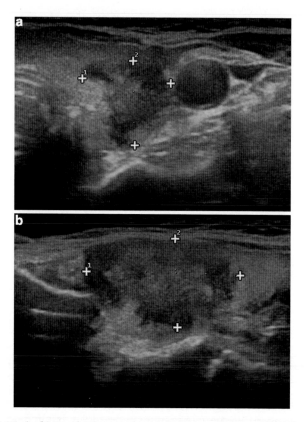

FIG. 6.25. (**a**, **b**) Focal subacute thyoiditis. This well-defined but lobulated and infiltrative appearing nodule was shown to be subacute thyroiditis by fine needle aspiration biopsy.

debris often with bright echoes from gas [19, 34]. Lymph nodes in the adjacent area enlarge significantly. The role of ultrasound is to detect an abscess, define the nearby anatomy including blood vessels, and guide drainage if necessary. It is sometimes difficult to distinguish acute suppurative thyroiditis from subacute granulomatous thyroiditis. This differentiation is important as the latter is often treated with corticosteroids, which would aggravate acute suppurative thyroiditis. CT scanning is a useful complement to ultrasound to define pharyngeal and mediastinal involvement and clarify the involved structures [35].

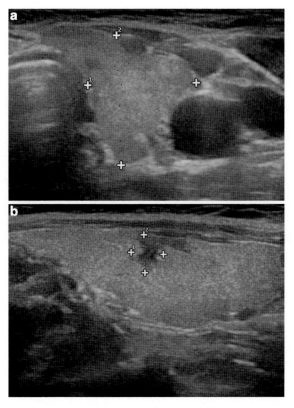

FIG. 6.26. (**a, b**) Focal subacute thyoiditis. An ultrasound performed 1 year after Fig. 6.25 shows near total resolution of the original area of inflamation.

Riedel's Thyroiditis

Also known as fibrous thyroiditis, Riedel's exhibits extensive fibrosis along with macrophage and eosinophil infiltration of the thyroid gland that extends into adjacent tissues. Patients present with enlarging, fixed, rock-hard, painless goiter with or without compressive symptoms. Ultrasound demonstrates an enlarged diffusely hypoechoic gland with fibrous septations and hypovascularity (Fig. 6.27). Unlike Hashimoto's thyroiditis, there may be carotid artery encasement. Elastography demonstrates significant stiffness [36].

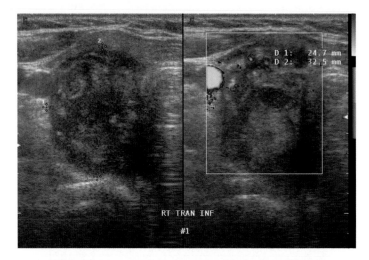

F IG. 6.27. Riedel's thyroiditis. This rapidly enlarging painless goiter was extremely hard on physical examination. Fine needle biopsy may be acellular or show macrophages and eosinophils.

Thyroid Amyloid

Systemic amyloidosis can cause infiltrative disease of any organ or gland. In the rare event that it involves the thyroid, the sonographic appearance is hyperechogenic with decreased sound penetration and a ground glass appearance [32].

DRUG-INDUCED THYROIDITIS

Patients treated with amiodarone, interleukin-2, interferon-alpha, ipilimumab, or tyrosine kinase inhibitors may develop destructive thyroiditis without pain. Drug therapy should be considered in evaluating all patients with diffuse thyroid enlargement.

SUMMARY

Diffuse thyroid enlargement may be due to one of several different varieties of thyroiditis. Autoimmune thyroid disease is by far the most common encountered in clinical practice. The sonographic hallmark of thyroid autoimmunity is diffuse hypoechogenicity and heterogeneity, with multiple variants as described. The role of ultrasound is to help confirm diagnosis, evaluate the size and vascularity of the gland, to identify any nonpalpable nodule that may require FNA biopsy, and to follow progress of the disease. Familiarity with the wide spectrum of presentation of thyroiditis helps to avoid unnecessary biopsy and surgery. In the hands of clinicians caring for the patients with thyroiditis, sonography is an efficient and cost-effective tool that complements the clinical evaluation of these patients.

References

1. Pearce E, Farwell A, Braverman L. Current concepts: thyroiditis. N Engl J Med. 2003;384(26):2646–55.
2. Pedersen OM, Aardal NP, Larssen TB, et al. The value of ultrasonography in predicting autoimmune thyroid disease. Thyroid. 2000;10(3):251–9.
3. Raber W, Gessi A, et al. Thyroid ultrasound versus antithyroid peroxidase antibody determination: a cohort study of four hundred fifty-one subjects. Thyroid. 2002;12(8):725–31.
4. Rago T, Chiovato L, Grasso L, et al. Thyroid ultrasonography as a tool for detecting thyroid autoimmune diseases and predicting thyroid dysfunction in apparently healthy subjects. J Endocrinol Invest. 2001;24:763–9.
5. Rotondi M, Cappelli C, Leporati P, et al. A hypoechoic pattern of the thyroid at ultrasound does not indicate autoimmune thyroid diseases in patients with morbid obesity. Eur J Endocrinol. 2010;163(1):105–9.
6. Loy M, Cianchetti ME, Cardia F, et al. Correlation of computerized gray-scale sonographic findings with thyroid function and thyroid autoimmune activity in patients with Hashimoto's thyroiditis. J Clin Ultrasound. 2004;32:136–40.
7. Livolsi VA. The pathology of autoimmune thyroid disease: a review. Thyroid. 1994;4(3):333–9.
8. Kwak JY, Kim EK, Hong SW, et al. Diffuse sclerosing variant of papillary carcinoma of the thyroid: ultrasound features with histopathological correlation. Clin Radiol. 2007;62(4):382–6.
9. Beland MD, Kwon L, Delellis RA, Cronin JJ, Grant EG. Nonshadowing echogenic foci in thyroid nodules. Are certain appearances enough to avoid thyroid biopsy? J Ultrasound Med. 2011;30:753–60.
10. Gul K, Dirikoc A, Kiyak G, et al. The association between thyroid carcinoma and Hashimoto's thyroiditis: the ultrasonographic and histopathologic characteristics of malignant nodules. Thyroid. 2010;20:873–8.
11. Fiore E, Rago T, Latrofa F, et al. Hashimoto's thyroiditis is associated with papillary thyroid carcinoma: role of TSH and of treatment with L-thyroxine. Endocr Relat Cancer. 2011;18(4):429–37.
12. Anil C, Goksel S, Gursoy A. Hashimoto's thyroiditis is not associated with increased risk of thyroid cancer in patients with thyroid nodules: a single-center prospective study. Thyroid. 2010;20(6):601–6.
13. Anderson L, Middleton W, et al. Hashimoto thyroiditis: Part 1, sonographic analysis of the nodular form of Hashimoto thyroiditis. AJR Am J Roentgenol. 2010;195:208–15.

14. Anderson L, Middleton W, et al. Hashimoto thyroiditis: Part 2, sonographic analysis of benign and malignant nodules in patients with diffuse Hashimoto thyroiditis. AJR Am J Roentgenol. 2010;195: 216–22.

15. Ohmori N, Miyakawa M, Ohmori K, et al. Ultrasonographic findings of papillary thyroid carcinoma with Hashimoto's thyroiditis. Intern Med. 2007;46(9):547–50.

16. Bonavita JA, Mayo J, Babb J, et al. Pattern recognition of benign nodules at ultrasound of the thyroid: which nodules can be left alone? AJR Am J Roentgenol. 2009;193:207–13.

17. Holm LE, Blomgren H, Lowhagen T. Cancer risks in patients with chronic lymphocytic thyroiditis. N Engl J Med. 1985;312:601–4.

18. Ota H, Ito Y, Matsuzuka F, et al. Usefulness of ultrasonography for diagnosis of malignant lymphoma of the thyroid. Thyroid. 2006;16:983.

19. Ahuja AT. The thyroid and parathyroids. In: Ahuja AT, Evans RM, editors. Practical head and neck ultrasound. London: Greenwich Medical Media Limited; 2000. p. 55–8.

20. Ralls PW, Mayekawa DS, Lee KP, et al. Color-flow Doppler sonography in Graves's disease: "thyroid inferno". AJR Am J Roentgenol. 1988;150(4):781–4.

21. Erdogan MF, Anil C, Cesur M, et al. Color flow Doppler sonography for the etiologic diagnosis of hyperthyroidism. Thyroid. 2007;17:223–8.

22. Kurita S, Sakurai M, Kita Y, et al. Measurement of thyroid blood flow area is useful for diagnosing the cause of thyrotoxicosis. Thyroid. 2005;15:1249–52.

23. Ota H, Amino N, Morita S, et al. Quantitative measurement of thyroid blood flow for differentiation of painless thyroiditis from Graves' disease. Clin Endocrinol (Oxf). 2007;67:41.

24. Bogazzi F, Vitti P. Could improved ultrasound and power Doppler replace thyroidal radioiodine uptake to assess thyroid disease? Nat Rev Endocrinol. 2008;4:70–1.

25. Bahn RS, Burch HB, Cooper DS, et al. Hyperthyroidism and other causes of thyrotoxicosis: management guidelines of the American Thyroid Association and American Association of Clinical Endocrinologists. Endocr Pract. 2011;17(3):456–520.

26. Cappelli C, Pirola I, de Martino E, et al. The role of imaging in Graves' disease: a cost-effectiveness analysis. Eur J Radiol. 2008;65:99–103.

27. Kahaly GJ, Bartalena L, Hegedüs L. The American Thyroid Association/American Association of Clinical Endocrinologists guidelines for hyperthyroidism and other causes of thyrotoxicosis: a European perspective. Thyroid. 2011;21(6):585–91.

28. Pellegriti G, Belfiore A, Giuffrida D, et al. Outcome of differentiated thyroid cancer in Graves' patients. J Clin Endocrinol Metab. 1998;83(8):2805–9.

29. Belfiore A, Russo D, Vigneri R, et al. Graves disease, thyroid nodules, and thyroid cancer. Clin Endocrinol (Oxf). 2001;55(6):711–8.

30. Yano Y, Shibuya H, Kitagawa W, et al. Recent outcome of Graves' disease patients with papillary thyroid cancer. Eur J Endocrinol. 2007;157(3):325–9.

31. Premawardhana LD, Parkes AB, Ammari F, et al. Postpartum thyroiditis and long-term thyroid status: prognostic influence of TPO antibody and US echogenicity. J Clin Endocrinol Metab. 2000;85:71–5.
32. Sholosh B, Borhani A. Thyroid ultrasound part 1: technique and diffuse disease. Radiol Clin North Am. 2011;49:393–416.
33. Park SY, Kim EK, Kim MJ, et al. Ultrasonographic characteristics of subacute granulomatous thyroiditis. Korean J Radiol. 2006;7:229–34.
34. Kim T, Orloff L. Thyroid ultrasonography. In: Orloff L, editor. Head and neck ultrasonography. Oxfordshire, UK: Plural Publishing; 2008. p. 69–114.
35. Masuoka H, Miyauchi A, Tomoda C, et al. Imaging studies in sixty patients with acute suppurative thyroiditis. Thyroid. 2011;21(10):1075–80.
36. Hennessey J. Riedel's thyroiditis: a clinical review. J Clin Endocrinol Metab. 2011;96(10):3031–41.

CHAPTER 7
Ultrasound of Nodular Thyroid Enlargement

Susan J. Mandel and Jill E. Langer

INTRODUCTION

Thyroid ultrasound is an exquisitely sensitive technique for the detection of thyroid nodules and is able to image nodules as small as 2–3 mm. The prevalence of sonographically detected nodules that cannot be palpated is up to 50–60% in individuals older than 60 [1]. Therefore, the challenge confronting the clinician is the identification of those nodules that have a higher probability of being a clinically relevant malignancy so that these can be targeted for fine-needle aspiration (FNA) biopsy and the recognition of those that may undergo sonographic surveillance. Furthermore, diffuse thyroid disorders, such as Graves' disease and Hashimoto's thyroiditis, image differently than the normal thyroid parenchyma, but it may be challenging to differentiate asymmetric involvement of the thyroid by one of these diffuse processes from a discrete thyroid nodule.

DIAGNOSTIC THYROID ULTRASOUND

The echotexture of the normal thyroid is homogeneous and brighter than the surrounding strap muscles. Usually the thyroid gland is outlined by a thin bright line that is thought to represent the thyroid capsule. The carotid arteries and jugular veins border the thyroid laterally and posteriorly, usually on the left, lies the air-containing esophagus with clear imaging of its muscular wall. The trachea, which is encircled by its cartilage rings, is situated posterior to the isthmus.

H.J. Baskin et al. (eds.), *Thyroid Ultrasound and Ultrasound-Guided FNA*, **127**
DOI 10.1007/978-1-4614-4785-6_7,
© Springer Science+Business Media, LLC 2013

Palpable thyroid nodules: After excluding those with low serum TSH levels, recently published evidence-based guidelines from the American Thyroid Association and the American Association of Clinical Endocrinologists recommend a diagnostic thyroid ultrasound for patients with palpable thyroid nodules [2, 3]. The rationale for this includes:

(a) *Confirmation of a sonographically identifiable nodule corresponding to the palpable abnormality.* A thyroid nodule is a discrete lesion in the thyroid that is distinct from the surrounding thyroid parenchyma. For one out of every six patients with a palpable thyroid nodule, ultrasound fails to demonstrate a corresponding nodule and, therefore, FNA biopsy is unnecessary [4, 5].

(b) *Detection of additional nonpalpable nodules for which FNA may be indicated.* Ultrasound identifies additional nonpalpable thyroid nodules in almost 50% of patients with an index palpable and sonographically confirmed thyroid nodule [4–6]. However, only about 20% of these nodules are supracentimeter in size.

(c) *Determination of accuracy of FNA by palpation.* For nodules that found to be more than 50% cystic [7] or are situated in the posterior aspect of the thyroid [8] palpation FNA is less accurate because of the potential for either nondiagnostic cytology or sampling error. Therefore, FNA with ultrasound guidance is the preferred technique.

(d) *Identification of the sonographic characteristics of the thyroid nodule(s).* Different sonographic features are associated with a higher likelihood of thyroid malignancy (see Table 7.1). Therefore, if a nodule is considered borderline in size for FNA or if several thyroid nodules are present, the sonographic appearance of a nodule may aid in decision-making about performance of FNA [9, 10].

Normal thyroid on physical examination. Thyroid ultrasound should neither be routinely performed in patients whose thyroid is normal by palpation nor be exploited as a substitute for physical examination. However, some exceptions exist. Diagnostic ultrasound should be considered in two groups of patients with a higher prevalence of thyroid cancer:

(a) *Prior history of head and neck irradiation.* Patients who received external beam radiation as children for benign conditions, such as thymic or tonsillar enlargement, acne, or birthmarks in infancy, childhood, or adolescence, more

Table 7.1 Grayscale sonographic features reported to be associated with thyroid cancer

	Median sensitivity (range) (%)	Median specificity (range) (%)
Hypoechoic c/w surrounding thyroid [9, 10, 20–24, 26, 27, 29–32]	81% (48–90%)	53% (36–92%)
Marked hypoechogenicity c/w strap muscle [25, 30, 32]	41% (27–59%)	94% (92–94%)
Microcalcifications [10, 20–22, 25–27, 29, 30, 32]	44% (26–73%)	89% (69–98%)
Macrocalcifications [22, 26, 27, 30, 32]	10% (2–17%)	94% (84–98%)
Absence of halo [22, 26, 27, 30, 32]	66% (33–100%)	43% (30–77%)
Irregular, microlobulated margins [9, 10, 20, 22, 26, 27, 29–32]	55% (17–84%)	80% (62–85%)
Solid consistency [9, 22, 26, 27, 32]	86% (78–91%)	48% (30–58%)
Taller-than-wide shape on transverse view [20, 25, 30, 32]	48% (33–84%)	92% (82–93%)

frequently develop both benign and malignant thyroid nodules and ultrasound detects these tumors and facilitates intervention [11]. Use of this therapy ceased in the early 1960s and current therapeutic radiation-related thyroid carcinoma typically occurs in patients who as children up to the age of 18 received treatment for malignancies that involved radiation to the head, neck, or upper mediastinum such as for Hodgkin's disease, preventive brain irradiation as in acute leukemias, or total body irradiation prior to bone marrow transplant. These predominantly papillary cancers are reported to occur in a median of 13–15 years after initial therapy, but thyroid cancers can be diagnosed up to three decades after the radiation exposure, emphasizing the need for a long-term surveillance strategy [12, 13]. In addition, because of the increased incidence of thyroid cancer in children younger than age 16 who were exposed to radiation after the Chernobyl accident, ultrasound has been instrumental for screening and identification of those affected [14].

(b) *Family history of thyroid cancer, including papillary thyroid cancer.* Recently emergent evidence reports that papillary cancer may be familial in up to 10% of cases [15, 16]. When family members from 53 families with nonmedullary thyroid cancer were examined by thyroid ultrasound, thyroid cancer (median size 10 mm, range 3–21 mm) was discovered in 10%, of which half were multifocal [17]. For familial medullary thyroid cancer (either isolated or as part of the multiple endocrine neoplasia II syndromes), thyroid ultrasound should be performed only in patients with mutations in the RET proto-oncogene to evaluate the thyroid and the cervical lymph nodes. In familial adenomatous polyposis and its variant, Gardner's syndrome, and in Cowden's disease, also called the multiple hamartoma syndrome, the prevalence of benign thyroid nodules and thyroid carcinoma is increased [18]. However, there are no current guidelines for screening sonography for this group of patients.

ULTRASOUND CHARACTERISTICS OF THYROID NODULES

Ultrasound not only detects the presence, location, and size of nodules within the thyroid gland, but it identifies imaging characteristics of these nodules. Over the last decade, multiple reports have evaluated sonographic features of thyroid nodules as predictors of malignancy. However, these studies neither utilize consistent methodologies nor uniformly address all characteristics. Some inconsistencies may be related to technical improvements in thyroid sonography, with earlier reports using a 7 MHz probe while more recent studies use a 12–14 MHz probe. But, differences in classification criteria account for largest proportion of variability among the studies [19]. For example, benign nodules may be identified by cytology or by histology; consequently, the proportion of thyroid cancers in these series varies from 4 to 32% [9, 10, 20–27]. Furthermore, classification of sonographic features differs among the series. Some only consider echogenicity for solid nodules; others include cystic nodules and echogenicity is determined by the solid portion. Most studies dichotomize a halo as absent or present, but some separate those with a partial halo from those with a complete halo [27]. Some series group all calcifications together [9, 20], others divide them into subtypes [26, 27]. Finally, identification of these qualitative ultrasound features is highly operator-dependent, especially for characterization of nodule margins [28].

A description of the individual sonographic characteristics of thyroid nodules follows, with a focus on the features that are associated with thyroid cancer. Table 7.1 lists these sonographic characteristics and summarizes their published median sensitivities and specificities for detection of malignancy summarized from 14 published reports [9, 10, 20–27, 29–32]. For inclusion in this analysis, each study must (1) contain at least 100 nodules; (2) analyze at least three sonographic characteristics; (3) report both sensitivity and specificity for thyroid cancer.

Echogenicity. The echogenicity of a thyroid nodule refers to its brightness compared to the normal thyroid parenchyma. The normal thyroid images as homogeneously hyperechoic and bright compared to the surrounding strap muscles of the neck. A nodule is generally characterized as hyper-, iso-, or hyperechoic. Hypoechogenicity is associated with thyroid malignancy and is thought to represent a microfollicular structure on histology, whereas macrofollicular lesions may image as iso- or hyperechoic [23] (Fig. 7.1).

Cystic fluid is classified as anechoic, with through transmission of sound waves and posterior acoustic enhancement. True cysts over 1.5–2 cm are rare, <2% of all lesions, but if present, these are reported to always be benign [27]. However, usually a solid component is present. Frequently, multiple small <1 cm cystic nodules may be imaged that are either simple cysts or may contain internal bright echogenic foci. The bright foci are often associated with "comet tail" or reverberation artifact within the cystic nodule (Fig. 7.2). With or without comet tail artifact, these small cysts are thought to represent nonneoplastic benign nodular hyperplasia with its associated colloid-filled cysts. In fact, the comet tail artifact is hypothesized to result from sound wave interaction with the condensed colloid protein [33].

For complex nodules that are predominantly cystic but have an associated solid component, the fluid represents degeneration and possible hemorrhage. There may be associated areas of internal debris that appear the same on grayscale imaging as viable tissue, but with color-flow Doppler (CFD), the debris is avascular. Aspiration of bloody fluid does not reliably differentiate benign from malignant lesions [34]. Although clear yellow fluid is more likely to be associated with a benign lesion, this can rarely be associated with thyroid cancer. From a recent Mayo clinic review of ultrasound findings in 360 consecutively operated thyroid cancers, only 9 (2.5%) were more than 50% cystic, and of these, all except one had another suspicious ultrasound feature that included either microcalcifications, intranodular vascularity, a mural nodule, or a thick irregular wall surrounding the cystic area [35] (Fig. 7.3). Therefore, for complex nodules with discrete solid

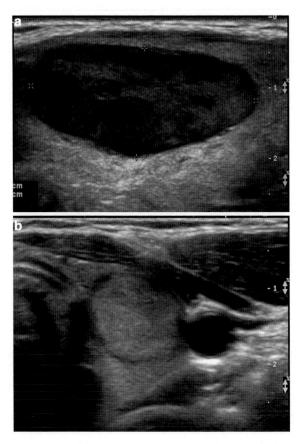

FIG. 7.1. (**a**) Hypoechoic solid nodule. (**b**) Iso- to hyperechoic solid nodule.

areas, sonographic features should be classified based upon these solid areas.

Nodule echogenicity may be challenging to determine in two situations. First, the extranodular thyroid may be affected by Hashimoto's thyroiditis and is therefore itself more heterogeneous in appearance, making classification of the nodule's echogenicity more difficult. Second, one-third of nodules are more than 25% cystic, and an additional quarter of nodules are up to 25% cystic [36]. Therefore, 55% of nodules have some cystic composition and the classification of echogenicity is made by examination of the solid component. This can be more straightforward if the cystic area is distinct from the solid area. However, some nodules

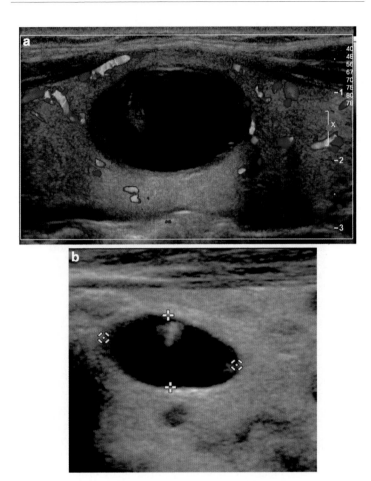

FIG. 7.2. (**a**) Pure cystic lesion without any internal vascular flow. (**b**) Cyst with comet tail artifact.

have mixed echogenicity throughout with minute <5 mm cystic areas separated by thin septations that are interspersed within solid tissue, a "spongiform" or "honeycomb" pattern [37, 38]. This appearance is often found in benign hyperplastic nodules (Fig. 7.4). These spongiform nodules may also have echogenic foci that are associated with the septations or the back wall of the small internal cystic spaces. These bright foci should not be confused with microcalcifications. In the suspicious hypoechoic solid nodules, the bright spots, representing calcifications, are located within the hypoechoic solid stroma itself (Fig. 7.5).

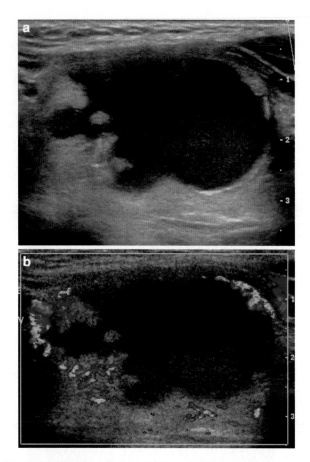

FIG. 7.3. Cystic Papillary Cancer. (**a**) Grayscale image of cystic papillary cancer. Note microcalcification in solid area. (**b**) Color flow Doppler (CFD) image of same nodule demonstrating increased vascularity in the papilliform solid area.

Furthermore, a spongiform nodule may relay the overall impression of iso- to hyperechogenicity. But, this must be distinguished from a complex nodule with discrete cystic areas where the solid components are otherwise iso- or hyperechoic. This second appearance may represent a true neoplastic growth, either follicular or Hürthle cell, and would require histology to discriminate between benign and malignant (Fig. 7.4b). A recent US-FNA series of 800 nodules reported that only pure cystic nodules had

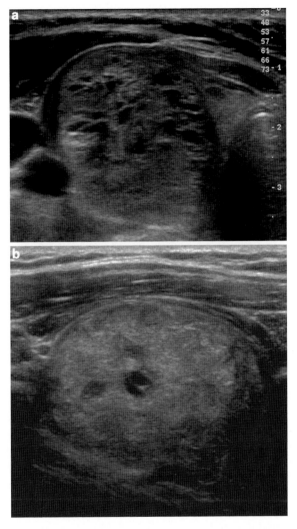

FIG. 7.4. (**a**) Spongiform nodule. Solid nodule with small interspersed cystic areas. Fine-needle aspiration (FNA) cytology is benign. (**b**) Predominantly solid nodule with discrete cystic area. FNA cytology is indeterminate, histology is benign follicular adenoma.

no risk of cancer, but that complex noncalcified nodules harbored a 3% risk of malignancy [27]. The distinction between complex nodules that were spongiform in appearance and those with isolated discrete cystic areas was not made however.

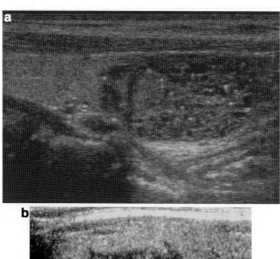

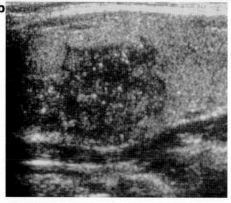

FIG. 7.5. (**a**) Echogenic foci (some with comet tail artifact) that are associated with the septations or the back wall of the small internal cystic spaces in a spongiform nodule. FNA cytology is benign. (**b**) Microcalcifications in the solid stroma of a hypoechoic solid nodule with irregular microlobulated margins. FNA cytology is papillary thyroid cancer.

Calcifications. Calcifications may be present in up to 30% of nodules and can be divided into different categories. Microcalcifications appear as small echogenic foci and are more specific (in some studies, up to 96%) than sensitive for thyroid cancer (Fig. 7.5b). Furthermore, the interobserver variability for the identification of microcalcifications is quite good [28]. It is hypothesized that these microcalcifications are the imaging equivalent of aggregates of psammoma bodies, the laminated spherical concretions characteristic of most papillary cancers, but occasionally found in benign nodules and Hashimoto's thyroiditis

[39]. Coarse or dense calcifications are larger than 2 mm and cause posterior acoustic shadowing. Occurring within either benign or malignant nodules, these dystrophic calcifications are present in areas of fibrosis and tissue degeneration and necrosis. However, coarse calcifications, either associated with microcalcifications or appearing in the center of a hypoechoic nodule, may be worrisome for malignancy [27, 37] (Fig. 7.6a). The third type of calcification is the peripheral or "egg-shell" calcification, once thought to indicate a benign nodule (Fig. 7.6b). However, this can be found in malignant nodules [39] and a particular worrisome finding is interruption of this rim calcification, indicating probable invasion by the cancer (Fig. 7.6c).

Margins. Sonography performed with high-frequency, high-resolution transducers allows detailed assessment of the interface of thyroid nodules with the surrounding parenchyma. Infiltrative, spiculated margins or a microlobular border (Figs. 7.5b, 7.6a) are therefore concerning for an unencapsulated invasive thyroid carcinoma. However, the distinction of infiltrative borders from indistinct borders is important because many small hyperplastic nodules will have poorly defined margins separating hyperplastic from normal tissue, but these are not infiltrative [30]. Interobserver variability for identification of this feature is the poorest [28], which may account for its reported lack of association with malignancy in several studies.

Halo. A halo is a sonolucent ring that surrounds a nodule and is thought to represent compressed perinodular blood vessels. Since benign hyperplastic nodules grow slowly and are generally not neoplastic, they displace the surrounding blood vessels as they expand. Lacking a true capsule, hyperplastic nodular tissue may even merge into the surrounding thyroid parenchyma in some areas. The thin halo, which demonstrates the nodule's peripheral vascularity on CFD, is found in about half of benign nodules, but is less common in thyroid cancer that is invasive (absent halo median 66% sensitivity for detection of thyroid cancer) (Fig. 7.7a,b). However, with high-resolution ultrasound, a second type of halo is now described, a thick irregular avascular halo [24], which may signify the fibrous capsule surrounding a neoplastic growth, either follicular or Hürthle cell, and is, therefore, more concerning (Fig. 7.7c).

Vascularity. The vascularity of a thyroid nodule is evident with CFD imaging. Based upon the mean Doppler shift, CFD is a measure of the directional component of the velocity of blood moving through the sample volume. The technical shortcomings of CFD include the interference by noise and angle dependence.

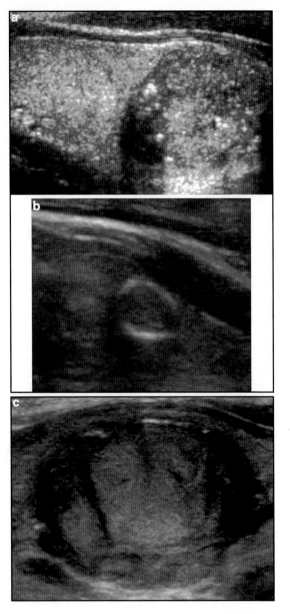

Fig. 7.6. (a) Hypoechoic solid nodule with irregular margins and micro- and macrocalcifications. The macrocalcification demonstrates posterior acoustic shadowing. This was a papillary thyroid cancer. (b) Eggshell calcifications. (c) Interrupted rim calcification in a follicular variant of papillary thyroid cancer. Note the interruption of the anterior calcified border that corresponded with localized invasion into the surrounding thyroid.

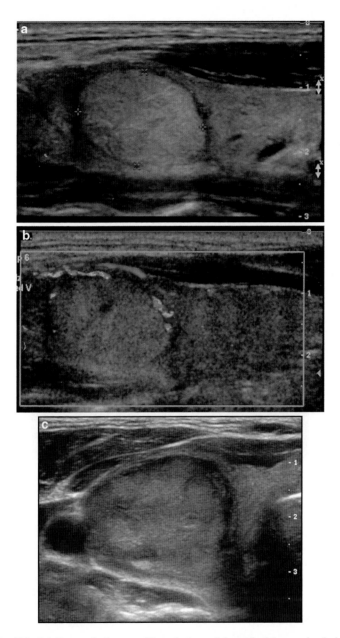

FIG. 7.7. (**a**) Grayscale image of isoechoic nodule with thin regular halo. Cytology is benign. (**b**) CFD image of same nodule indicating the halo corresponds with peripheral vascularity. (**c**) Thick, irregular, and incomplete halo surrounding solid iso- to hyperechoic nodule. Histology is Hürthle cell cancer.

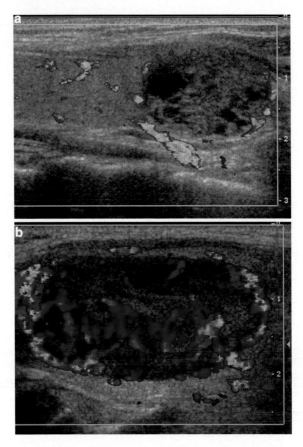

FIG. 7.8. (**a**) Peripheral vascularity in spongiform nodule. Cytology is benign. (**b**) Increased intranodular vascularity in hypoechoic nodule.

More recently, power Doppler (PD) analysis has been applied to nodule assessment. By amplification of the Doppler shift signal, it can record information about the Doppler signal amplitude. PD is more sensitive for detection of flow in small vessels that would not be detected by CFD. Furthermore, PD imaging is relatively independent of the angle of the probe and the sound beam and noise can be assigned to a homogeneous background rather than appearing as random color on CFD [24].

Using CFD, nodule vascularity is categorized as absent (type I), perinodular (type II) (Figs. 7.7b, 7.8a), or peri- and intranodular (type III) (Fig. 7.8b). Although increased intranodular vascularity has been reported by earlier studies to be a worrisome feature, a recent report analyzing over 1,000 nodules did not confirm its independent association with papillary thyroid cancer, after accounting for grayscale features of hypoechogenicity, taller-than-wide shape, and noncircumscribed margins. Intranodular vascularity was observed in 31% of benign nodules and only 17% of papillary cancers [40]. One possible explanation for the discrepancy in reports on vascularity may be related to the specific type of thyroid cancer. Small papillary cancers, such as analyzed by Moon et al., may lack vascularity [40], whereas intranodular vascularity may more commonly be associated with follicular cancers [41].

Taller than wide. Thyroid cancer has been associated with a nodule's anterioposterior to transverse diameter ratio (A/T) greater than 1 as measured on the transverse view, a feature which has been evaluated by several series [20, 25, 30, 32]. This finding replicates the results in the sonographic literature evaluating breast carcinomas [25]. Disproportionate growth in the anterioposterior dimension is considered an aggressive growth pattern across rather than within the normal tissue planes. This finding may not be very sensitive for thyroid cancer, but it has a specificity ranging from 82 to 93% and is most commonly noted in smaller cancers, under 1 cm [32].

Elastography. US elastography is a recently developed dynamic technique that provides an estimate of tissue stiffness by measuring its degree of distortion under the application of an external force. This technology is based upon the principle that the softer areas of tissue deform more easily than the harder parts under compression, thus allowing an objective determination of tissue consistency. Because of the observation that malignant lesions are often associated with changes in tissue mechanical properties that render it stiffer, elastography may have potential as an adjunctive tool for the diagnosis of thyroid cancer, especially for indeterminate cytology nodules (see Chap. 15).

Other features. There are two other grayscale imaging findings that are highly suggestive of malignancy. The first is the detection of abnormal cervical lymph nodes. Both the ATA [2] and AACE [3] Guidelines for evaluating patients with thyroid nodules state that sonographic evaluation of the cervical lymph nodes should be part of a standard diagnostic thyroid US if a nodule has suspicious US features. Cervical lymph node metastases may have a variety of abnormal findings including cystic regions, punctuate calcifications, hyperechoic foci, increased peripheral vascularity, and a rounded shape [42] (see Chap. 8). Because of the presence of the thyroid, it is more difficult to evaluate the central neck or paratracheal lymph nodes.

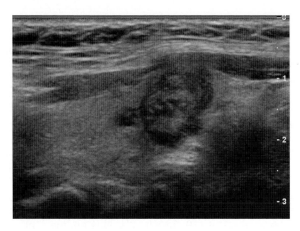

Fɪɢ. 7.9. Hypoechoic solid nodule with irregular borders. Note anterior border of lesion penetrates through anterior thyroid capsule into surrounding tissue.

Second, extrathyroidal invasion may be occasionally seen when the tumor growth extends through either the anterior or posterior thyroid capsule, which normally appears as a bright white outline surrounding the thyroid. In such instances, the margin of the tumor has an ill-defined edge that interrupts this capsule [43] (Fig. 7.9). Only rarely is intratracheal growth seen.

Limitations of sonography. Recognizing the limitations of individual sonographic features for prediction of thyroid cancer, some series have explored the association of combinations of these features with cancer risk. In general, as the specificity increases, the sensitivity decreases. For example, although very few (<4%) benign nodules will be hypoechoic with microcalcifications, only a minority of thyroid cancers (26–31%) will have this appearance [10, 21, 26]. Therefore, if only such nodules were to be aspirated, over 70% of cancers would be missed. The combination of sonographic features that maximizes sensitivity and specificity is a solid hypoechoic nodule, which identifies ~65% of all cancers, but still describes the appearance of 30% of benign nodules [9, 22, 26] and excludes any attempt at classification of complex nodules. Additionally, as many as 66% of papillary thyroid cancers have at least one sonographic feature not typically associated with malignancy and 69% of benign nodules have one sonographic predictor of malignancy [28, 44].

In addition, some of the variability associated with the reported sensitivities of individual sonographic features for prediction of thyroid malignancy may depend upon the histology of the thyroid cancer. Papillary thyroid cancers are more likely to be solid, hypoechoic, and lack a halo compared with follicular thyroid cancers. Follicular cancers most commonly have a halo (90%), which is irregular (60%), and are iso- to hyperechoic [45]. In addition, the two most common histological subtypes of papillary thyroid cancer, follicular variant and classic, also have different US profiles. The classic variant is more likely to be hypoechoic with microcalcifications and spiculated margins [46].

Benign sonographic appearance. Another way to utilize sonographic features as predictors of malignancy is to identify nodules that lack all reported grayscale suspicious characteristics. Using Bayes' theorem to determine what is termed posttest probability, that is, the probability of disease that is recalculated after the results of a diagnostic test, the risk of malignancy can be calculated for a nodule without hypoechogenicity, taller-than-wide shape, infiltrative margins, and calcifications (both microcalcifications and macrocalcifications) [30]. Given a 7–9% population prevalence of thyroid cancer, for every 1,000 nodules that have such a benign appearance, only nine would be malignant. Therefore, one would have to perform 1,000 FNAs on nodules lacking these four US features to identify nine cancers.

There are two sonographic appearances that meet the criteria of ABSENCE of these four suspicious features. One appearance is the previously described spongiform nodule (Figs. 4 and 6). In the report of Bonavita et al. [31], all 210 nonvascular nodules with this US appearance were benign, and in that of Moon et al. [30], only 1 of the 360 thyroid cancers appeared spongiform on US. The second sonographic appearance of a thyroid nodule that is equated with benignity is that of a pure cyst, which although rare, <2%, is virtually always benign. Both ATA and AACE guidelines recognize pure cystic and spongiform nodules as low risk for malignancy and the size cutoff for FNA of such lesions is more lenient (if performed at all) than for intermediate and high-risk sonographically appearing nodules [2, 3].

The role of US is to confer a degree of risk to a thyroid nodule to aid in clinical decision-making about whether FNA is indicated especially for smaller nodules, where the vast majority of microcarcinomas are clinically indolent. Therefore, using constellations of US features, the high-risk nodule would image on grayscale US as solid, markedly hypoechoic, with microcalcifications, and an infiltrative border with a taller-than-wide shape. An intermediate risk nodule might be a hypoechoic nodule lacking microcalcifications, with smooth borders or an iso- to hyperechoic predominantly solid nodule [31, 37]. Therefore, it is critical to recognize that ultrasound does not replace FNA cytology, rather the two modalities are complementary.

Two clinical scenarios illustrate the synergy of these modalities in clinical decision-making. First, for nodules less than 2 cm, both the ATA and AACE guidelines recommend size threshold cutoffs for FNA based upon sonographic features [2, 3]. In fact, for small nodules <1.5 cm where the cost-benefit analysis of FNA is unclear, decision-making based upon suspicious sonographic features of hypoechogenicity, microcalcifications, irregular margins, or increased vascularity is superior to using an arbitrary size cutoff of >1 cm to identify thyroid cancers [9, 10] Second, if multiple thyroid nodules are present as potential candidates for FNA, sonographic appearance should guide in nodule selection. For example, FNA would be first performed for a 1.6 cm hypoechoic solid vascular nodule, even in the presence of a larger 3.7 cm mixed echogenicity nonvascular nodule.

Change in size. After a benign FNA cytology result, surveillance recommendations include periodic assessment of nodule size with reaspiration if growth is observed. Since ultrasound is superior to physical examination for nodule size determination, size changes should be determined by serial sonography. However, agreement does not exist for definition of nodule growth by US, and the recent consensus statement on thyroid nodules published by the Society of Radiologists in Ultrasound acknowledged that "the panelists did not come to a consensus on how to define substantial nor on how to monitor growth." [38] Some groups have suggested a 15% increase in nodule volume [36]. However, interobserver variation for ultrasound determination of nodule volume is reported to be about 45–50% [47]. Reproduction of the same planar image of the nodule for follow-up may be difficult. The American Thyroid Association guidelines propose as a reasonable definition of growth a 20% increase in two of the three nodule diameters, with a minimum increase of at least 2 mm^2. This methodology is actually quite useful because it equates with at least a 44% increase in nodule volume, which would overcome the reported interobserver variability allowing for determination of true change in size.

No single sonographic feature or combination of features is adequately sensitive to identify all malignant nodules. However, certain features and combination of features have high predictive value to indicate if a nodule is likely to be malignant or benign. Clinical judgment, assessment of personal risk factors, and ultrasound appearance combined with FNA cytology provide the optimal process for nodule diagnosis.

References

1. Mazzaferri EL. Management of a solitary thyroid nodule. N Engl J Med. 1993;328:553–9.
2. Cooper DS, Doherty GM, Haugen BR, et al. Revised American Thyroid Association management guidelines for patients with thyroid nodules and differentiated thyroid cancer. Thyroid. 2009;19:1167–214.
3. Gharib H, Papini E, Paschke R, et al. American Association of Clinical Endocrinologists, Associazione Medici Endocrinologi, and European Thyroid Association medical guidelines for clinical practice for the diagnosis and management of thyroid nodules: executive summary of recommendations. Endocr Pract. 2010;16:468–75.
4. Marqusee E, Benson CB, Frates MC, et al. Usefulness of ultrasonography in the management of nodular thyroid disease. Ann Intern Med. 2000;133:696–700.
5. Brander A, Viikinkoski P, Tuuhea J, Voutilainen L, Kivisaari L. Clinical versus ultrasound examination of the thyroid gland in common clinical practice. J Clin Ultrasound. 1992;20:37–42.
6. Tan GH, Gharib H, Reading CC. Solitary thyroid nodule. Comparison between palpation and ultrasonography. Arch Intern Med. 1995;155:2418–23.
7. Alexander EK, Heering JP, Benson CB, et al. Assessment of nondiagnostic ultrasound-guided fine needle aspirations of thyroid nodules. J Clin Endocrinol Metab. 2002;87:4924–7.
8. Hall TL, Layfield LJ, Philippe A, Rosenthal DL. Sources of diagnostic error in fine needle aspiration of the thyroid. Cancer. 1989;63:718–25.
9. Leenhardt L, Hejblum G, Franc B, et al. Indications and limits of ultrasound-guided cytology in the management of nonpalpable thyroid nodules. J Clin Endocrinol Metab. 1999;84:24–8.
10. Papini E, Guglielmi R, Bianchini A, et al. Risk of malignancy in nonpalpable thyroid nodules: predictive value of ultrasound and color-Doppler features. J Clin Endocrinol Metab. 2002;87:1941–6.
11. Schneider AB, Ron E, Lubin J, Stovall M, Gierlowski TC. Dose–response relationships for radiation-induced thyroid cancer and thyroid nodules: evidence for the prolonged effects of radiation on the thyroid. J Clin Endocrinol Metab. 1993;77:362–9.
12. Brignardello E, Corrias A, Isolato G, et al. Ultrasound screening for thyroid carcinoma in childhood cancer survivors: a case series. J Clin Endocrinol Metab. 2008;93:4840–3.
13. Acharya S, Sarafoglou K, LaQuaglia M, et al. Thyroid neoplasms after therapeutic radiation for malignancies during childhood or adolescence. Cancer. 2003;97:2397–403.
14. Shibata Y, Yamashita S, Masyakin VB, Panasyuk GD, Nagataki S. 15 years after Chernobyl: new evidence of thyroid cancer. Lancet. 2001;358:1965–6.
15. Hemminki K, Eng C, Chen B. Familial risks for nonmedullary thyroid cancer. J Clin Endocrinol Metab. 2005;90:5747–53.
16. Malchoff CD, Malchoff DM. The genetics of hereditary nonmedullary thyroid carcinoma. J Clin Endocrinol Metab. 2002;87:2455–9.

17. Uchino S, Noguchi S, Yamashita H, et al. Detection of asymptomatic differentiated thyroid carcinoma by neck ultrasonographic screening for familial nonmedullary thyroid carcinoma. World J Surg. 2004;28: 1099–102.

18. Sturgeon C, Clark OH. Familial nonmedullary thyroid cancer. Thyroid. 2005;15:588–93.

19. Langer JE, Mandel SJ. Thyroid nodule sonography: assessment for risk of malignancy. Imaging Med. 2011;3:513–24.

20. Cappelli C, Pirola I, Cumetti D, et al. Is the anteroposterior and transverse diameter ratio of nonpalpable thyroid nodules a sonographic criteria for recommending fine-needle aspiration cytology? Clin Endocrinol (Oxf). 2005;63:689–93.

21. Rago T, Vitti P, Chiovato L, et al. Role of conventional ultrasonography and color flow-doppler sonography in predicting malignancy in 'cold' thyroid nodules. Eur J Endocrinol. 1998;138:41–6.

22. Takashima S, Fukuda H, Nomura N, Kishimoto H, Kim T, Kobayashi T. Thyroid nodules: re-evaluation with ultrasound. J Clin Ultrasound. 1995;23:179–84.

23. Brkljacic B, Cuk V, Tomic-Brzac H, Bence-Zigman Z, Delic-Brkljacic D, Drinkovic I. Ultrasonic evaluation of benign and malignant nodules in echographically multinodular thyroids. J Clin Ultrasound. 1994;22:71–6.

24. Cerbone G, Spiezia S, Colao A, et al. Power Doppler improves the diagnostic accuracy of color Doppler ultrasonography in cold thyroid nodules: follow-up results. Horm Res. 1999;52:19–24.

25. Kim EK, Park CS, Chung WY, et al. New sonographic criteria for recommending fine-needle aspiration biopsy of nonpalpable solid nodules of the thyroid. AJR Am J Roentgenol. 2002;178:687–91.

26. Nam-Goong IS, Kim HY, Gong G, et al. Ultrasonography-guided fine-needle aspiration of thyroid incidentaloma: correlation with pathological findings. Clin Endocrinol (Oxf). 2004;60:21–8.

27. Frates MC, Benson CB, Doubilet PM, et al. Prevalence and distribution of carcinoma in patients with solitary and multiple thyroid nodules on sonography. J Clin Endocrinol Metab. 2006;91:3411–7.

28. Wienke JR, Chong WK, Fielding JR, Zou KH, Mittelstaedt CA. Sonographic features of benign thyroid nodules: interobserver reliability and overlap with malignancy. J Ultrasound Med. 2003;22:1027–31.

29. Kovacevic O, Skurla MS. Sonographic diagnosis of thyroid nodules: correlation with the results of sonographically guided fine-needle aspiration biopsy. J Clin Ultrasound. 2007;35:63–7.

30. Moon WJ, Jung SL, Lee JH, et al. Benign and malignant thyroid nodules: US differentiation–multicenter retrospective study. Radiology. 2008;247:762–70.

31. Bonavita JA, Mayo J, Babb J, et al. Pattern recognition of benign nodules at ultrasound of the thyroid: which nodules can be left alone? AJR Am J Roentgenol. 2009;193:207–13.

32. Ahn SS, Kim EK, Kang DR, Lim SK, Kwak JY, Kim MJ. Biopsy of thyroid nodules: comparison of three sets of guidelines. AJR Am J Roentgenol. 2010;194:31–7.

33. Ahuja A, Chick W, King W, Metreweli C. Clinical significance of the comet-tail artifact in thyroid ultrasound. J Clin Ultrasound. 1996;24:129–33.

34. de los Santos ET, Keyhani-Rofagha S, Cunningham JJ, Mazzaferri EL. Cystic thyroid nodules. The dilemma of malignant lesions. Arch Intern Med. 1990;150:1422–7.

35. Henrichsen TL, Reading CC, Charboneau JW, Donovan DJ, Sebo TJ, Hay ID. Cystic change in thyroid carcinoma: Prevalence and estimated volume in 360 carcinomas. J Clin Ultrasound. 2010;38:361–6.

36. Alexander EK, Hurwitz S, Heering JP, et al. Natural history of benign solid and cystic thyroid nodules. Ann Intern Med. 2003;138:315–8.

37. Reading CC, Charboneau JW, Hay ID, Sebo TJ. Sonography of thyroid nodules: a "classic pattern" diagnostic approach. Ultrasound Q. 2005;21:157–65.

38. Frates MC, Benson CB, Charboneau JW, et al. Management of thyroid nodules detected at US: Society of Radiologists in Ultrasound consensus conference statement. Radiology. 2005;237:794–800.

39. Taki S, Terahata S, Yamashita R, et al. Thyroid calcifications: sonographic patterns and incidence of cancer. Clin Imaging. 2004;28:368–71.

40. Moon HJ, Kwak JY, Kim MJ, Son EJ, Kim EK. Can vascularity at power Doppler US help predict thyroid malignancy? Radiology. 2010;255:260–9.

41. Fukunari N, Nagahama M, Sugino K, Mimura T, Ito K. Clinical evaluation of color Doppler imaging for the differential diagnosis of thyroid follicular lesions. World J Surg. 2004;28:1261–5.

42. Langer JE, Mandel SJ. Sonographic imaging of cervical lymph nodes in patients with thyroid cancer. Neuroimaging Clin N Am 2008;18:479–89, vii-viii.

43. Ito Y, Kobayashi K, Tomoda C, et al. Ill-defined edge on ultrasonographic examination can be a marker of aggressive characteristic of papillary thyroid microcarcinoma. World J Surg 2005;29:1007–11; discussion 11–2.

44. Chan BK, Desser TS, McDougall IR, Weigel RJ, Jeffrey Jr RB. Common and uncommon sonographic features of papillary thyroid carcinoma. J Ultrasound Med. 2003;22:1083–90.

45. Jeh SK, Jung SL, Kim BS, Lee YS. Evaluating the degree of conformity of papillary carcinoma and follicular carcinoma to the reported ultrasonographic findings of malignant thyroid tumor. Korean J Radiol. 2007;8:192–7.

46. Kim DS, Kim JH, Na DG, et al. Sonographic features of follicular variant papillary thyroid carcinomas in comparison with conventional papillary thyroid carcinomas. J Ultrasound Med. 2009;28:1685–92.

47. Brauer VF, Eder P, Miehle K, Wiesner TD, Hasenclever H, Paschke R. Interobserver variation for ultrasound determination of thyroid nodule volumes. Thyroid. 2005;15:1169–75.

CHAPTER 8
Ultrasound and Mapping of Neck Lymph Nodes

Gregory Randolph, Barry Sacks, and H. Jack Baskin, Sr

INTRODUCTION

The strategic value of ultrasound imaging in both treating and following patients with thyroid cancer has become increasingly appreciated over the past decade. Ultrasound has been incorporated into the American Thyroid Association's *Guidelines for Patients with Thyroid Nodules and Differentiated Thyroid Cancer*. Neck sonography has become pivotal in planning the preoperative surgical approach in patients undergoing initial thyroid cancer surgery as well as in the postoperative surveillance of patients with thyroid cancer. The key to determining the extent of the appropriate initial surgery as well as the recognition of recurrent cancer is ultrasound's ability to detect early malignancy in the surrounding neck lymph nodes.

In this chapter we will begin by discussing the surgical levels and compartments of the neck. It is critical that the endocrinologist performing the ultrasound examination understands this division of the neck into spaces so that there is accurate communication of the ultrasound findings to the operating surgeon. Next we will focus on ultrasound characteristics that separate benign from malignant lymph nodes and how this may be confirmed by ultrasound-guided FNA (UG FNA). We will then discuss the method of preoperative ultrasound evaluation and its ramifications regarding the optimization of surgery. Finally, we will focus on how ultrasound, in conjunction with thyroglobulin, is used in a cost-effective manner for the long-term surveillance and early detection of residual, recurrent or metastatic thyroid cancer.

H.J. Baskin et al. (eds.), *Thyroid Ultrasound and Ultrasound-Guided FNA*, **149**
DOI 10.1007/978-1-4614-4785-6_8,
© Springer Science+Business Media, LLC 2013

SURGICAL LEVELS AND COMPARTMENTS OF THE NECK

The neck is a large three-dimensional structure. Lymphatic metastasis from thyroid cancer tends to segregate into specific regions of the neck. Because of this localization of the majority of thyroid cancer nodal metastasis and pursuant to communication among treating physicians, neck subregions have been defined and have great utility in the preoperative evaluation of patients with nodal disease. One must not underestimate the importance of accurate three-dimensional communication between treating physicians in the identification of nodal metastasis for accurate surgery.

The neck is subdivided into six basic regions or Levels (Fig. 8.1). Level I constitutes lymph nodes above the anterior and posterior bellies of the digastric muscle cephalad to the hyoid bone and inferior to the inferior border of the mandible and includes the submental group of nodes. Level II or upper jugular region extends from the skull base and spinal accessory nerve downward to the hyoid bone. Level II is subdivided into IIA below the spinal accessory nerve and IIB above the spinal accessory nerve. The mid-jugular group is Level III which extends on the carotid sheath and laterally from the hyoid down to the cricoid cartilage. Level IV or lower jugular group includes nodes on the carotid sheath and laterally extending on the fasical carpet from the cricoid cartilage

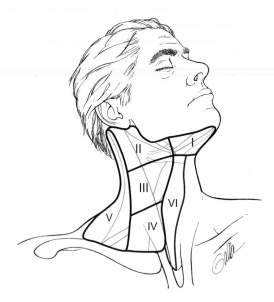

FIG. 8.1. Surgical levels of the neck.

down to the clavicle. Level V is a triangular region formed by the posterior edge of the sternocleidomastoid muscle (SCM) and anterior edge of the trapezius muscle and is subdivided into the region 5A above the level of the cricoid cartilage and 5B or supra-clavicular region below the level of the cricoid cartilage. Level VI or central compartment is composed of four subcompartments: (1) prelaryngeal (aka Delphian nodal group), (2) pretracheal, (3) left paratracheal, and (4) right paratracheal. A Level VII or superior mediastinal group has also been described but is felt to be encompassed in the lower portions of the ATA's central neck dissection grouping [1]. Typically standard neck dissection for papillary carcinoma of the thyroid excludes Levels I, IIB, and V due to the low prevalence of disease in the subareas. An exception to this is in a patient with bulky lateral neck nodal disease where these areas may require dissection.

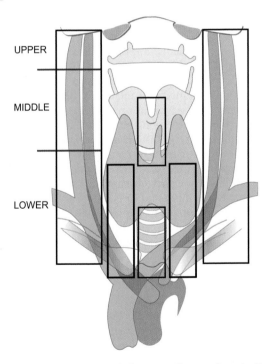

FIG. 8.2. "Compartment oriented dissection." Lateral neck dissection is divided into *Upper* (Level II lymph nodes), *Middle* (Level III lymph nodes) and *Lower* (Level IV lymph nodes). Central neck dissection encompasses the pretracheal region, the prelaryngeal region, and at least one paratracheal region.

These nodal subgroups are further segregated into surgical neck dissection units of the lateral or central neck. The current prevailing philosophy in surgical management of nodal disease is a "compartment oriented dissection philosophy." The result of these compartmental definitions and surgical subgroupings is that, typically for papillary carcinoma of the thyroid, nodal surgical procedures are defined as either lateral neck dissection which encompasses Levels II, III, and IV or a central neck dissection which encompasses prelaryngeal, pretracheal, and at least one paratracheal region (Fig. 8.2). Note that occasionally, especially in patients with aggressive subtypes of thyroid cancer, patients may present with nodal metastases which are outside of these known neck regions. However the vast majority of patients with well-differentiated nodal metastasis can be described with this terminology.

ULTRASOUND FEATURES OF BENIGN VS. MALIGNANT LYMPH NODES

The normal neck contains approximately 300 lymph nodes. Benign nodes are typically flattened or slightly oval in shape and most are less than 0.5 cm in size in their *short axis*. However, they frequently become inflamed and enlarged. This is particularly true for the nodes in the pharyngeal area where nodes up to 0.8 cm are commonly seen. Therefore, the overall size of a lymph node is of little benefit in determining if a lymph node is malignant or benign. Because malignant nodes start out small and nonmalignant nodes can be enlarged, we must use ultrasound criteria other than size to differentiate these benign hyperplastic lymph nodes from those that are malignant.

In imaging lymph nodes in the neck, the transducer is held in the transverse position and measurement of the node is made of the *short axis* (usually near the anterior–posterior plane) and the *long axis* (usually near the transverse plane). Benign lymph nodes are flattened and have a *short/long axis ratio* less than 0.5. If they become inflamed and hyperplastic, they enlarge but generally maintain their flattened shape (*short/long axis ratio* <0.5). Malignant lymph nodes generally have a fuller more rounded appearance in the transverse view with a *short/long axis ratio* greater than 0.5. Measuring in the longitudinal plane is of little or no benefit since benign nodes can be elongated several cm in this view. Because lymph node hyperplasia is so common in the neck, only those lymph nodes whose *short axis* is >0.5 cm (0.8 cm in Levels I and II) and *short/long axis ratio* >0.5 are usually biopsied. Others can have their location mapped and be reexamined in 6 months.

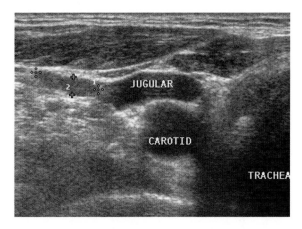

FᴵG. 8.3. Benign lymph node. The normal neck contains scores of lymph nodes some of which are easily seen with ultrasound. This lymph node (calipers) appears benign because it is flat with a short/long axis ratio <0.5.

A normal lymph node has a hypoechoic cortex but often shows a central hyperechoic hilum containing fat and intranodal blood vessels referred to as a hilar line. The hilar line is present in most benign lymph nodes with a *short axis* >0.5 cm and is more prominent in older patients. Malignant lymph nodes in the neck whether they are metastatic from the thyroid or elsewhere (i.e., squamous cell carcinoma) or lymphoma will seldom show a hilar line. When ultrasound is performed on a patient with nodular goiter, or a patient with a history of thyroid cancer and a rising thyroglobulin; finding a lymph node with a short axis >0.5 cm with a rounded shape (*short/long axis ratio* >0.5) and absent hilar line warrants an ultrasound-guided FNA of the node (Figs. 8.3, 8.4, 8.5, 8.6, and 8.7).

Other ultrasound findings, when found, are even more likely to indicate malignancy in a lymph node [2] (Table 8.1). Any calcification, either microcalcifications or amorphous calcifications with posterior acoustic shadowing, in a lymph node is indicative of malignancy. Cystic necrosis within a lymph node, often recognized because of posterior acoustic enhancement is another sign of malignancy. Although cystic necrosis may occasionally be seen with tuberculosis of lymph nodes, in the western world it is far more commonly seen in malignant lymph nodes (Figs. 8.8, 8.9, 8.10, 8.11, 8.12, 8.13, 8.14, 8.15, 8.16, 8.17, 8.18, 8.19, and 8.20).

Power Doppler is preferred over color Doppler in evaluating lymph nodes because of its sensitivity to arteriolar blood flow.

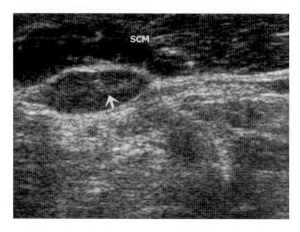

FIG. 8.4. This lymph node beneath the sternocleidomastoid muscle (SCM) is slightly more oval but still maintains a short/long axis ratio <0.5. It also has a distinct hilar line (*arrow*), a strong indication that it is benign.

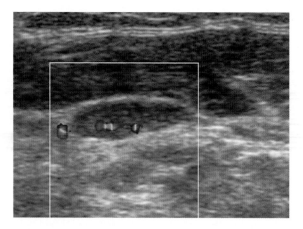

FIG. 8.5. Power Doppler of the previous lymph node shows vascularization of the hilum which contains small arterioles. Note there is no vascularization seen in the periphery of the node.

Normal nodes generally show vascularization along the hilum, but malignant lymph nodes often have chaotic vascularization throughout the cortex due to recruitment of vessels into the periphery of the node [3, 4] (Figs. 8.21, 8.22, 8.23, 8.24, and 8.25).

The internal jugular vein is adjacent to and follows the course of the carotid artery. Since metastatic nodes commonly occur

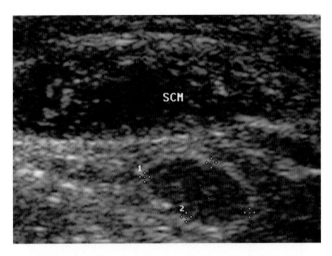

FIG. 8.6. Malignant lymph node. This lymph node (calipers) is slightly more rounded with a short/long axis ratio >0.5 in the transverse view. Note the absence of a hilar line which makes this node suspicious. A UG FNA was needed to confirm malignancy.

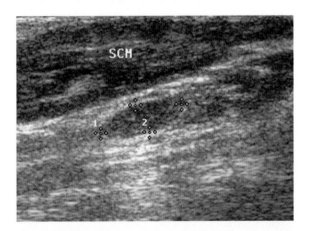

FIG. 8.7. Same lymph node in longitudinal view. It appears more benign in this view because it is flatter; even malignant lymph nodes can be long in longitudinal view. Therefore, always take the short/long axis measurement in the transverse view.

Table 8.1 Neck lymph node characteristics

	Benign	Malignant
Short/long axis	<0.5	>0.5
Hilar line	Present	Absent
Jugular deviation or compression	Absent	Present
Microcalcifications	Absent	Present
Cystic necrosis	Absent	Present
Vascularity	Central	Chaotic/peripheral

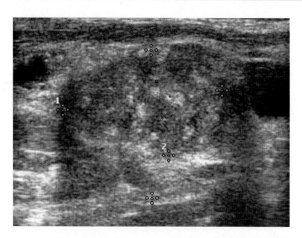

Fig. 8.8. This markedly heterogeneous lymph node (calipers) contains scattered calcifications indicating metastatic papillary carcinoma.

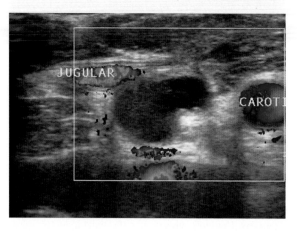

Fig. 8.9. This 2 cm rounded lymph node in the right neck is 80% cystic; note the distal enhancement. Although occasionally seen in tuberculosis, cyst formation within a lymph node usually indicates metastatic papillary carcinoma.

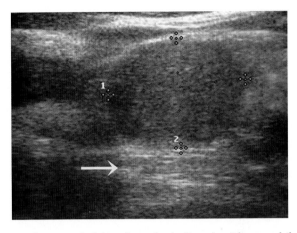

FIG. 8.10. This rounded lymph node (calipers) without a hilar line is hypoechoic and has begun to develop cystic necrosis. Liquid formation within a solid lymph node is often first suspected because of distal enhancement (*arrow*).

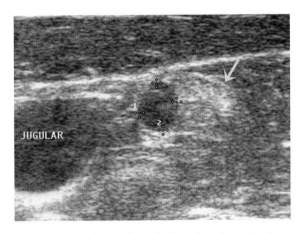

FIG. 8.11. This metastatic lymph node, less than 1 cm in size, contains cystic necrosis on the medial side which is hypoechoic (calipers) and shows enhancement. The other side (*arrow*) is solid and hyperechoic. UG FNA of the hypoechoic area yielded negative cytology but high levels of Tg in needle washout—a finding not unusual if there is cystic necrosis.

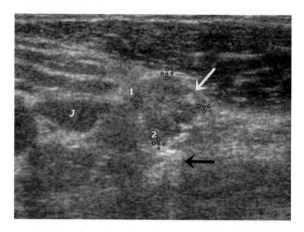

FIG. 8.12. Typical small metastatic lymph node (calipers) near the jugular vein (*J*). Note the rounded shape with a short/long axis of 1, absence of a hilar line, calcification (*white arrow*), and enhancement (*black arrow*) indicating early cystic necrosis.

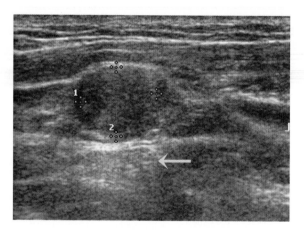

FIG. 8.13. Two centimeter non-palpable lymph node (calipers) in 47 year old male 7 years post-thyroidectomy. Enhancement distal to the node (*arrow*) indicates cystic necrosis has started. FNA found negative cytology but very high levels of Tg in the needle washout.

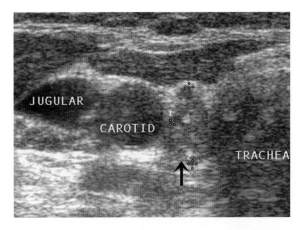

FIG. 8.14. Ultrasound of 54-year-old female 36 years after her thyroidectomy reveals a paratracheal lymph node (*arrow*) in the right central compartment. Note the short/long axis is >1 and several calcifications are seen indicating malignancy. FNA showed positive cytology, but Tg in needle washout was negative demonstrating the need to do both tests when lymph nodes are biopsied.

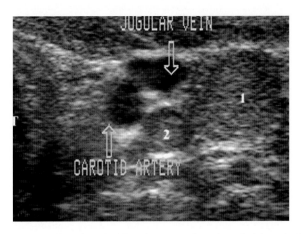

FIG. 8.15. A 1 cm lymph node (*1*) and a 0.5 cm lymph node (*2*) in the lateral neck are both rounded without a hilar line. Both nodes had papillary cancer at surgery.

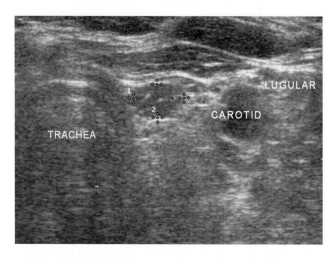

Fig. 8.16. Ultrasound of a 57-year-old female 13 years after a thyroidectomy shows a small oval node (calipers) in the left central compartment that is suspicious.

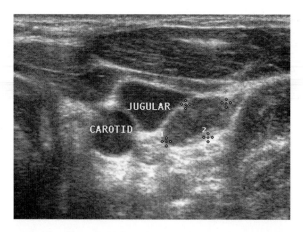

Fig. 8.17. This lymph node (calipers) was suspicious because of its borderline short/long axis of 0.5 and absent hilum. Surgery confirmed metastatic papillary cancer.

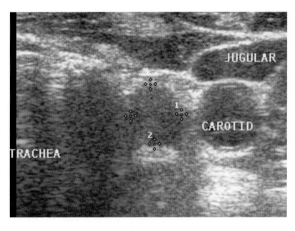

FIG. 8.18. Metastatic lymph node (calipers) in left central compartment with short/long axis >1 and no hilar line.

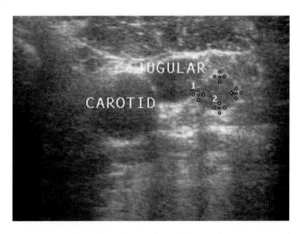

FIG. 8.19. Another lymph node (calipers) less than 0.5 cm that was biopsied because of its shape and location. FNA cytology showed papillary carcinoma.

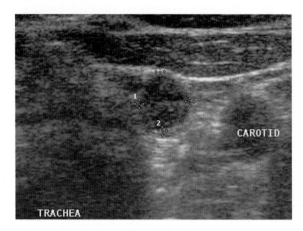

FIG. 8.20. Ultrasound of a 50-year-old female 18 years after total thyroidectomy revealed a paratracheal lymph node (calipers) in the central compartment with a short/long axis of 1.

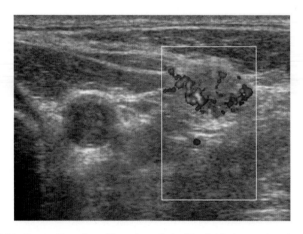

FIG. 8.21. Power Doppler of lymph node in Fig. 8.12 shows chaotic vascularization of the periphery of the node rather than the normal hilar vascular pattern. Although cytology from the FNA was negative, a high level of Tg was found in the needle washout.

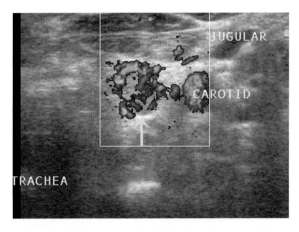

FIG. 8.22. Ultrasound of a 16-year-old female 1 year post-thyroidectomy. Power Doppler of a small lymph node (*arrow*) found in the central compartment between the trachea and the left carotid shows chaotic vascularization.

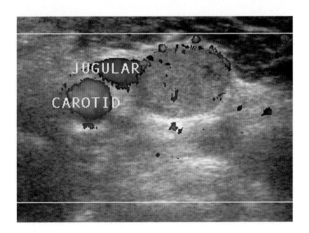

FIG. 8.23. Larger lymph node found in the lateral compartment of the same patient. Power Doppler again shows an abnormal pattern with recruitment of vessels into the cortex of the lymph node.

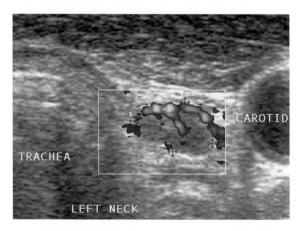

FIG. 8.24. Power Doppler of lymph node in Fig. 8.16 shows a malignant vascular pattern. Cytology was negative on FNA but Tg in needle washout was high confirming malignancy.

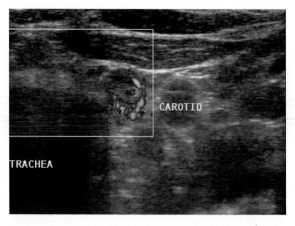

FIG. 8.25. Power Doppler of lymph node in Fig. 8.20 shows peripheral vascular pattern of malignancy. FNA cytology was positive and Tg in the needle washout was >10,000.

in proximity with the jugular vein or in the carotid sheath, any deviation of the jugular vein away from the carotid artery strongly suggest the presence of a malignant lymph node. Sometimes it requires moving the transducer around in various planes in order

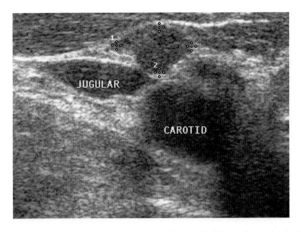

Fig. 8.26. On transverse view, this small rounded lymph node (calipers) without a hilar line is in close proximity to the great vessels.

to reveal an obscure node. The entire length of the vessels should be surveyed closely with particular attention given to any area where the artery and vein diverge.

In addition to causing deviation of the internal jugular vein, malignant lymph nodes tend to compress the vein and cause partial obstruction to blood flow. Color Doppler is better for demonstrating the impeded blood flow in the jugular vein. Benign lymph nodes rarely deviate or obstruct the jugular unless they become very large (Figs. 8.26, 8.27, 8.28, 8.29, 8.30, 8.31, and 8.32).

It is important to remember that the ultrasound characteristics that are helpful in deciding if a thyroid nodule is benign or malignant may not apply to lymph nodes. For example, metastatic lymph nodes can have well-defined borders until they become quite large. While malignant thyroid nodules are almost never hyperechoic, both normal and malignant lymph nodes are generally hypoechoic compared to thyroid, but they have varying degrees of echogenicity. For example early papillary metastases are sometimes dense and may be relatively hyperechoic. As they enlarge up to 1 cm they develop cystic necrosis and become hypoechoic. Therefore, echogenicity may not be helpful in determining if a lymph node is malignant. Matting of lymph nodes occurs with malignancy but is not a helpful sign since it is also seen with inflammation or in patients who have had radiation.

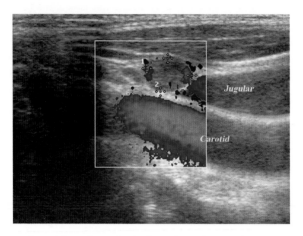

FIG. 8.27. Same lymph node (calipers) in longitudinal view shows compression of the jugular vein against the carotid. UG FNA confirmed malignancy.

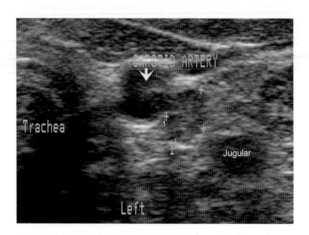

FIG. 8.28. This 0.5 cm lymph node (calipers) lies between the carotid and jugular. Its location and shape (short/long axis ratio >1) strongly suggest that it is malignant which was confirmed by UG FNA.

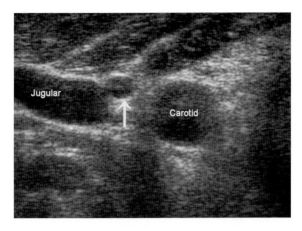

FIG. 8.29. Although this lymph node (*arrow*) measures only 2.5 mm, its location and shape lead to UG FNA, and Tg was found in the needle washout confirming metastatic thyroid cancer.

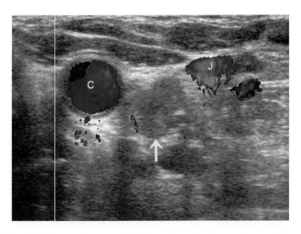

FIG. 8.30. This irregular rounded lymph node (*arrow*) was discovered because of the separation of the jugular from the carotid. The calcification at 3 o'clock indicates it is malignant, but UG FNA is necessary before surgery.

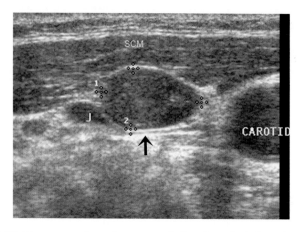

FIG. 8.31. Transverse view of a metastatic lymph node (calipers) in right neck beneath the SCM and lateral to the carotid artery. The node is impinging upon the jugular vein (*J*) at the arrow. The short/long axis ratio is >0.5 and no hilar line is seen. UG FNA had positive cytology and Tg was found in the needle washout.

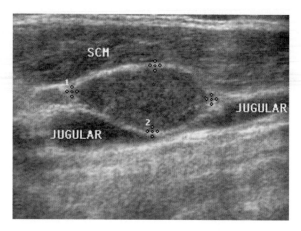

FIG. 8.32. Longitudinal view of the same lymph node (calipers) showing partial obstruction of the jugular vein. In this view the short/long axis ratio is <0.5, emphasizing the need to measure the short/long ratio in the transverse view.

ULTRASOUND-GUIDED FNA OF LYMPH NODES

Because the sonographic features of malignant lymph nodes are not always present and there is overlap in the ultrasound appearance of benign and malignant lymph nodes, UG FNA of suspicious nodes is often required for a definitive diagnosis before recommending surgery.

UG FNA of lymph nodes is carried out in the same manner as a UG FNA of a thyroid nodule with aspirate slides prepared and sent for cytology interpretation. Lymph node cytology is sometimes difficult to interpret [5]. However, differentiated thyroid cancer metastases contain thyroglobulin (Tg) which can be measured and used as a tissue marker. Therefore after making the slide, the biopsy needle(s) is then flushed with 1 cc normal saline and the washout sent for Tg assay [6, 7]. A normal saline control is also sent for Tg assay. The material in the needle is diluted approximately 100–1,000-fold; therefore, a Tg > 10 in the needle washout is considered positive for malignancy. Because the intracellular Tg is not exposed to circulating anti-TgAB, a positive test for anti-TgAB in the serum does not interfere with measurement of Tg obtained from lymph nodes as it does with serum Tg [8]. Either a positive cytology report or finding Tg in the needle washout confirms the lymph node is malignant. Using either positive cytology or the presence of Tg as proof of cancer, Lee et al. reported 100% sensitivity and specificity in detecting metastatic thyroid cancer [9]. Studies have found the Tg in the needle washout to be more sensitive than cytology in detecting malignancy [10]. This is likely due to poor cellular material in lymph nodes having cystic necrosis (see Fig. 8.9). If medullary thyroid cancer is suspected, calcitonin can be used as the tissue marker.

PREOPERATIVE ULTRASOUND AND SURGICAL MANAGEMENT

Papillary thyroid carcinoma (PTC) is a disease characterized by lymph node metastases. Clinically evident nodes are defined as nodes evident by (1) preoperative physical exam, (2) preoperative radiographic evaluation, or (3) intraoperative detection by the surgeon and are present in *35%* of patients presenting with PTC [11–13]. However small volume microscopic lymph nodes may be present in up to *80%* of patients diagnosed with PTC [14–23]. The main prognostic significance of the presence of nodal disease in the patient with papillary carcinoma lies in the risk of recurrence rather than in survival. In patients with small volume nodal disease, locoregional recurrence rates in treated patients range from 2 to 6% regardless of whether lymph node dissection is performed

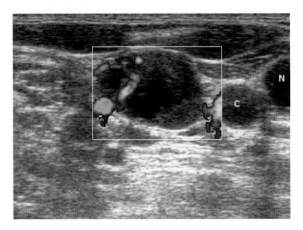

FIG. 8.33. Preoperative ultrasound of a patient seen for a thyroid nodule in the right lobe (*N*) revealed a large cystic lymph node in the right lateral neck (*box*). Note the short/long axis >0.5, absent hilum, and abnormal vascularity. Although FNA of the lymph node had negative cytology, Tg in needle washout was positive.

or RAI is given [24–36]. Such microscopic nodal disease is of little if any clinical significance. In contrast neck lymph nodes detected on preoperative neck US (i.e., clinically apparent macroscopic nodal disease) convey a higher risk of recurrence (>20%), even when treated with therapeutic neck dissection and/or RAI ablation, than either clinical N0 necks or pathologically proven N1a disease [37, 38]. Nodal surgery should be based on the detection and treatment of gross clinically apparent macroscopic disease. The ATA Management Guidelines recommends preoperative neck ultrasound for all patients undergoing surgery for thyroid cancer (Recommendation 21). Given this cumulative data all patients with papillary carcinoma of thyroid should have a robust radiographic map to identify and to elucidate the distribution of macroscopic nodal disease preoperatively (Figs. 8.33 and 8.34).

The Problem of the Central Neck

Evidence of the value of preoperative ultrasound of the central compartment is less conclusive. It may be less important because most endocrine surgeons now routinely perform a central node dissection at the time of the thyroidectomy. Preoperative ultrasound of the central compartment is much less sensitive than it is in the lateral neck because even macroscopic lymph nodes may be obscured by the thyroid gland. Preoperative FNA of central

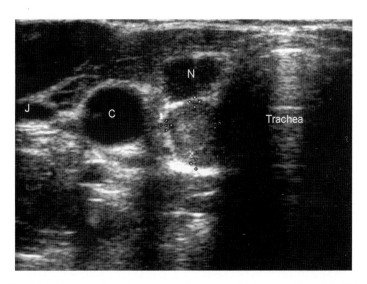

FIG. 8.34. Preoperative ultrasound of patient with a thyroid nodule (N) whose FNA was positive for papillary cancer shows a suspicious lymph node (calipers) adjacent to the lower pole of the thyroid. A central node dissection at the time of surgery revealed that this was metastatic papillary cancer.

compartment lymph nodes is fraught with the risk of contamination if the needle inadvertently passes through the thyroid which might cause a false positive cytology and/or Tg in the washout. It is still recommended that the central compartment be examined at the time of lateral neck ultrasound and that any suspicious lymph nodes be mapped for the surgeon. Because 70–90% of positive lymph nodes in the central neck are not seen by ultrasound before the thyroid is removed, a "negative" ultrasound examination is of no value.

Axial CT scan with contrast may provide improvement in detection of central neck nodal disease. In one recent study ultrasound detection of central neck nodal disease sensitivity in primary papillary carcinoma patients was 26% whereas combined radiographic mapping through ultrasound and axial CT scan with contrast improved sensitivity to 54% with a negative predictive value in the central compartment of 75%. In this study overall CT scan was found to improve macroscopic nodal dissection and identified compartments that required dissection for macroscopic nodal disease that had been missed on ultrasound in 25% of primary patients with papillary carcinoma of thyroid allowing appropriate expansion of the nodal surgical plan. Most consider the minimal delay due to CT contrast for possible radio-active iodine treatment is of little significance as compared to the accurate preoperative mapping of macroscopic nodal disease and appropriately tuned surgery to the individual patient's pattern of nodal disease [39].

POSTOPERATIVE ULTRASOUND AND SURGICAL MANAGEMENT

Ultrasound has assumed a primary role in the surveillance of patients who have been treated for thyroid cancer. Because of its propensity to occur at any age, even in the very young, and to recur many years later, thyroid cancer must be monitored for the life-time of the patient. To do this in a cost-effective manner has been a challenge. Until the 1990s the only diagnostic tool available was a ^{131}I whole body scan (WBS) done after withdrawing the patient from their thyroid hormone replacement. The sensitivity of a WBS in the early detection of residual, recurrent, or metastatic thyroid cancer is poor. This is apparent from the many patients who have increased thyroglobulin (Tg) but negative diagnostic scans that are treated with ^{131}I and have positive posttreatment scans [40–42]. Park et al. has also shown that the doses of ^{131}I used for WBS can stun the uptake of iodine in metastatic lesions and interfere with the subsequent treatment dose of ^{131}I [43]. The expense, poor sensitivity, and risk of stunning with a WBS make it an unsatisfac-tory test with which to follow patients with thyroid cancer.

In the last decade two new probes have become widely avail-able that aid in the early detection of recurrent thyroid cancer. The first is a sensitive, reliable, reproducible Tg assay that bio-chemically detects the earliest sign of cancer recurrence. The second is high-resolution ultrasound of the postoperative neck to identify early lymph node recurrence. Using these new tools, especially neck ultrasound combined with UG FNA of suspicious lymph nodes, has greatly improved the sensitivity of cancer surveillance in these patients.

Physical examination of the neck of a patient who has under-gone a thyroidectomy for thyroid cancer is seldom helpful in the *early* detection of a recurrence. The scar tissue following surgery combined with the propensity of metastatic lymph nodes to lie deep in the neck beneath the SCM make palpation of enlarged lymph nodes in the neck difficult. Even lymph nodes several centimeters in diameter are often not palpable. High-resolution ultrasound has proven to be a very sensitive method to find and locate early recur-rent cancer and lymph node metastasis. Frasoldati et al. studied

494 patients with a history of low risk well-differentiated thyroid cancer by a withdrawal WBS, stimulated Tg, and ultrasound and found that 51 patients had a recurrence by at least one test [44]. The WBS was positive in 23 patients (45%), the stimulated Tg was positive in 34 patients (67%), and the ultrasound with FNA was positive in 48 patients (94%). Since most thyroid cancer initially metastasizes to the neck, it is rare for thyroid cancer to spread elsewhere without neck lymph node involvement. Therefore, neck ultrasound has proven to be the most sensitive test available in locating early recurrent disease even before serum Tg is elevated.

Identifying and evaluating lymph nodes should be done with high-resolution ultrasound using a 10–15 MHz transducer with power Doppler capability to assess vascularity. When performing ultrasound of the neck in a patient who has undergone a thyroidectomy, one sees that the carotid artery and jugular vein have migrated medially close to the trachea. Someone unfamiliar with the ultrasound appearance of the postoperative neck should begin by examining the neck of someone who underwent a thyroidectomy or hemithyroidectomy for benign disease. This allows one to become accustom to the neck structures and the altered anatomy of the postoperative neck without worrying about recurrent thyroid cancer. Following a thyroidectomy the thyroid bed is filled with a varying amount of hyperechoic connective tissue that appears white (dense) on ultrasound. This serves well in demarcating a recurrence of cancer or a metastatic lymph node, which will appear dark or hypoechoic. The criteria discussed earlier are used to determine when to perform a UG FNA with both cytology and assay for Tg in the needle washout.

The decision to move forward with post-thyroidectomy nodal surgery must be a multidisciplinary decision made in the setting of a thorough discussion between endocrinology, surgery and importantly the patient. The risks of revision surgery are very substantial and include but are not restricted to unilateral or bilateral recurrent laryngeal nerve paralysis with paralytic dysphonia, dysphagia, and potentially respiratory distress as well as permanent hypoparathyroidism. Substantial thyroid cancer experience and experience with the revision cervical surgery are prerequisite for successful outcomes.

Central neck thyroid cancer recurrence may demonstrate invasive disease and the downward spiraling to the patient's clinical course. More typically however revision nodal surgery goals do not include improvement in survival but are more typically measured in improvements in a laboratory test, thyroglobulin. We must be careful to make sure what price the patient pays for this laboratory value improvement. Surgery must have clear-cut and definable goals. Rondeau recently showed small central neck nodal recurrences can be stable in the setting of TSH suppression without other treatment [45].

Several recent studies note that thyroglobulin can be rendered undetectable with revision papillary carcinoma nodal surgery in up to 40% of patient [46–48].

Given the distortion of neck anatomy and the need for accurate nodal localization during revision surgery we have investigated the use of CT scanning as an adjunct to ultrasound in the preoperative evaluation of patients with recurrent nodal disease and found that CT scanning added to ultrasound in terms of macroscopic nodal disease localization in 27% of such revision patients [39].

References

1. Carty SE, Cooper DS, et al. Consensus statement on the terminology and classification of central neck dissection for thyroid cancer. Thyroid. 2009;19(11):1153–8.

2. Ahuja A, Ying M, Phil M, King A, Yuen HY. Lymph node hilus—gray scale and power Doppler sonography of cervical nodes. J Ultrasound Med. 2001;20:987–92.

3. Ahuja A, Ying M, Yuen H, Metreweli C. Power Doppler sonography of metastatic nodes from papillary carcinoma of the thyroid. Clin Radiol. 2001;56:284–8.

4. Ahuja A, Ying M. An overview of neck node sonography. Invest Radiol. 2002;37:333–42.

5. Ballantone R, Lombardi C, Raffaelli M, Traini E, Crea C, Rossi E, et al. Management of cystic thyroid nodules: the role of ultrasound-guided fine-needle aspiration biopsy. Thyroid. 2004;14:43–7.

6. Frasoldati A, Toschi E, Zini M, Flora M, Caroggio A, Dotti C, et al. Role of thyroglobulin measurement in fine-needle aspiration biopsies of cervical lymph nodes in patients with differentiated thyroid cancer. Thyroid. 1999;9:105–11.

7. Pacini F, Fugazzola L, Lippi F, Ceccarelli C, Centoni R, Miccoli P, Elisei R, Pinchera A. Detection of thyroglobulin the needle aspirates of non-thyroidal neck masses: a clue to the diagnosis of metastatic differentiated thyroid cancer. J Clin Endocrinol Metab. 1992;74:1401–4.

8. Baskin HJ. Detection of recurrent papillary thyroid carcinoma by thyroglobulin assessment in the needle washout after fine-needle aspiration of suspicious lymph nodes. Thyroid. 2004;14:959–63.

9. Lee M, Ross D, Mueller P, Daniels G, Dawson S, Simeone J. Fine-needle biopsy of cervical lymph nodes in patients with thyroid cancer: a prospective comparison of cytopathologic and tissue marker analysis. Radiology. 1993;187:851–4.

10. Cignarelli M, Ambrosi A, Marino A, Lamacchia O, Campo M, Picca G. Diagnostic utility of thyroglobulin detection in fine-needle aspiration of cervical cystic metastatic lymph nodes from papillary thyroid cancer with negative cytology. Thyroid. 2003;13:1163–7.

11. Gemsenjager E, Perren A, et al. Lymph node surgery in papillary thyroid carcinoma. J Am Coll Surg. 2003;197(2):182–90.

12. Bardet S, Malville E, et al. Macroscopic lymph-node involvement and neck dissection predict lymph-node recurrence in papillary thyroid carcinoma. Eur J Endocrinol. 2008;158(4):551–60.

13. Cranshaw IM, Carnaille B. Micrometastases in thyroid cancer. An important finding? Surg Oncol. 2008;17(3):253–8.

14. Noguchi M, Hashimoto T, et al. Indications for bilateral neck dissection in well-differentiated carcinoma of the thyroid. Jpn J Surg. 1987;17(6):439–44.

15. Noguchi S, Murakami N. The value of lymph-node dissection in patients with differentiated thyroid cancer. Surg Clin North Am. 1987;67(2):251–61.

16. Mirallie E, Visset J, et al. Localization of cervical node metastasis of papillary thyroid carcinoma. World J Surg. 1999;23(9):970–3; discussion 973–4.

17. Qubain SW, Nakano S, et al. Distribution of lymph node micrometastasis in pN0 well-differentiated thyroid carcinoma. Surgery. 2002;131(3):249–56.

18. Wang TS, Dubner S, et al. Incidence of metastatic well-differentiated thyroid cancer in cervical lymph nodes. Arch Otolaryngol Head Neck Surg. 2004;130(1):110–3.

19. Triponez F, Poder L, et al. Hook needle-guided excision of recurrent differentiated thyroid cancer in previously operated neck compartments: a safe technique for small, nonpalpable recurrent disease. J Clin Endocrinol Metab. 2006;91(12):4943–7.

20. Ito Y, Higashiyama T, et al. Risk factors for recurrence to the lymph node in papillary thyroid carcinoma patients without preoperatively detectable lateral node metastasis: validity of prophylactic modified radical neck dissection. World J Surg. 2007;31(11):2085–91.

21. Lee SK, Choi JH, et al. Sentinel lymph node biopsy in papillary thyroid cancer: comparison study of blue dye method and combined radioisotope and blue dye method in papillary thyroid cancer. Eur J Surg Oncol. 2009;35(9):974–9.

22. Lim YC, Choi EC, et al. Central lymph node metastases in unilateral papillary thyroid microcarcinoma. Br J Surg. 2009;96(3):253–7.

23. Ross DS, Litofsky D, et al. Recurrence after treatment of micropapillary thyroid cancer. Thyroid. 2009;19(10):1043–8.

24. Baudin E, Travagli JP, et al. Microcarcinoma of the thyroid gland: the Gustave-Roussy Institute experience. Cancer. 1998;83(3):553–9.

25. Yamashita H, Noguchi S, et al. Extracapsular invasion of lymph node metastasis. A good indicator of disease recurrence and poor prognosis in patients with thyroid microcarcinoma. Cancer. 1999;86(5):842–9.

26. Chow SM, Law SC, et al. Papillary microcarcinoma of the thyroid—prognostic significance of lymph node metastasis and multifocality. Cancer. 2003;98(1):31–40.

27. Ito Y, Uruno T, et al. An observation trial without surgical treatment in patients with papillary microcarcinoma of the thyroid. Thyroid. 2003;13(4):381–7.

28. Wada N, Duh QY, et al. Lymph node metastasis from 259 papillary thyroid microcarcinomas: frequency, pattern of occurrence and recurrence, and optimal strategy for neck dissection. Ann Surg. 2003;237(3):399–407.

29. Roti E, Rossi R, et al. Clinical and histological characteristics of papillary thyroid microcarcinoma: results of a retrospective study in 243 patients. J Clin Endocrinol Metab. 2006;91(6):2171–8.

30. Hay ID. Management of patients with low-risk papillary thyroid carcinoma. Endocr Pract. 2007;13(5):521–33.

31. Mazzaferri EL. Management of low-risk differentiated thyroid cancer. Endocr Pract. 2007;13(5):498–512.

32. Hay ID, Hutchinson ME, et al. Papillary thyroid microcarcinoma: a study of 900 cases observed in a 60-year period. Surgery. 2008;144(6):980–7; discussion 987–8.

33. Noguchi S, Yamashita H, et al. Papillary microcarcinoma. World J Surg. 2008;32(5):747–53.

34. Giordano D, Gradoni P, et al. Treatment and prognostic factors of papillary. Clin Otolaryngol. 2010;35(2):118–24.

35. So YK, Son YI, et al. Subclinical lymph node metastasis in papillary microcarcinoma: a study of 551 resections. Surgery. 2010;148(3):526–31.

36. Zetoune T, Keutgen X, et al. Prophylactic central neck dissection and local recurrence in papillary thyroid cancer: a meta-analysis. Ann Surg Oncol. 2010;17(12):3287–93.

37. Moreno MA, Agarwal G, et al. Preoperative lateral neck ultrasonography as a long-term outcome predictor in papillary thyroid cancer. Arch Otolaryngol Head Neck Surg. 2011;137(2):157–62.

38. Ito Y, Jikuzono T, et al. Clinical significance of lymph node metastasis of thyroid papillary carcinoma located in one lobe. World J Surg. 2006;30(10):1821–8.

39. Lesnik, Randolph, et al. Papillary thyroid carcinoma nodal surgery directed by a preoperative radiographic map utilizing CT scan and ultrasound in all primary and reoperative patients. WJS (submitted).

40. Pineda J, Lee T, Ain K, et al. Iodine-131 therapy for thyroid cancer patients with elevated thyroglobulin and negative diagnostic scan. J Clin Endocrinol Metab. 1995;80:1488–92.

41. Schumberger M, Arcangioli O, Piekarski J, et al. Detection and treatment of lung metastases of differentiated thyroid carcinoma in patients with normal chest x-ray. J Nucl Med. 1988;29:1790–4.

42. Torre E, Carballo M, Erdozain R, Lienas L, Iriarte M, Layana J. Prognostic value of thyroglobulin and I-131 whole-body scan after initial treatment of low-risk differentiated thyroid cancer. Thyroid. 2004;14:301–6.

43. Park H, Perkins O, Edmondson J. Influence of diagnostic radioiodines on the uptake of ablative dose of iodine-131. Thyroid. 1994;4:49–54.

44. Frasoldati A, Presenti M, Gallo M, Coroggio A, Salvo D, Valcavi R. Diagnosis of neck recurrences in patients with differentiated thyroid carcinoma. Cancer. 2003;97:90–6.

45. Rondeau G, Fish S, et al. Ultrasonographically detected small thyroid bed nodules identified after total thyroidectomy for differentiated thyroid cancer seldom show clinically significant structural progression. Thyroid. 2011;21(8):845–53.
46. Al-Saif O, Farrar WB, et al. Long-term efficacy of lymph node reoperation for persistent papillary thyroid cancer. J Clin Endocrinol Metab. 2010;95(5):2187–94.
47. Schuff KG, Weber SM, et al. Efficacy of nodal dissection for treatment of persistent/recurrent papillary thyroid cancer. Laryngoscope. 2008;118(5):768–75.
48. Clayman GL, Shellenberger TD, et al. Approach and safety of comprehensive central compartment dissection in patients with recurrent papillary thyroid carcinoma. Head Neck. 2009;31(9):1152–63.

CHAPTER 9
Ultrasonography of the Parathyroid Glands

Dev Abraham

INTRODUCTION

Primary hyperparathyroidism (PHPT) is a common condition affecting approximately 100,000 new patients each year in the USA [1]. An apparent increase in the incidence was traced to the wide availability and the use of multichannel analyzers for routine testing. This has resulted in the early detection of subclinical disease since 1970[2]. The technological advancement in multichannel analyzers and the easy availability of biochemical testing have changed the disease presentation of PTHP. The majority of subjects presents well before onset of symptoms or end organ damage. In more than 85% of these cases, a solitary adenoma is the cause of the problem. Accurate localization of the adenoma enables minimally invasive surgery to be performed, often as an outpatient surgery or with shortened hospitalization and recuperative times [3].

SURGICAL ANATOMY OF THE PARATHYROID GLANDS

The parathyroid glands were described in 1852 by Sir. Richard Owen, when he performed the first recorded postmortem dissection of an Indian Rhinoceros [4]. Normal parathyroid glands are ovoid or bean-shaped and measure approximately 3 mm in size. The superior parathyroid glands are smaller than the lower located counterparts. The parathyroid glands have an anatomically distinct vascular supply from that of the thyroid gland and are enveloped in a pad of fibro-fatty capsule [5]. In subjects with

H.J. Baskin et al. (eds.), *Thyroid Ultrasound and Ultrasound-Guided FNA*, **179**
DOI 10.1007/978-1-4614-4785-6_9,
© Springer Science+Business Media, LLC 2013

normal calcium homeostasis; due to its small size, non-enlarged parathyroid glands cannot usually be visualized by ultrasound despite the considerable advancements made in today's ultrasound machines. Precise understanding of the typical location and the normal anatomical variations of parathyroid glands is the cornerstone to the successful identification and removal of glands that develop adenomas or hyperplasia.

One postmortem series revealed the presence of four glands in 91% of the subjects, three glands in 5%, and five glands in 4% [6]. Supernumerary glands are found in less than 5% of individuals and are very rare [7]. The locations of parathyroid glands vary widely due to their embryonic origination from the third and fourth pharyngeal pouches with eventual migration to the lower neck. The superior parathyroid glands develop in the fourth pharyngeal pouch and migrate caudally along with the ultimo branchial bodies, which give rise to parafollicular-C cells of the thyroid gland. The superior pair is commonly located along the upper two third of the posterior margin of the thyroid lobes. The superior parathyroid glands are relatively constant in their location, compared to the inferior pair. Anomalous locations of the superior glands include posterior pharyngeal and trachea-esophageal grooves. The third branchial pouches give rise to the inferior pair of parathyroid glands and the thymus, together they migrate to the lower neck. Forty-four percent of these glands are located within 1 cm of the inferior pole of the thyroid gland, 17% are in close proximity to the inferior margin of the thyroid gland, 26% are found close to the superior portion of the thymus along the thyro-thymic ligament and 2% are found within the mediastinal portion of the thymus [8]. Unusual variations in the site of location of the parathyroid glands include the carotid bifurcation, within the carotid sheath, intra-thyroidal and retropharyngeal locations. Due to these anatomical variations, accurate localization becomes crucial to the success of minimally invasive parathyroid surgery.

LOCALIZATION STUDIES

Ultrasound evaluation of the parathyroid glands should not be performed to diagnose PHPT. Its use should be reserved strictly for localization purposes. Appropriate biochemical testing should be conducted and surgical indication(s) established in each patient, prior to proceeding to any type of localization studies.

The two most widely used studies to locate the abnormal parathyroid gland(s) are 99 Tc MIBI (functional study) and ultrasonography (anatomical study). The respective localization techniques have their strengths and weaknesses and equally efficacious [9]. Most isotope-based studies "lateralize" the lesion, whereas, US studied provide precise localization information. To a practicing endocrinologist, the use of ultrasonography to study a patient with suspected parathyroid adenoma poses several advantages. The most important of these are the proven safety, ease of availability of ultrasound equipment, the lack of ionizing irradiation, short duration of the study, and the potential cost savings. The limitations of parathyroid localization using ultrasonography include operator variability and experience.

The procedure of ultrasonography, imaging features of parathyroid adenomas, the indication and technique of performing parathyroid biopsy will be discussed hence forth.

THE TECHNIQUE OF PERFORMING ULTRASONOGRAPHY OF PARATHYROID GLANDS

Proper positioning of the patient is crucial to the successful visualization of enlarged parathyroid gland(s). The patient should be made to lie flat on a firm table with one or two pillows placed underneath the posterior upper torso and the shoulders to enable full extension of the neck. The head should be supported with folded towel to enhance patient tolerance. Patients with cervical spine diseases such as ankylosing spodylosis may have very limited neck extension, making it impossible to conduct an adequate study.

The linear transducer (3–5 cm) is applied to the anterior neck along with adequate amount of coupling gel and the thyroid gland is located. The structures of the neck should be carefully studied in multiple axis and at different levels of the neck. Most clinicians use multifrequency transducers (5–15 MHz) to study the thyroid gland. Parathyroid ultrasonography does not require different equipment. The lower frequency settings are more effective at visualizing the deeper reaches of the neck. The most common sites of location such as the posterior margin of the thyroid capsule and the regions caudal to the thyroid lobes are inspected first, looking for a lesion(s) with features of enlarged parathyroid gland. Due to the inherent mobility of parathyroid adenomas, the tumor may not be visualized readily, particularly the superior adenomas located within the trachea-esophageal groove or intra-thoracic inferior gland adenomas. Asking such subjects to cough, strain, turn the head from side to side and or taking deep breaths in and out can "bring out" such an adenoma to enable visualization (Fig. 9.1). These maneuvers can provide a transient glimpse of a mobile adenoma, which may otherwise go unnoticed.

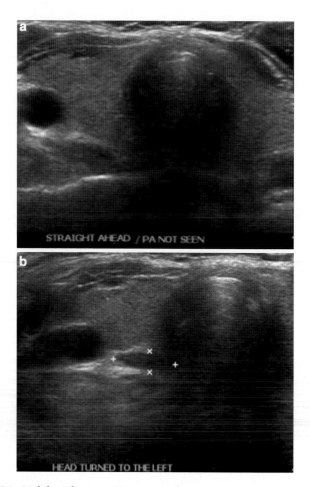

FIG. 9.1. Mobile right upper TE groove adenoma.

ULTRASOUND EVALUATION IN MEN SYNDROMES AND CHRONIC RENAL FAILURE PATIENTS

1. Multiple Endocrine Neoplasia: PHPT occurs in MEN 1 and MEN 2a syndromes. In these syndromes, multi-gland disease is very common. All gland inspection is required during surgery even if localization studies reveal unilateral abnormality, therefore, US or 99 Tc MIBI localization is of little value. However, there is a role for performing US evaluation in MEN subjects who have had unsuccessful surgeries.

2. Renal failure: In subjects with chronic renal failure, most often than not, all glands are involved to a variable degree. Surgical intervention should involve inspection of all parathyroid glands; therefore, localization is of limited value. However, if percutaneous ETOH ablation is considered in a poor surgical candidate, US evaluation is valuable. Also, due to the enlargement of multiple glands, renal patients present an excellent opportunity to practice parathyroid ultrasonography.

ULTRASOUND FEATURES OF THE PARATHYROID ADENOMAS

The following are the distinct ultrasonographic features of parathyroid adenomas:

Refer to Figs. 9.2, 9.3, 9.4, 9.5, 9.6, 9.7, 9.8, 9.9, and 9.10 for correlation.

1. Extra thyroidal location and indentation sign: The majority of parathyroid adenomas are located outside the posterior capsule of the thyroid gland [10–12]. These lesions are located in close relation to the posterior capsule of the thyroid gland [10]. The visualization of a lesion along the posterior aspect of thyroid gland in the clinical context of hypercalcemia makes the possibility of a parathyroid gland very likely. It is quite common to see an indentation made by the parathyroid adenoma on the posterior capsule of the thyroid gland: "The indentation sign". There is a noticeable echogenic line observed, separating the parathyroid and the thyroid glands, which represents the fibro-fatty capsule. Parathyroid adenomas are embedded within the thyroid gland in about 2–5% of cases [11, 12], when it is indistinguishable in appearance from a thyroid nodule. The incidence of intra-glandular location was higher in patients with multi-gland disease in one series, 3% in patients with uniglandular disease versus 15% in those with hyperplasia [12].

2. Homogenously hypoechoic texture: This is the most distinguishing imaging characteristic of parathyroid adenomas. The enlarged parathyroid glands are most often homogeneously hypoechoic echotexture in relation to the thyroid gland [13].

3. Vascular pedicle and blood flow: The presence of an independent artery (polar artery) feeding an adenoma was found in 83% of parathyroid adenomas [14]. Besides the visualization of the polar artery other patterns such as the "vascular arc" pattern and diffuse flow within the adenoma [15] have also been described (Fig. 9.6).

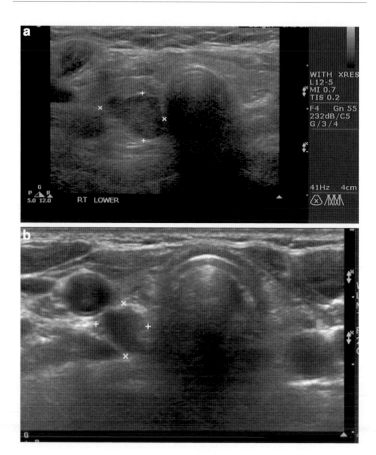

FIG. 9.2. (**a**, **b**) Inferior parathyroid adenoma in transverse view.

4. Variable shapes: Parathyroid adenomas conform to the anatomical pressures of surrounding structures, therefore, considerable variations in shapes is observed (Fig. 9.11).

LACK OF VISUALIZATION OF PARATHYROID LESION(S) IN HYPERCALCEMIC SUBJECTS

In the hands of experienced operators, parathyroid ultrasonography has high level of sensitivity and specificity. Despite the best of efforts, in about 10–20% of the subjects, no lesion could be visualized. The likely cause includes posterior located lesions, retropharyngeal superior adenomas, inferior intra-thoracic lesions and or

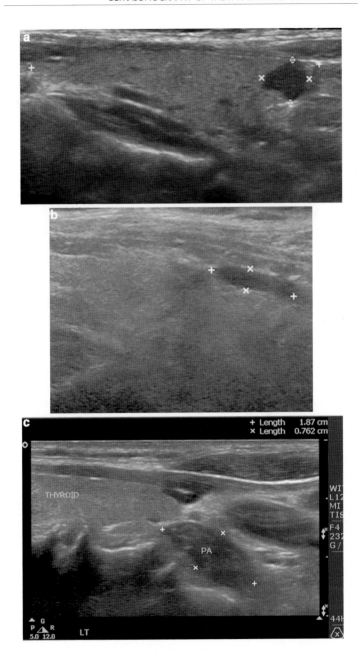

FIG. 9.3. (**a**, **b**, **c**) Inferior parathyroid adenoma seen in longitudinal view.

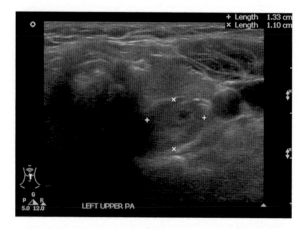

FIG. 9.4. Superior parathyroid adenoma seen in transverse view.

parathyroid hyperplasia. In one study, posterior located parathyroid adenoma was observed in 58% of subjects with negative US and Tc99MIBI scans [16].

PARATHYROID INDCIDENTALOMA

Subclinical parathyroid tumors can be discovered incidentally during neck ultrasonography. The frequency of observing these incidental tumors is rare [17, 18]. Fine needle aspiration with parathormone (PTH) estimation in syringe washings can identify these lesions as parathyroid tumors.

CYSTIC PARATHYROID ADENOMAS

Cystic parathyroid adenomas are very rare. Simple cysts of the parathyroid glands without hypercalcemia are occasionally encountered during assessment of suspected thyroid cysts. Partial cystic change of an adenoma is depicted in Fig. 9.16. Syringe washout PTH estimation is useful to prove the origin of these cysts (Fig. 9.12).

BIOPSY OF PARATHYROID LESIONS

Biopsy of suspected parathyroid lesions can be safely performed in the office setting and syringe washings analyzed for PTH [19, 20] (Fig. 9.13). Elevation of PTH in syringe washings provides confirmation with high degree of specificity and differentiates from coexistent posterior located thyroid nodules (Fig. 9.14) [20]. A lesion larger than > 1.5 cm with obvious ultrasound features

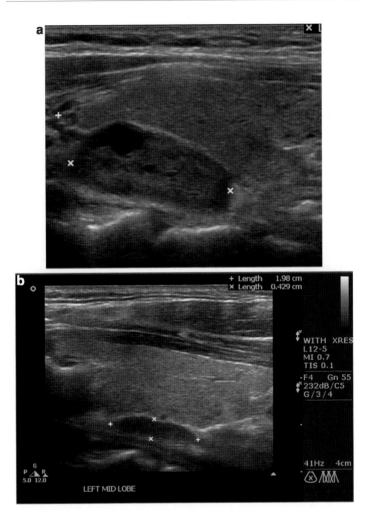

FIG. 9.5. (**a, b**) Superior parathyroid adenoma seen in longitudinal view. Indentation sign.

of a solitary parathyroid adenoma does not require biopsy confirmation. Subjects with bilateral or multiple lesions, patients who received unsuccessful surgery, negative Tc99MIBI study, atypical location, coexistent multinodular goiter and prior to percutaneous interventions are some of the indications to perform biopsy confirmation. Parathyroid incidentaloma observed during cervical ultrasonography can also be sampled for diagnosis.

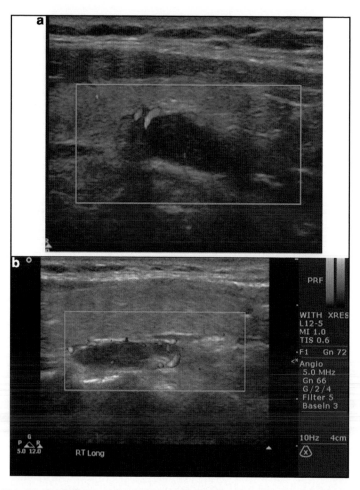

FIG. 9.6. (**a**) Polar vascular pedicle color Doppler. (**b**) Polar vessels depicted by power Doppler. (**c**) Arc pattern of blood flow. (**d**) Diffuse blood flow seen within adenoma.

Central compartment lymph nodes are often seen in subjects with Hashimoto's disease (Fig. 9.15). These reactive appearing lymph nodes should not be confused with parathyroid incidentalomas. The texture of the thyroid gland can provide clues to the diagnosis of Hashimoto's disease in undiagnosed subjects. The reactive lymphadenopathy is often multiple and observed in several areas in the perithyroidal region and may have a hilum.

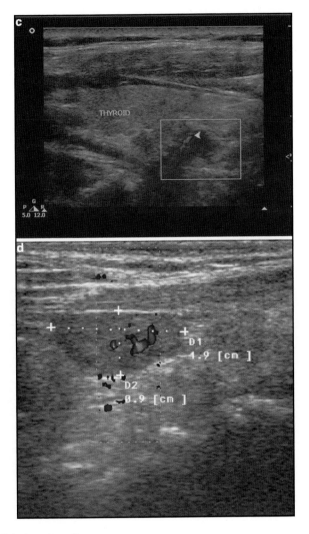

FIG. 9.6. (continued)

The technique of biopsy is similar to that of thyroid FNA with a few differences. We advocate the use of 27 or 25 G needles and to attempt fewer passes. Also vigorous "jabbing" technique is best avoided. The use of larger needles with multiple passes can lead to fibrosis of the gland or capsule, complicating subsequent surgical

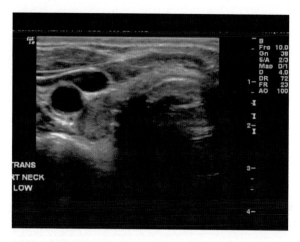

FIG. 9.7. Adenoma within the carotid sheath during surgery.

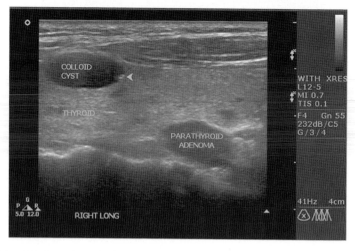

FIG. 9.8. Parathyroid adenoma visualized along side of incidental thyroid disease.

excision [21]. Biopsy induced histological changes have not been universally observed by others when appropriate smaller bore needles are used for sampling [22]. Due to the deep location of parathyroid lesions, longer needles may be required to enable biopsy to be performed. Parathyroid tumors can be mobile and may

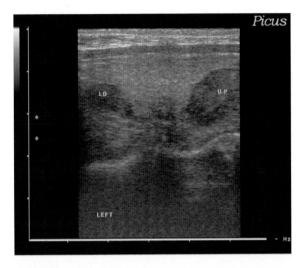

Fig. 9.9. Double adenoma visualized in longitudinal view. Note also PA located within the thyroid gland capsule.

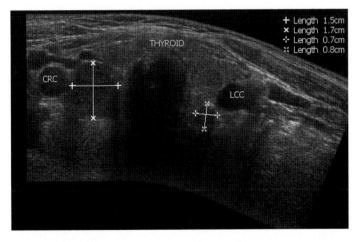

FIG. 9.10. Double inferior parathyroid adenoma in panoramic view. The findings were confirmed during surgery.

need a sharp and abrupt jab to penetrate the capsule. Parathyroid lesions provide bloody aspirates and suction is applied to enable the bloody fluid to enter the hub of the needle. The primary object

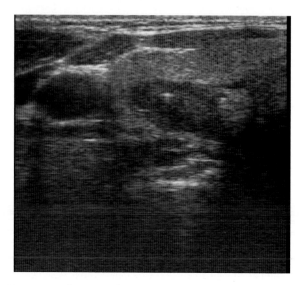

FIG. 9.11. Biopsy of suspected PA.

is to obtain specimen for PTH estimation. Absence of bloody aspirate is typically encountered with non-parathyroid lesions, most often, a central compartment lymph node.

The syringe aspirate can be processed in the following manner:

1. Prepare one or two slides with the specimen obtained during parathyroid FNA and rinse the reminder of the specimen in 2 mL of normal saline.
2. The fluid is centrifuged immediately, separate the supernatant from the cellular debris and freeze before transporting to the laboratory.
3. It is not necessary to submit the slides for cytological evaluation until the syringe washing PTH results become available. If the PTH level is low in the syringe aspirate, the prepared slides are submitted for cytological analysis. The latter technique ensures a certain level of safety against the chance sampling of posteriorly located coincidental metastatic lymph nodes. Metastatic lymph nodes in the central compartments are often multiple, unlike parathyroid adenoma.

Most laboratories in the USA are willing to perform intact PTH estimations in tissue specimens if prior arrangements are made

FIG. 9.12. Parathyroid cyst and aspirate.

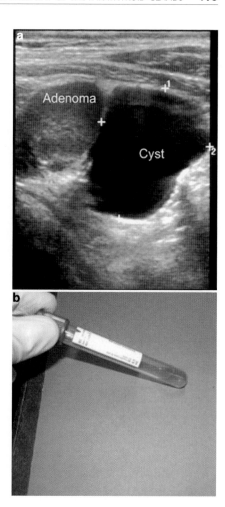

with the lab supervisor. It is good practice to freeze and save the leftover cell pellet. This can be reconstituted in saline and used as a second specimen in the event of loss of the primary specimen. In our laboratory, the phenomenon of "hook effect" has not been observed during **PTH** estimation by the above described technique despite the **PTH** levels being enormously elevated [20]. Parathyroid cytology is not useful during evaluation for parathyroid adenomas. Irrespective of the presence or absence of parathyroid cells, the

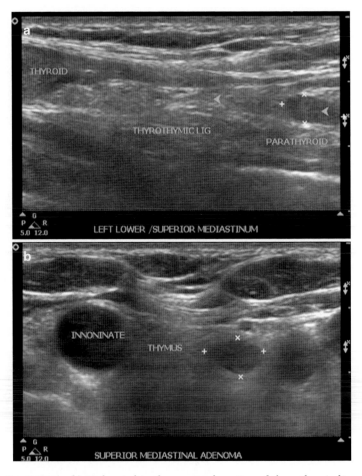

FIG. 9.13. (**a**, **b**) PA located in the proximal portion of thyro-thymic ligament and within thymus.

PTH levels in FNA fluid was elevated in all specimens obtained from parathyroid tissue. Also, thyroid cells can be observed in 30% of FNA specimens when posteriorly located lesions are biopsied through the thyroid lobe [23].

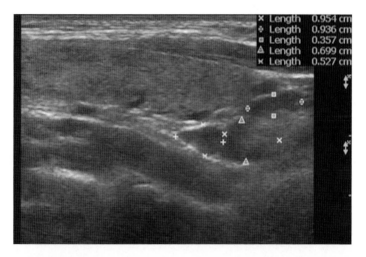

FIG. 9.14. Multiple reactive lymphadenopathy at the location of an inferior parathyroid gland.

ETOH ABLATION OF PARATHYROID GLANDS AND ADENOMAS

The primary therapy for parathyroid adenomas is surgical excision of the affected gland(s). In subjects who have undergone multiple unsuccessful surgeries or considered too high of an anesthesia risk, US guided ETOH ablation can be attempted. Injection is performed using 27 or 25 g needle. The immediate loss of Doppler vascular signal and opacification of the hypoechoic adenoma can be observed in Fig. 9.15, indicating successful intervention.

COEXISTENT THYROID DISEASE

Parathyroid ultrasonography provides the additional advantage of identifying coexistent thyroid nodules and cancers [20, 23, 24]. This alerts the surgeon to the presence of thyroid pathology that can be addressed during the same surgery. Not all thyroid lesions can be visualized during surgery and none by Tc 99MIBI imaging.

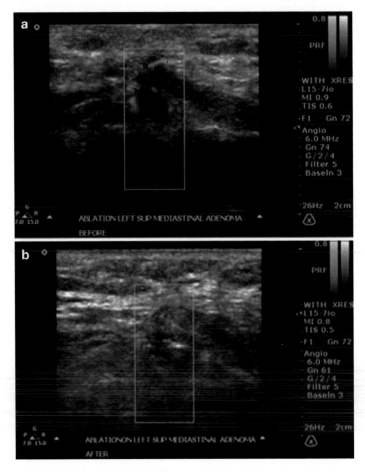

FIG. 9.15. Parathyroid ethanol ablation. Note the disappearance of vascular signal and opacification of the hypoechoic texture.

CONCLUSION

The use of ultrasongraphic evaluation of parathyroid adenomas provides several advantages. These include, the lack of radiation, time and cost efficiency. Also, it allows carefully conducted biopsy to be performed under guidance and ablation in selected subjects.

It is important to identify coexistent thyroid nodules and cancers in subjects undergoing parathyroid surgery. Just as important is the pre-operative calcium estimation in subjects undergoing thyroid surgery due to common coexistence of these two conditions.

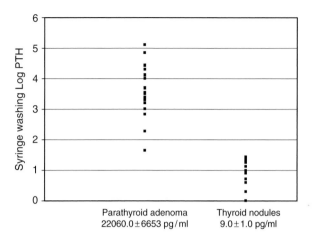

FIG. 9.16. PTH levels in syringe washing samples obtained from PA and thyroid nodules. Reproduced with permission from: Endocrine Practice Vol 13 No.4 July/ Aug 2007.

References

1. Kebebew E, Clark OH. Parathyroid adenoma, hyperplasia and carcinoma: localization, technical details of primary neck exploration and treatment of hypercalcemic crisis. Surg Oncol Clin N Am. 1998;7:721–48.

2. Heath III H, Hodgson SF, Kennedy M. Primary hyperparathyroidism: incidence, morbidity and potential economic impact in a community. N Engl J Med. 1980;302:189–93.

3. Udelsman R, Donovan PI. Open minimally invasive parathyroid surgery. World J Surg. 2004;28(12):1224–6.

4. Owen R. On the anatomy of the Indian Rhinoceros (Rh. Unicornis L.). Trans Zool Soc Lond. 1862;4:31–58.

5. Gilmore JR. The gross anatomy of parathyroid glands. J Pathol. 1938;46:133.

6. Alveryd A. Parathyroid glands in thyroid surgery. Acta Chir Scand. 1968;389:1.

7. Wang CA, Mahaffey JE, Axelrod L, et al. Hyperfunctioning supernumerary parathyroid glands. Surg Gynecol Obstet. 1979;148:711.

8. Akerstrom G, Malmaeus J, Bergstrom R. Surgical anatomy of human parathyroid glands. Surgery. 1984;95:14.

9. Cheung K, Wang TS, Farrokhyar F, Roman SA, Sosa JA. A meta-analysis of preoperative localization techniques for patients with primary hyperparathyroidism. Ann Surg Oncol. 2012;19(2):577–83.

10. Yeh MW, Barraclough BM, Sidhu SB, Sywak MS, Barraclough BH, Delbridge LW. Two hundred consecutive parathyroid ultrasound studies by a single clinician: the impact of experience. Endocr Pract. 2006;12(3):257–63.

11. Andre V, Andre M, Le Dreff P, Granier H, Forlodou P, Garcia JF. Intrathyroid parathyroid adenoma. J Radiol. 1999;80(6):591–2.

12. McIntyre Jr R, Eisenach J, Pearlman N, Ridgeway C, Dale Liechty R. Intrathyroidal parathyroid glands can be a cause of failed cervical exploration for hyperparathyroidism. Am J Surg. 1997;174(6):750–4.

13. Kamaya A, Quon A, Jeffrey RB. Sonography of the abnormal parathyroid gland. Ultrasound Q. 2006;22(4):253–62.

14. Lane MJ, Desser TS, Weigel RJ, Jeffrey Jr RB. Use of color and power Doppler sonography to identify feeding arteries associated with parathyroid adenomas. AJR Am J Roentgenol. 1998;171(3):819–23.

15. Wolf RJ, Cronan JJ, Monchik JM. Color Doppler sonography: an adjunctive technique in assessment of parathyroid adenomas. J Ultrasound Med. 1994;13(4):303–8.

16. Harari A, Mitmaker E, Grogan RH, Lee J, Shen W, Gosnell J, et al. Primary hyperparathyroidism patients with positive preoperative sestamibi scan and negative ultrasound are more likely to have posteriorly located upper gland adenomas (PLUGs). Ann Surg Oncol. 2011;18(6):1717–22.

17. Pesenti M, Frasoldati A, Azzarito C, Valcavi R. Parathyroid incidentaloma discovered during thyroid ultrasound imaging. J Endocrinol Invest. 1999;22(10):796–9.

18. Frasoldati A, Pesenti M, Toschi E, Azzarito C, Zini M, Valcavi R. Detection and diagnosis of parathyroid incidentalomas during thyroid sonography. J Clin Ultrasound. 1999;27(9):492–8.

19. Doppman JL, Krudy AG, Marx SJ, Saxe A, Schneider P, Norton JA, et al. Aspiration of enlarged parathyroid glands for parathyroid hormone assay. Radiology. 1983;148(1):31–5.

20. Abraham D, Sharma PK, Bentz J, Gault PM, Neumayer L, McClain DA. The utility of ultrasound guided FNA of parathyroid adenomas for preoperative localization prior to minimally invasive parathyroidectomy. Endocr Pract. 2007;13(4):333–7.

21. Norman J, Politz D, Browarski E. Diagnostic aspiration of parathyroid adenomas causes severe fibrosis complicating surgery and final histologic diagnosis. Thyroid. 2007;17(12):1251–5.

22. Abraham D, Duick AS, Baskin HJ. Appropriate administration of fine-needle aspiration (FNA) biopsy on selective parathyroid adenomas is safe. Thyroid. 2008;18(5):581–2.

23. Agarwal AM, Bentz JS, Hungerford R, Abraham D. Parathyroid fine-needle aspiration cytology in the evaluation of parathyroid adenoma: cytologic findings from 53 patients. Diagn Cytopathol. 2009;37:407–10.

24. Krause UC, Friedrich JH, Olbricht T, Metz K. Association of primary hyperparathyroidism and non-medullary thyroid cancer. Eur J Surg. 1996;162(9):685–9.

CHAPTER 10
Surgical Trends in Treatment of Thyroid Nodules, Thyroid Cancer, and Parathyroid Disease

Haengrang Ryu, Rachel Harris, and Nancy D. Perrier

INTRODUCTION

Operative intervention on the thyroid and parathyroid glands has been increasingly performed with minimally invasive and selective techniques over the past decade. This often requires a high-quality, preoperative imaging evaluation that provides tumor localization and knowledge of the relevant anatomical considerations. In this chapter imaging modalities are discussed with regards to benign and malignant disease. Indications for thyroid lobectomy, total thyroidectomy, neck dissection, minimally invasive parathyroidectomy, and standard cervical exploration (SCE) are discussed.

Surgery is a critical discipline involved in the treatment of thyroid and parathyroid gland disease. "Glandulae laryngis" was first described in 1543 by the anatomist Andrea Vesalius (1514–1564), and the first distinct image of the thyroid gland with the typical horseshoe shape dates back to the work of Julius Casserius (1545–1616) [1]. Since then, many surgeons have strived to reduce the mortality and morbidity associated with thyroid gland resection. Theodor Kocher (1841–1917), a noted surgeon, established the standard cervical approach technique for thyroidectomy, and he was awarded the Nobel Prize for physiology and medicine in 1909 [2].

With the development of modern medical technology, most notably surgical instrumentation and radiography, techniques for surgical resection of the thyroid and parathyroid glands have

H.J. Baskin et al. (eds.), *Thyroid Ultrasound and Ultrasound-Guided FNA*, **199**
DOI 10.1007/978-1-4614-4785-6_10,
© Springer Science+Business Media, LLC 2013

evolved. However, a thorough understanding of the underlying disease remains the most important aspect of surgical decision-making. In this chapter, we discuss the types of surgical procedures currently used to treat thyroid and parathyroid disease and the methods used to determine which procedure is most appropriate for each patient.

THYROID AND PARATHYROID SURGICAL PROCEDURES

Below is a list of the types of surgical procedures used to treat thyroid and parathyroid disease.

Subtotal thyroidectomy: Bilateral removal of thyroid tissue with the intent of leaving tissue in situ. This procedure is not commonly performed in contemporary endocrine surgery.

Lobectomy or hemithyroidectomy: Complete removal of one thyroid lobe, which also usually includes the isthmus.

Near-total thyroidectomy: Total extracapsular removal of one lobe, including the isthmus, with less than 5% of the contralateral lobe remaining in situ. This is an intended total thyroidectomy in which, at the surgeon's discretion, a remnant of the thyroid parenchyma is left intact near the ligament of berry or superior pole to maintain vascularity of the parathyroid gland(s) or to preserve the recurrent laryngeal nerve.

Total thyroidectomy: Complete removal of both lobes and the isthmus, leaving behind only viable parathyroid glands.

Central neck dissection: Bilateral removal of all lymph nodes of level VI (central position in the neck). The superior border is the hyoid bone, the inferior border is the suprasternal notch, and the lateral borders are the common carotid arteries.

Compartment-oriented, modified lateral neck dissection: Removal of all soft tissue from level IIa to Vb. The superior border is the digastric muscle, the inferior border is the clavicle, the lateral border is the spinal accessory nerve, and the medial border is the common carotid artery.

Minimally invasive parathyroidectomy: Removal of one parathyroid gland without exploration of the cervical region or identification of other glands. Preoperative imaging suggests where to start the operation and intraoperative parathyroid hormone assays selectively suggest when to stop the operation.

Standard cervical exploration (SCE): An exploration and inspection of both sides of the neck. With reference to parathyroid surgery,

Table 10.1 Complications of thyroid and parathyroid surgery

General complications

Wound infection

Laryngotracheal edema

Bleeding

Specific surgical complications

Recurrent laryngeal nerve injury

Superior laryngeal nerve injury

Lymphatic leak

Hypoparathyroidism

Thyroid storm

this is usually with the intent of identifying all four parathyroid glands and removing those that appear abnormally enlarged and hyperfunctional.

Subtotal parathyroidectomy: Removal of three parathyroid glands and portion of the fourth for multigland primary parathyroid disease or secondary hyperparathyroidism.

Table 10.1 shows a list of complications associated with these procedures.

SURGICAL PLANNING

Routine Preoperative Imaging

Prior to surgical intervention, the entire thyroid gland and central and lateral cervical compartments require radiologic evaluation. For benign disease, radiologic evaluation can reveal thyroiditis, reactive lymph nodes, enlarged parathyroid glands, and the presence of an aberrant right subclavian artery or concomitant malignancy. In thyroid cancer, metastasis is common but physical examination has poor sensitivity to detect lymph node disease; thus, radiologic evaluation is needed.

Ultrasonography is the imaging modality of choice for initially examining the thyroid gland. Although user-dependent, it is also noninvasive and inexpensive. Not only does it provide information about nodal status, but it also reveals the size and location of the tumor in the contralateral lobe and detects the presence of extrathyroidal extension. The overall accuracy of ultrasonography was found to be 67 and 71.3% for tumor and nodal staging, respectively [16]. Thus, ultrasound-guided fine-needle aspiration (FNA) biopsy of sonographically suspicious lymph nodes should be performed to confirm malignancy if this would change disease management [9]. If extrathyroidal tumor extension or advanced disease is suspected, computed tomographic study is needed to evaluate occult areas that are poorly assessed with ultrasonography (such as level VII), as well as tumor extension into adjacent structures, including the esophagus and trachea [17, 18].

Ultrasound-Guided FNA Biopsy of Thyroid Nodules
Thyroid nodules are common; prevalence ranges from 30 to 60% in autopsy reports of the general population [8]. Preoperative determination of which nodules require surgical intervention is necessary to avoid unnecessary operations. Ultrasound-guided FNA is an excellent means of determining whether a nodule is malignant.

The American Thyroid Association recommends FNA biopsy for thyroid nodules that are predominantly cystic, located posteriorly to the thyroid gland, or have suspicious sonographic appearance (microcalcifications, hypoechoic, increased nodular vascularity, infiltrative margins, or taller than wide on transverse view). If more than two nodules are noted, the most worrisome should be preferentially aspirated. If the patient has a high risk for malignancy, such as a history of exposure to ionizing radiation in childhood or adolescence, one or more first-degree relatives with thyroid cancer, [18] F-fluorodeoxyglucose avidity on positron emission tomographic study, or a *MEN2* or familial medullary *RET* protooncogene mutation, FNA is recommended regardless of the size of the nodule. Additionally, if there is evidence of nodule growth either by palpation or on sonographic findings (more than a 50% change in volume or a 20% increase in at least two nodule dimensions, with a minimal increase of 2 mm in solid nodules or in the solid portion of mixed cystic–solid nodules), the FNA should be repeated, preferably with ultrasound guidance [9]. Biopsy-proven thyroid cancer requires total thyroidectomy.

Role of Intraoperative Ultrasound
Intraoperative ultrasound helps determine the anatomy and map the extent of the operation. This is particularly true in reoperative surgery [19]. Ultrasound can be performed in the operating room after the patients is properly positioned but before incision

[20]. Intraoperative ultrasound can provide information about the extent (level II, Vb) of nonpalpable lymph node metastasis in relation to surrounding structures. Ultrasound-guided dye injection or wire localization can also be used in this setting [20].

THYROID DISEASE

Indications for Total Thyroidectomy for Benign Thyroid Disease

Because of the associated complications, total thyroidectomy was rarely performed until the late nineteenth century [3]. Since the beginning of the twentieth century, improved understanding of how to prevent hypoparathyroidism and postoperative tetany, as well as improved anesthesia, have led to the use of thyroidectomy for management of benign thyroid disease. Indications for total thyroidectomy include not only thyroid cancer but also Graves' disease and both multinodular toxic and symptomatic nontoxic goiter (Fig. 10.1) [4–6]. Total thyroidectomy allows immediate and complete eradication of the disease and helps the patient avoid reoperative surgery [4–6]. Because thyrotoxicosis has a modestly high recurrence rate after medical therapy or radioactive iodine ablation and total thyroidectomy is an effective and immediate, it may be considered a first-line treatment in certain cases of Graves' disease [7].

Indications for Total Thyroidectomy vs Lobectomy for Thyroid Cancer

The advantage of thyroid lobectomy is that if the final pathologic review determines that malignancy is not present, the patient will likely not require lifelong thyroid hormone replacement therapy if the residual lobe remains intact. The risk, however, is that the patient will require a second trip to the operating room for completion thyroidectomy if malignancy is found. In addition, a bilateral lobectomy procedure exposes the patient to twice the risk (albeit low) of hypoparathyroidism and nerve injury compared with a total thyroidectomy.

Total thyroidectomy is indicated for patients with indeterminate nodules that are large (>4 cm), have marked atypia, are "suspicious for papillary carcinoma," or if the patient has a family history of thyroid carcinoma or personal history of radiation exposure. For patients with proven thyroid cancer >1 cm, a near-total or total thyroidectomy should be considered for the initial surgical procedure unless the patient has known contralateral recurrent laryngeal nerve injury or is unable to undergo general anesthesia or anticoagulation therapy. Thyroid lobectomy may

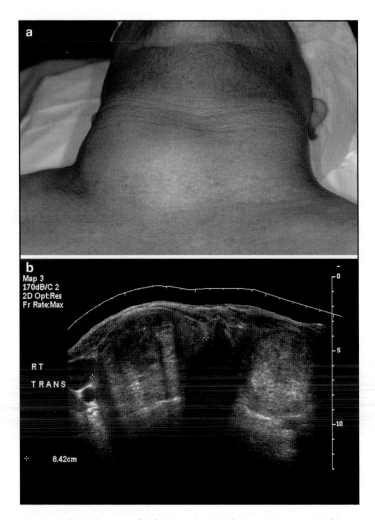

FIG. 10.1. Thyroidectomy for benign thyroid disease in a 72-year-old man. An anterior mass on his neck had increased in size over the past 2 years and he experienced dysphagia (**a**). Ultrasound images (**b**) revealed that the right lobe measured 10.2 × 6.4 × 8.4 cm and the left lobe measured 9.0 × 5.0 × 5.9 cm. The patient underwent a total thyroidectomy for multinodular goiter. The gross specimen is shown of the *right* lobe (**c**). The weight of the specimen was 510 g. The bivalved specimen shows typical thyroid goitrous parenchyma (**d**).

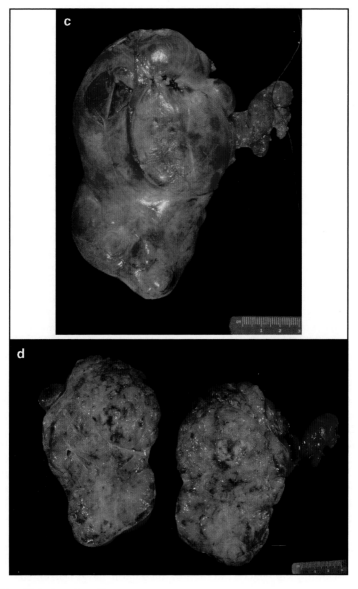

Fig. 10.1. (continued)

be sufficient treatment for small (<1 cm), low-risk, unifocal, intrathyroidal papillary carcinomas in the absence of prior head and neck irradiation or radiologically or clinically involved cervical nodal metastases [9].

FNA biopsy is often used to determine whether suspicious thyroid nodules are malignant (see above). However, up to 11% of patients have an inconclusive cytologic evaluation [10]. Because the rate of malignancy can be as high as 20% for solitary nodules whose biopsy results are indeterminant (follicular neoplasm or Hurthle cell neoplasm) [11], a lobectomy or thyroidectomy should be performed for indeterminate nodules.

Indications for Central Neck Dissection for Thyroid Cancer

Identification of central neck lymph node disease, either by palpation or by imaging, indicates that a therapeutic central neck dissection (level VI) should accompany total thyroidectomy. However, even if metastatic nodal disease is not detected, it may still be present: the incidence of central lymph node metastasis in clinically node-negative patients is approximately 30–60% [12, 13]. Because of high rate of concomitant microscopic disease, some surgeons advocate for the role of prophylactic central compartment neck dissection. This is controversial because concomitant central neck dissection with total thyroidectomy increases the risk of postoperative hypoparathyroidism and recurrent laryngeal nerve injury [14]. These complications can be devastating to a patient's quality of life. Because of this, the procedure is recommended only when the potential benefits outweigh the risks. It is not recommended routinely for differentiated thyroid carcinoma but may be performed if the surgeon feels that it can be done safely [13]. Prophylactic central neck dissection should be considered in the presence of advanced papillary thyroid carcinoma (T3 or T4) and it is recommended for preoperatively determined medullary thyroid carcinoma [15]. For small (T1 or T2), noninvasive, clinically node-negative, differentiated thyroid cancers and most follicular cancer, a near-total or total thyroidectomy without prophylactic central neck dissection may be most appropriate.

Therapeutic lateral neck node dissection should be performed for patients with biopsy-proven lateral neck metastasis [9]. However, prophylactic lateral neck dissection is not warranted for any disease type.

Conventional Open Thyroidectomy Procedure

Because volume and experience have bearing on outcomes, thyroidectomy should be performed by an experienced surgeon to reduce the risk of complications [7]. After safe induction of general anesthesia, the patient is placed in a supine position with the neck mildly hyperextended and both arms tucked (Fig. 10.2). A 4–5-cm transverse incision is made approximately two finger breadths above the sternal notch. Subplatysmal skin flaps are made to the thyroid cartilage superiorly, to the sternal notch inferiorly, and to the medial side of the anterior border of the sternocleidomastoid muscles laterally. The strap muscles are divided at the midline, and the thyroid gland is exposed. Inferior and superior parathyroid glands are identified and protected with gentle dissection, avoiding disruption of the lateral vascular pedicle. The recurrent laryngeal nerve is identified in the tracheoesophageal groove and traced carefully to its insertion into the cricothyroid muscle. The inferior thyroidal vessels and middle thyroidal vein are individually isolated and ligated, and the thyroid gland is dissected off the tracheal cartilage with care to prevent injury to the superior laryngeal nerve. Next, the superior thyroidal vessels are divided and ligated as they enter the thyroid parenchyma and the gland is mobilized medially off of the anterior surface of the trachea. If a total thyroidectomy is needed, a contralateral lobectomy is performed using a symmetric, mirror-like technique. After the specimen is delivered out of the wound, the strap muscles and skin are closed with absorbable sutures.

Robot-Assisted Transaxillary Thyroid Surgery

Robot-assisted transaxillary thyroid surgery (RATS) is a minimally invasive technique popularized in South Korea due to the desire to avoid an obvious cervical scar. RATS may offer a reasonable alternative for patients with the appropriate body habitus and gland size who are interested in avoiding a cervical scar. Currently we reserve this technique for patients with benign disease. This approach involves a 5-cm incision in the ipsilateral axilla. The initial dissection is from the lateral border of the pectoralis major muscle to the heads of the sternocleidomastoid muscle. A space behind the strap muscles is created to expose the lateral aspect of the thyroid gland. The DaVinci robot is then employed. The three-dimensional visualization and magnification of the equipment is used to perform the thyroid lobe dissection. Gas insufflation is not required. Based on preoperative workup, patients are selected who have lesions of low malignant potential, thyroid lobe size <6 cm, BMI <36 and no prior neck surgery. Operative time for RATS lobectomy is longer than standard open thyroidectomy and there is additional risk of brachial plexus praxia, likely due to extension and positioning of the ipsilateral arm. Patients are also more likely to have numbness.

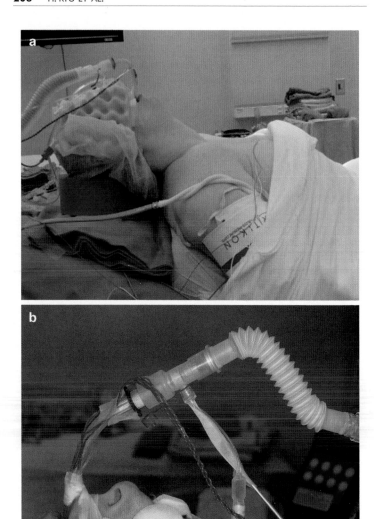

FIG. 10.2. (**a**) Patient positioning for thyroidectomy. The patient is placed in a supine, semi-Fowler's position, which includes elevation of the head of the bed. The head is slightly hyperextended via roll behind the clavicles. The arms are tucked to the side of the bed. (**b**) An intubated patient with an endotracheal tube placed for selective intraoperative nerve monitoring. During the thyroidectomy, selective nerve monitoring is useful to confirm function of the recurrent laryngeal nerve. Bipolar stainless steel contact electrodes are embedded in the endotracheal tube and properly aligned to monitor the innervation of both vocal cords.

PARATHYROID DISEASE

Primary hyperparathyroidism is a common endocrine disorder with prevalence rate of 1–4 per 1,000 in the general population and the incidence of the disease increases with age. Osteoporosis, nephrolithiasis, fatigue, insomnia, difficulty with concentration and memory are symptoms associated with the disease. A parathyroid adenoma is the most common cause of primary hyperparathyroidism.

Surgical removal of the parathyroid adenoma is the only definitive treatment known for the disease. In the hands of an experienced surgeon, the cure rate is more than 95%. Since the first parathyroidectomy in the USA was reported in 1926, and until the mid-1990s, a standard cervical operation with wide exploration was the technique of choice. This operation offered the surgeon the opportunity to inspect all four parathyroid glands and to resect the largest offending gland. Three factors drove the change from wide cervical exploration to selective minimally invasive dissections. First, the advent of rapid intraoperative biochemical testing, which provided rapid feedback to the surgeon as to when the correct gland was removed, as removal of all hyperfunctioning tissue gives rise to a very rapid and measurable drop in peripheral blood PTH levels. Second, the modern surgical practice is increasingly interested in reducing the amount of dissection, size of incision, operative time, postoperative pain, and hospitalization. Third, improved imaging technology now allows accurate localization of parathyroid adenomas, which allows better surgical targeting and, thus, smaller operations [8–12].

Locating the Parathyroid Adenoma

Critical to the success of minimally invasive parathyroidectomy is the need for accurate preoperative localization of adenomas. The traditional imaging modalities utilized for this purpose were Sestamibi scanning and ultrasonography. The Sestamibi radionuclide accumulates in the mitochondria of hyperfunctioning parathyroid tissue and this accumulation renders the adenoma visible to nuclear scintigraphy. Ultrasonography can identify the physical nodule of the adenoma in the necks of patients with favorable anatomy. Preoperative imaging suggests where to start the dissection and intraoperative parathyroid hormone monitoring suggests when to stop the dissection by suggesting that all hyperfunctional parathyroid tissue has been removed. The goal is to perform a safe resection and minimize dissection, which causes scarring.

Resection of an enlarged solitary parathyroid gland by an experienced surgeon is 95% curative for primary hyperparathyroidism.

However, the success rate of reoperations is approximately 70%; recurrent and persistent disease is reported in up to 30% of patients who undergo a reoperation for persistent disease. Thus, accurately locating the gland before the procedure is important in the setting of both primary and recurrent disease.

To improve communication between specialists involved in the treatment (endocrinologists, radiologists, surgeons, and pathologists) and to avoid ambiguity, a standardized system was developed to succinctly describe parathyroid gland location (Fig. 10.3) [21].

Role of FNA in Parathyroid Disease

Rarely is FNA indicated to confirm the presence of a parathyroid adenoma. Usually the size, blood flow, and pedicle clearly distinguish the parathyroid gland from a thyroid nodule or lymph node. In addition, the anatomy can be confirmed with complementary radiographic studies that identify hyperfunctional parathyroid tissue (Sestamibi or four-dimensional computed tomographic scans). FNA can cause bleeding or an inflammatory reaction around the adenoma, which results in a more difficult surgical dissection. As such, we do not recommend routine biopsy of the parathyroid glands except under special circumstances, which should be discussed with the operating surgeon. In particular for reoperative parathyroid surgery, biopsy may be needed when no definitive target lesion has been identified, the disease is escalating, and when discordant imaging studies show more than one suspicious mass.

Immunohistochemical stains of ultrasound-guided FNA biopsy specimens are one means of confirming that a nodular structure is of parathyroid origin. However, in difficult reoperative cases in which a scar is present, immunohistochemical stains may not be definitive because the specimen may appear to be of follicular cell origin. This can be confusing for the pathologist and the surgeon. In these cases, parathyroid hormone assay can be utilized [22]. This requires planning and preparation. The aspirate or needle rinse can be suspended in 1.0 mL of saline and sent for assessment. This technique has a sensitivity and specificity of 91 and 95%, respectively [23]. The assay will reveal excessively high parathyroid hormone levels if the specimen is from parathyroid tissue and low levels if it is from thyroid or lymph node tissue. The parathyroid hormone assay cannot determine whether tissue is hypercellular, but it can determine whether it is of parathyroid origin.

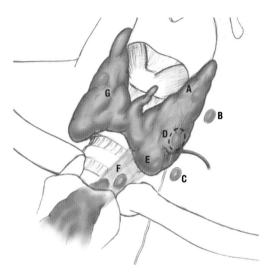

FIG. 10.3. Illustration depicting the common locations of parathyroid glands. Type A: Adherent to the posterior thyroid parenchyma. This is the expected location of a normal gland. Type B: Behind the thyroid parenchyma—exophytic to the thyroid parenchyma and lying posteriorly in the tracheoesophageal groove. An undescended gland high in the neck near the carotid bifurcation or mandible is classified as a type B + gland. Type C: Caudal to the thyroid parenchyma, in the tracheoesophageal groove. This gland is commonly missed; it could be mistaken for the esophagus when palpated. It is located inferior to the inferior pole of the thyroid parenchyma, nearer or closer to the clavicle. Type D: Dangerously close to the recurrent laryngeal nerve, on the mid-posterior surface of the thyroid parenchyma, this may make dissection difficult. Because of its location, the embryologic origin of this gland is unknown. Type E: External to the thyroid, near the inferior pole, and in medial aspect of the recurrent laryngeal nerve. This gland is relatively easy to resect because it is in the paratracheal region. Type F: Has fallen into the thyrothymic ligament. This gland is referred to as an "ectopic" gland. It can usually be retrieved from the superior portion of the thymus; however, it sometimes requires delivery from the anterior mediastinum via the neck. Type G: Intrathyroidal lesion (gated in thyroid tissue), a "gauche," rare gland.

Suspicious thyroid lesions are often identified in the preoperative workup for parathyroid disease, and the presence of concomitant thyroid cancer would obviously alter the surgical approach. Thus, although ultrasound-guided FNA biopsy is not recommended for parathyroid nodules, it is a useful adjunct for evaluating thyroid nodules [24].

Minimally Invasive Parathyroidectomy

Preoperative workup of an adenoma to a specific quadrant allows the surgeon to plan the incision site and minimize both dissection and operative time. Superior glands are excised via a lateral approach, whereas inferior glands are excised via an anterior approach. In the lateral approach, a 2-cm incision is made anterior to the medial border of the sternocleidomastoid muscle (Fig. 10.4). The lateral borders of the strap muscles are separated longitudinally from the sternocleidomastoid. The lateral border of the thyroid parenchyma is noted and the thyroid gland is retracted medially. Manual palpation can facilitate identification of the adenoma. If necessary, the thyroid capsule is meticulously incised. The gland is circumferentially dissected and vascular pedicle is divided. Care is taken to avoid injury to the recurrent laryngeal nerve.

The surgical approach for a suspected inferior gland is a 2-cm incision made towards the ipsilateral side from the midline. The strap muscles are identified, separated longitudinally, and retracted laterally. The inferior pole of the thyroid is retracted medially. The dorsal, inferior side of the thyroid gland and the superior thyrothymic ligament are carefully dissected. If necessary the thyroid capsule is incised. The adenoma is identified and removed in a similar fashion as above. Intraoperative decrease of serum PTH (IOPTH) by greater than 50% at either 5 or 10 min after excision suggests that all hyperfunctional tissue has been removed. It is imperative to remember that the purpose of the IOPTH decline is to suggest to the surgeon when to stop the operation.

Standard Cervical Exploration

SCE is indicated in patients with familial, suspected multigland or secondary parathyroid disease. A 2–3 cm incision is made just caudal to the cricoid cartilage. The initial dissection is similar to that of a thyroidectomy. After the strap muscles are separated longitudinally, an ipsilateral dissection is ensued. The thyroid gland is retracted medially and the tracheoesophageal groove is inspected. The recurrent laryngeal nerve is identified and preserved as are normal parathyroid glands. Normal parathyroid glands are approximately 30 mg in weight and 1×3 mm in size. They are subtle and have a golden peanut-buttery hue. Care is taken to avoid devascularization of the parathyroid pedicle. Normal glands should not be biopsied. A mirror-like procedure is performed on the contralateral side. An obvious, asymmetrically enlarged parathyroid gland can be identified in most cases. The color, contours, shape, consistency, and size are all important delineating features that separate normal from abnormal glands.

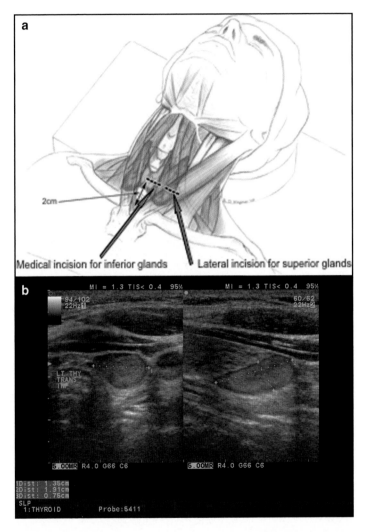

FIG. 10.4. Minimally invasive parathyroidectomy performed on a patient with a left inferior parathyroid adenoma. The patient was a 30-year-old woman with an 8-month history of recurrent nephrolithiasis. Preoperative biochemical tests showed synchronous elevation of calcium levels to 11.2 mg/dL (normal range: 8.4–10.2 mg/dL) and parathyroid hormone levels of 166 pg/mL (normal range: 9–80 pg/mL). (**a**) Preoperative ultrasound images.

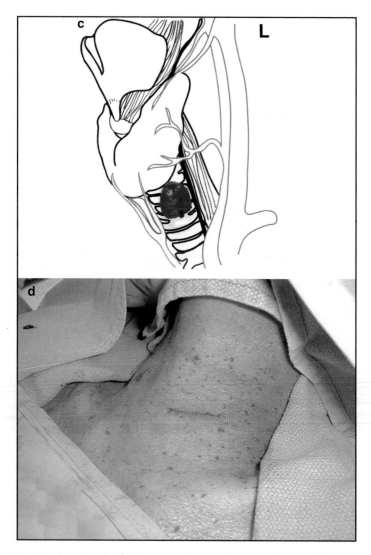

FIG. 10.4. (continued) (**b**) Gross specimen on the operative template representing the classic type E *left* position. (**c**) Diagram showing planned location of the incision. (**d**) Sutured wound after the procedure.

If an obvious enlarged parathyroid adenoma is not found in the standard locations described, the thyrothymic ligament and superior portion of the cervical thymus should be mobilized. If the preoperative diagnosis is familial disease, or multiple enlarged glands are identified, then a 3.5 gland resection should be performed. Confirmation of viability of the chosen remnant is critical prior to resection of other glands.

SUMMARY

Contemporary thyroid and parathyroid surgical techniques are safe and effective. A multidisciplinary approach that involves preoperative planning with information gleaned from colleagues in radiology, nuclear medicine, pathology, and endocrinology is crucial for surgical success. A confident preoperative diagnosis should be important to minimize unnecessary reoperations and increased risk of complications. A thorough understanding of the disease process is a key element needed for the endocrine surgeon.

References

1. Hast M. The anatomy of the larynx: an aspect of renaissance anatomy by Julius Casserius. Proc Inst Med Chic. 1970;28:64.
2. Kocher T. Über Kropfextirpation und ihre Folgen. Arch Klin Chir. 1883;29:254.
3. Gough IR, Wilkinson D. Total thyroidectomy for management of thyroid disease. World J Surg. 2000;24:962–5.
4. Wheeler MH. Total thyroidectomy for benign thyroid disease. Lancet. 1998;351:1526–7.
5. Barczyński M, Konturek A, Hubalewska-Dydejczyk A, et al. Five-year follow-up of a randomized clinical trial of total thyroidectomy versus Dunhill operation versus bilateral subtotal thyroidectomy for multinodular nontoxic goiter. World J Surg. 2010;34:1203–13.
6. Barczy ski M, Konturek A, Stopa M, et al. Total thyroidectomy for benign thyroid disease: is it really worthwhile? Ann Surg. 2011; 254(5):724–30.
7. Bahn Chair RS, Burch HB, Cooper DS, et al. Hyperthyroidism and other causes of thyrotoxicosis: management guidelines of the American Thyroid Association and American Association of Clinical Endocrinologists. Thyroid. 2011;21(6):593–646.
8. Tan GH, Gharib H. Thyroid incidentalomas: management approaches to nonpalpable nodules discovered incidentally on thyroid imaging. Ann Intern Med. 1997;126(3):226–31.
9. Cooper DS, Doherty GM, Haugen BR, et al. Revised American Thyroid Association management guidelines for patients with thyroid nodules and differentiated thyroid cancer. Thyroid. 2009; 19(11):1167–214.
10. García-Pascual L, Barahona M-J, Balsells M, at el. (2011) Complex thyroid nodules with nondiagnostic fine needle aspiration cytology: histopathologic outcomes and comparison of the cytologic variants (cystic vs. acellular). Endocrine 39(1):33–40.

11. Gharib H, Goellner JR, Zinsmeister AR, Grant CS, Van Heerden JA. Fine-needle aspiration biopsy of the thyroid. The problem of suspicious cytologic findings. Ann Intern Med. 1984;101:25–8.

12. Koo BS, Choi EC, Yoon YH, Kim DH, Kim EH, Lim YC. Predictive factors for ipsilateral or contralateral central lymph node metastasis in unilateral papillary thyroid carcinoma. Ann Surg. 2009;249(5):840–4.

13. Roh JL, Park JY, Park CI. Total thyroidectomy plus neck dissection in differentiated papillary thyroid carcinoma patients: pattern of nodal metastasis, morbidity, recurrence, and postoperative levels of serum parathyroid hormone. Ann Surg. 2007;245:604–10.

14. Cavicchi O, Piccin O, Caliceti U, et al. Transient hypoparathyroidism following thyroidectomy: a prospective study and multivariate analysis of 604 consecutive patients. Otolaryngol Head Neck Surg. 2007;137:654–8.

15. Kloos RT, Eng C, Evans DB, et al. Medullary thyroid cancer: management guidelines of the American Thyroid Association. Thyroid. 2009;19(6):565–612.

16. Park JS, Son KR, Na DG, Kim E, Kim S. Performance of preoperative sonographic staging of papillary thyroid carcinoma based on the sixth edition of the AJCC/UICC TNM classification system. Am J Roentgenol. 2009;192(1):66–72.

17. Soler ZM, Hamilton BE, Schuff KG, Samuels MH, Cohen JI. Utility of computed tomography in the detection of subclinical nodal disease in papillary thyroid carcinoma. Arch Otolaryngol Head Neck Surg. 2008;134:973–8.

18. Choi JS, Kim J, Kwak JY, Kim MJ, Chang HS, Kim EK. Preoperative staging of papillary thyroid carcinoma: comparison of ultrasound imaging and CT. Am J Roentgenol. 2009;193(3):871–8.

19. Karwowski JK, Jeffrey RB, McDougall IR, et al. Intraoperative ultrasonography improves identification of recurrent thyroid cancer. Surgery. 2002;132:924–9.

20. Sippel RS, Elaraj DM, Poder L, et al. Localization of recurrent thyroid cancer using intraoperative ultrasound-guided dye injection. World J Surg. 2009;33:434–9.

21. Perrier ND, Edeiken B, Nunez R, Gayed I, Jimenez C, Busaidy N, Potylchansky E, Kee S, Vu T. A novel nomenclature to classify parathyroid adenomas. World J Surg. 2009;33(3):412–6.

22. Maser C, Donovan P, Santos F, Donabedian R, Rinder C, Scoutt L, Udelsman R. (2006) Sonographically guided fine needle aspiration with rapid parathyroid hormone assay. Ann Surg Oncol 13(12):1690–1695. Epub 2006 Sep 29.

23. Erbil Y, Salmashoglu A, Kabul E, et al. Use of preoperative parathyroid fine-needle aspiration and parathormone assay in the primary hyperparathyroidism with concomitant thyroid nodules. Am J Surg. 2007;193:665–71.

24. Owens CL, Rekhtman N, Sokoll L, Ali SZ. Parathyroid hormone assay in fine-needle aspirate is useful in differentiating inadvertently sample parathyroid tissue from thyroid lesions. Diagn Cytopathol. 2008;36:227–31.

CHAPTER 11
Ultrasound of Salivary Glands and the Non-endocrine Neck

Robert A. Sofferman

The thyroid gland is situated in the lower mid neck but both inflammatory and malignant conditions of this organ system may involve other adjacent and distant cervical regions. In order to understand these relationships, it is instructive to subdivide the neck into sections. In the demonstration and reporting of the position of metastatic lymphadenopathy the neck is classically separated into six zones or levels (Fig. 11.1). Level I is triangular in shape bounded by the anterior and posterior bellies of the digastric muscle and superiorly by the inferior rim of the mandible. Levels II–IV are situated along the internal jugular vein (IJV) with each third designated as a separate zone. Level II begins at the skull base and ends inferiorly at the level of the hyoid bone. Level III is the middle third of the IJV approximately between the hyoid bone and cricoid cartilage. Level IV is the lower third of the IJV between cricoid cartilage and clavicle. Level V is triangular in shape, bordered by the posterior aspect of the sternocleidomastoid muscle, anterior aspect of the trapezius muscle, and the clavicle and is often referred to as the posterior cervical triangle. Lastly Level VI is a midline rectangular region from the hyoid to sternal manubrium and lateral extent to both carotid arteries. There are approximately 200–300 lymph nodes in the neck and facial region [1] and these are distributed among each zone. Head and neck specialists must understand the relationship between lymph nodes and which

H.J. Baskin et al. (eds.), *Thyroid Ultrasound and Ultrasound-Guided FNA*, **219**
DOI 10.1007/978-1-4614-4785-6_11,
© Springer Science+Business Media, LLC 2013

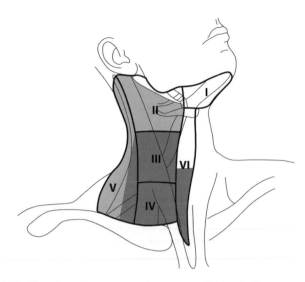

Fig. 11.1. The six neck zones are demonstrated. The *darker areas* are the likely sites for metastatic papillary and medullary carcinoma.

structures or areas they reference. With this knowledge, the primary malignancy or source of inflammatory lymphadenopathy can be localized even before imaging. Metastatic lymphadenopathy to level I arises from primary lesions in the anterior and mid oral cavity, sublingual and submandibular salivary glands, and facial skin. The regional sources for level II adenopathy are posterior oral cavity, i.e., soft palate, tonsil, tongue base, hypopharynx, and parotid. Level III is the regional distribution from the larynx and adjacent mucosal structures and the thyroid gland. Level IV drains lymphatics from the hypopharynx and esophagus as well as thyroid gland. Levels IV and V may be indicators from malignancy of the lower esophagus, upper GI tract and pancreas especially on the left and Pancoast tumors from the lung may present as malignant lymphadenopathy inferiorly in level V. The thyroid gland may involve lymph nodes in levels II to VI. Lastly, inflammatory and malignant lesions of the skin such as melanoma may produce lymph node enlargement in zones adjacent to the respective primary skin site.

LEVEL I

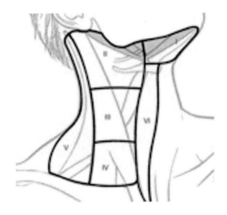

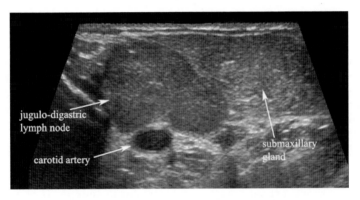

jugulo-digastric
lymph node

submaxillary
gland

carotid artery

Fig. 11.2. This gray scale transverse ultrasound in zone I–IIa demonstrates a hypertrophied jugulodigastric lymph node superficial to the carotid artery.

This level has a close relationship to the oral cavity. As such, lymphatic and vascular conditions of the floor of mouth and submandibular gland demonstrate mass lesions in this area. Although it is rare for thyroid carcinoma to metastasize to level I, in the survey of the neck with ultrasound this region should be examined. Lymph nodes are commonly enlarged in level I, especially the jugulodigastric node which is just craniad and superficial to the carotid bulb (Fig. 11.2). It may be considered in the posterior aspect of zone I or in the craniad portion of level II. Its name derives

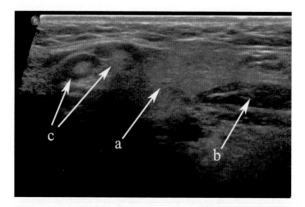

Fig. 11.3. The submandibular gland (**a**), anterior belly of digastric (**b**), and subcapsular lymph nodes (**c**) are demonstrated in this transverse gray scale ultrasound.

from the fact that it is located at the place where the posterior belly of the digastric muscle passes over the IJV. While present in most individuals this commonly hypertrophied lymph node is particularly notable in adolescents and young adults who have experienced recent episodes of tonsillopharyngitis.

Submandibular Gland

The submandibular gland has a homogeneous ground-glass appearance on ultrasound. It is a discrete structure with a deep lobe which extends deep to the mylohyoid muscle. It is the most recognizable structure in level I and often demonstrates adjacent benign hypertrophic lymph nodes (Fig. 11.3). The duct structure is not generally identified unless there is an obstructing calculus.

An obstructing calculus of the main (Wharthin's) duct produces ectasia and an appearance which could suggest a vascular structure (Fig. 11.4). Doppler is a useful tool to determine that the tubular structure is not vascular. One or more stones can be identified by the presence of posterior shadowing artifact along the duct structure.

A mass within the submandibular gland may be benign or malignant. The sonographic features which favor a benign lesion are a discrete homogeneous mass and a surrounding capsule which clearly separates the lesion from surrounding submandibular

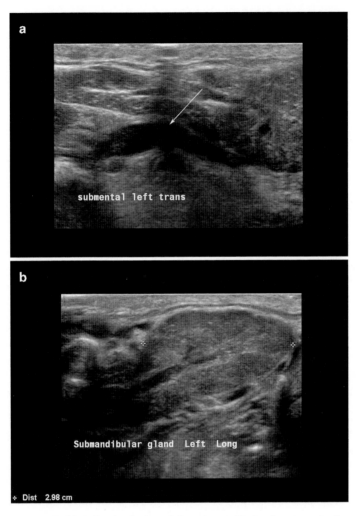

FIG. 11.4. (**a**, **b**) A distal calculus of the submandibular duct into the floor of mouth produces dilation of the entire ductal architecture as designated by the *arrow* (**a**). This ductal ectasia can be identified even within the gland parenchyma (**b**).

parenchyma. The most common benign lesion is a pleomorphic adenoma [2] which demonstrates posterior enhancement, one of the few tumors which demonstrate this characteristic so often seen in cysts (Fig. 11.5).

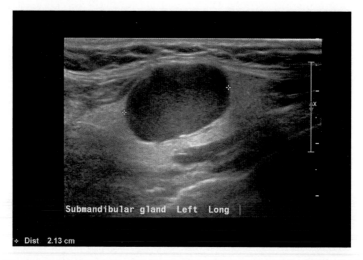

Submandibular gland Left Long

✛ Dist 2.13 cm

FIG. 11.5. A benign mixed tumor (also known as pleomorphic adenoma) of the submandibular gland is demonstrated with gray scale ultrasound.

Ranula

A ranula is a cystic enlargement of a portion of the sublingual gland [3]. It may remain situated in the floor of the mouth or can extend posteriorly deep to the mylohyoid muscle and as such is then designated a "plunging ranula (Fig. 11.6)." It is due to an outflow obstruction of one of the sublingual gland ducts. On aspiration, the fluid is relatively clear and has the consistency of saliva. It usually produces a cystic swelling of the floor of mouth and may elevate the mobile tongue.

Lymphangioma

In contrast to the ranula, a lymphangioma [4] can also produce a cystic mass lesion in level I or floor of mouth. It is primarily cystic but there are septations which indicate a macrocystic lesion. Power Doppler is essential to differentiate the lymphangioma from its mate, a hemangioma (Fig. 11.7). A lymphangioma

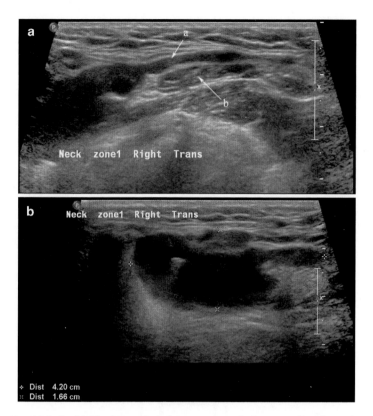

FIG. 11.6. (**a**, **b**) The hypoechoic homogeneous lesion extending from the sublingual region posteriorly (*a*) deep to the mylohyoid muscle (*b*) ends adjacent to the submandibular gland as a dilated cystic structure. The cystic extension adjacent to the submandibular gland is demonstrated in (**b**) and is what designates it as a "plunging ranula".

demonstrates its vasculature within the septae rather than within the lesion's parenchyma. Hemangiomas [5] are also found in the parotid gland and it is the most common parotid mass lesion in children (Fig. 11.8).

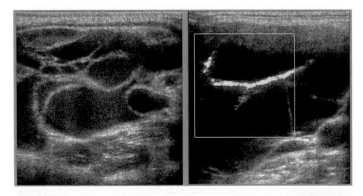

FIG. 11.7. Septations within this lesion are indicative of a vascular lesion. Power Doppler demonstrates that the contributory vessels are only within the septae, indicating that the lesion is relatively avascular and consistent with a lymphangioma.

LEVEL II

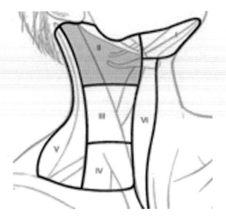

Level II is the most common location for a number of lesions which often cannot be differentiated from one another on physical examination alone. As mentioned previously, the jugulodigastric lymph node is commonly palpated and demonstrated with ultrasound. Usually, sonography demonstrates an appropriate hilum with corresponding hilar vascularity on Doppler both of which suggest likely nodal hypertrophy. When cystic without the usual vascular pattern, a second branchial cleft cyst [6, 7] must be considered in

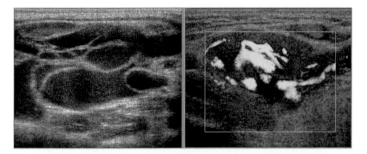

FIG. 11.8. Septations within this lesion suggest a vascular lesion, but the differential between a lymphangioma and hemangioma cannot be made without Doppler. Power Doppler on the *right* proves that this lesion is highly vascular and therefore more consistent with a hemangioma.

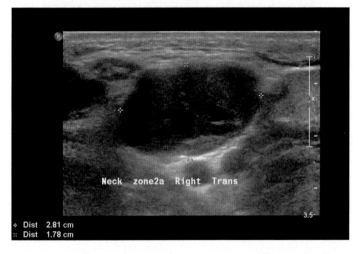

FIG. 11.9. A purely cystic lesion within zone IIa is usually considered a second branchial cleft cyst. This hypoechoic mass proved to be cystic on FNA, but cytology demonstrated metastatic squamous cell carcinoma.

the differential and fine-needle aspiration cytology is required to make differential determinations. However, any cystic node in the head and neck must be suspect for metastatic lymphadenopathy (Fig. 11.9). The most common primary origin of a cystic squamous cell carcinomatous node in level II might be tonsil or tongue base. Although rare, papillary carcinoma of the thyroid gland may present as a cystic mass in the neck and even as a solitary mass in level

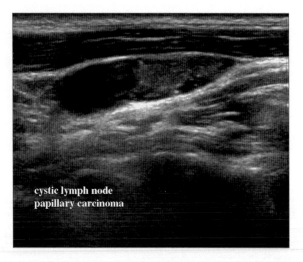

cystic lymph node
papillary carcinoma

FIG. 11.10. Sagittal view of a lymph node in zone IIa demonstrates cystic changes in its superior region and microcalcifications. This node was proven to be replaced by metastatic papillary carcinoma.

II (Figs. 11.10 and 11.11). The key is to both examine the entire thyroid gland with ultrasound and add thyroglobulin to the assay of the cystic fluid. This is especially important when the cyst is in the mid-lower neck.

A solid mass in Level II may displace the carotid artery into an anterior location. In this circumstance, a lesion of neurogenic origin should be suspected [8–10]. The cervical plexus or sympathetic chain may be the source of this type of lesion (Fig. 11.12). If a Horner syndrome is identified, the lesion is most likely to have originated from the sympathetic autonomic system (Figs. 11.13 and 11.14). If the patient has hoarseness and a vocal cord paralysis, the lesion may have originated from the vagus nerve. In circumstances where a mass resides at the carotid bulb and separates the internal and external carotid arteries, a carotid body tumor or chemodectoma would be realistic considerations [11, 12] (Fig. 11.15). In this circumstance, Doppler demonstrates both the intense vascularity of the mass which is not noted in a schwannoma [13] (Fig. 11.16). The vascular supply to the mass is actually from the ascending pharyngeal artery which can be seen in the lateral Doppler image in this sagittal image (Fig. 11.17) Although none of these lesions are malignant and failure to identify and manage them has limited clinical consequences, it is important to understand how to separate them from the more important clinical conditions.

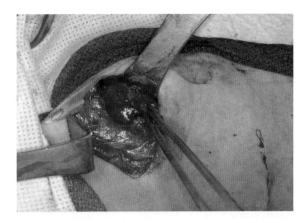

FIG. 11.11. The surgical field during total thyroidectomy and supraomohyoid neck dissection of the zone IIa papillary carcinoma from the previous ultrasound is demonstrated. The only abnormal node identified both grossly and after full pathologic assessment of the specimen was the cystic lymph node in zone IIa.

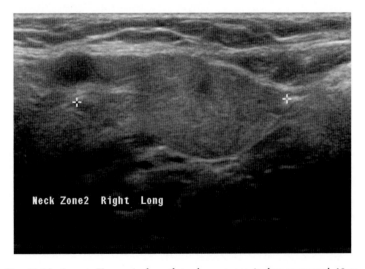

FIG. 11.12. A zone IIa cervical rootlet schwannoma is demonstrated. Note the taper of the mass inferiorly which is typical of a neurogenic lesion.

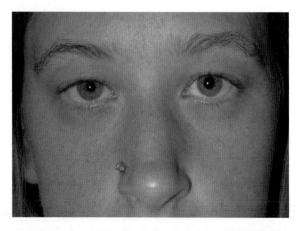

FIG. 11.13. A patient with a sympathetic chain neurofibroma presents with a Horner's syndrome.

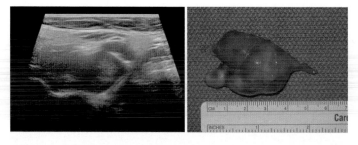

FIG. 11.14. This composite image of a cervical plexus schwannoma demonstrates that the actual gross image of the surgical specimen is identically reflected in the preoperative sagittal ultrasound.

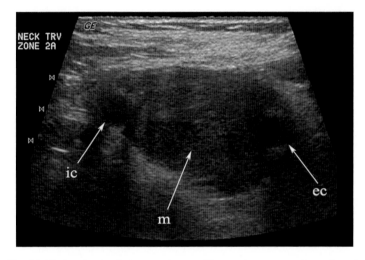

FIG. 11.15. Any hypoechoic mass in zone IIa may be construed as a lymph node or schwannoma. When the mass (*m*) separates the internal (*ic*) and external (*ec*) carotid arteries a chemodectoma or carotid body tumor must be suspected.

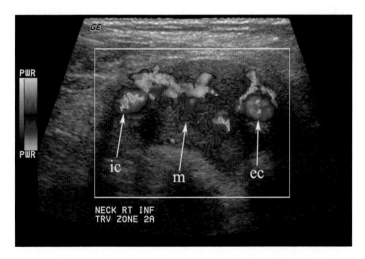

FIG. 11.16. This carotid body tumor located in zone IIa at the carotid bifurcation is clearly defined with color Doppler. The internal (*ic*) and external (*ec*) carotid arteries are splayed apart by the vascular mass (*m*).

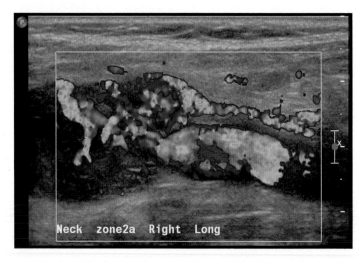

FIG. 11.17. Sagittal color Doppler image of a carotid body tumor demonstrates its vascular supply from a vessel separate from the common carotid artery. This ascending pharyngeal artery is a branch of the external carotid system.

LEVEL III

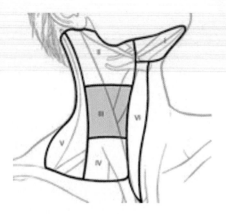

This region along with level IV is most often associated with conditions relative to the thyroid gland. Although extremely rare, lateral aberrant thyroid tissue [14] may be misinterpreted as metastatic lymphadenopathy (Fig. 11.18). These lesions are separate from the main gland and are homogeneous and more rounded in

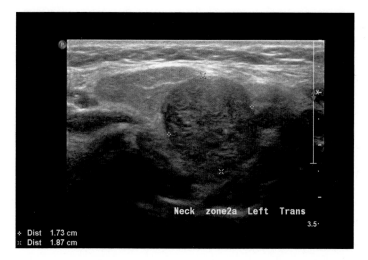

Neck zone2a Left Trans
3.5·

⊹ Dist 1.73 cm
∷ Dist 1.87 cm

Fig. 11.18. A rounded mass in zone IIa is demonstrated in transverse gray scale ultrasound. This proved to be one of two lateral thyroid rests which were completely separate from the thyroid gland. This mass is adjacent to the normal submandibular gland.

structure than a lymph node (Fig. 11.19). However, in the context of a mass lesion adjacent to the thyroid gland which is suspect for metastasis, a thyroglobulin would be recommended in addition to cytology. If the cytology is benign, no mass lesion of the thyroid gland is identified, and the thyroglobulin is positive one still must suspect this is a metastatic node from an occult papillary thyroid carcinoma. A formal excision of the mass will be required and in this rare circumstance would confirm this lesion as benign thyroid tissue (Figs. 11.20 and 11.21).

Patients with recurrent suppurative thyroiditis, especially left-sided, may actually have a congenital fistula which extends from the apex of the pyriform sinus ending in the thyroid parenchyma [15–17] (Fig. 11.22). Episodes may actually begin in children as young as 3 months and present as recurrent retropharyngeal abscess. Neck ultrasound may reveal an inflammatory process overlying the thyroid cartilage in addition to the changes in the adjacent thyroid gland (Fig. 11.23). In some cases, an actual fistulous tract can be identified.

The esophagus is an easily recognizable structure deep to the left lobe of the thyroid gland and adjacent to the trachea. Both the muscular and mucosal layers can be identified in the

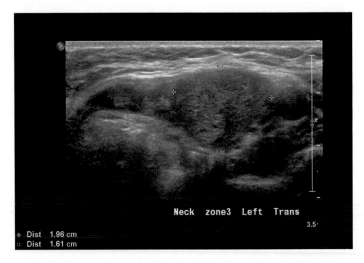

FIG. 11.19. A separate zone III mass is identified and also proven to be a lateral thyroid rest in this same patient.

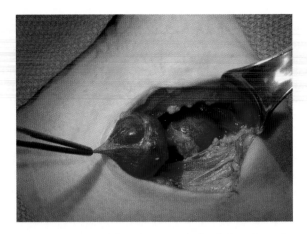

FIG. 11.20. At upper cervical exploration, both of these lateral rests are demonstrated during the process of removal.

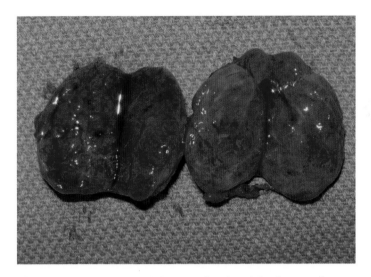

FIG. 11.21. After resection and division of each nodule, the typical cut surface appearance of normal thyroid tissue is demonstrated.

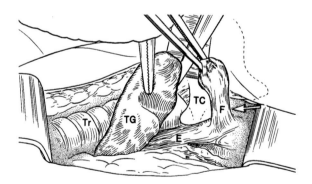

FIG. 11.22. This artistic rendering demonstrates a fistula (*F*) arising from the esophagus (*E*) and positioned just lateral to the thyroid cartilage (TC). The fistula is invariably left-sided and extends to the thyroid gland, frequently into its parenchyma.

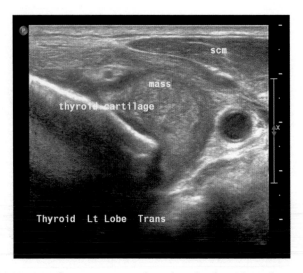

FIG. 11.23. An inflammatory mass lateral to the thyroid cartilage extending into the thyroid gland is secondary to a fistula extending from the esophagus (fourth branchial pouch sinus). Note the small circular structure superficial and to the left of the inflammatory mass; this is the actual fistula.

normal state. A Zenker's diverticulum is a mucosal hernia between the cricopharyngeus and inferior constrictor muscles allowing a pouch to form which traps food and fluid [18–20]. It may be mistaken for a mass lesion and occasionally has been submitted to FNA. The sonographic features are loss of these specific layers, some enlargement of the apparent esophageal structure, and internal, refractile debris (Figs. 11.24 and 11.25). Either on cine loop or sequential post-swallow static images the debris often evacuates to some degree. Of course, the ultrasound is simply a means to suspect this lesion and esophagram is the definitive required imaging study.

Finally, in today's management scheme patients with primary hyperparathyroidism require a nuclear medicine study and ultrasound. Usually enlarged single hypoechoic lesions suggestive of an adenoma or multiple lesions indicating diffuse hyperplasia are self-explanatory. When this is noted in the context of hypercalcemia, there is very little confusion about what the images represent. Occasionally, a level III nodule is identified in patients in whom primary hyperparathyroidism is not suspected (Figs. 11.26 and 11.27). Although the cytology may not define

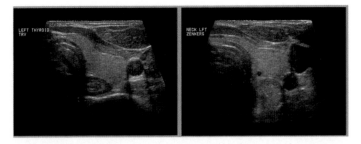

FIG. 11.24. The *left* demonstrates the normal esophagus and the *right* an expanded esophagus consistent with a Zenker's diverticulum.

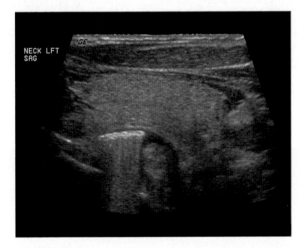

FIG. 11.25. The sagittal view of this Zenker's diverticulum demonstrates food debris which demonstrate refractile sound waves. Note the posterior position of the diverticulum relative to the left lobe of the thyroid gland.

the precise nature of the lesion the differential diagnosis always includes lymphadenopathy. The vascularity of a parathyroid adenoma [21] differs from that of a lymph node (Figs. 11.28 and 11.29) and the absence of lymphocytes on aspiration cytology suggests that the lesion is unusual. Certainly a calcium and intact PTH would give a very accurate direction of analysis. An aspirate for PTH will identify the lesion as ectopic parathyroid.

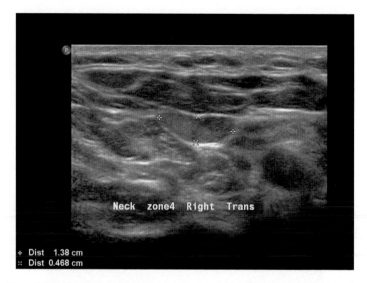

FIG. 11.26. A parathyroid adenoma may occasionally be ectopic within the lateral neck, in this instance level III.

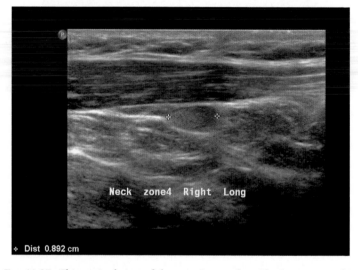

FIG. 11.27. This sagittal view of the ectopic parathyroid adenoma noted in Fig. 11.26 demonstrates its ovoid shape.

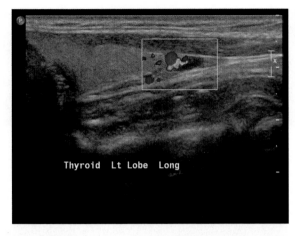

Fig. 11.28. The blood supply to a parathyroid adenoma ends bluntly in the parenchyma without arborization. This small adenoma has the characteristic vascular supply.

LEVEL IV

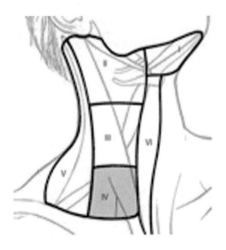

Any mass or cystic structure in level IV is suspect for metastatic thyroid carcinoma. The thoracic duct usually enters the venous system on the left side at the posterior junction of the internal jugular and innominate veins. Due to this special anatomical

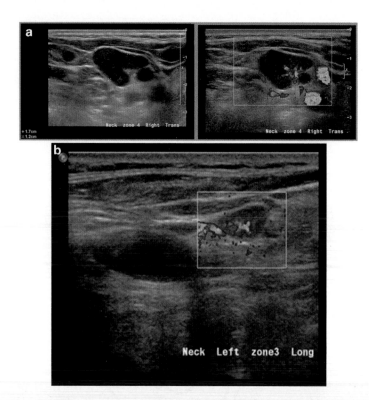

FIG. 11.29. (**a**, **b**) The arborized pattern of vascularity of a hyperplastic lymph node is demonstrated with color Doppler. Note the axial vasculature entering at the nodal hilum which is nicely shown in gray scale on the *left* of (**a**). (**b**) The small vessel pattern in a lymph node which in gray scale alone has the same size and appearance of a possible ectopic parathyroid adenoma.

relationship, metastatic malignancy can be identified in this medial location at the junction of level IV and medial level V. These malignancies are invariably adenocarcinomas whose origin is from the structures below the clavicle. More specifically, the gastrointestinal tract from esophagus to colon may send malignant cells through the thoracic duct to the neck. In addition, other abdominal organs such as the pancreas can produce the same metastatic result. Metastatic squamous cell carcinoma is always suspected when a partially or completely cystic mass is identified in the upper neck

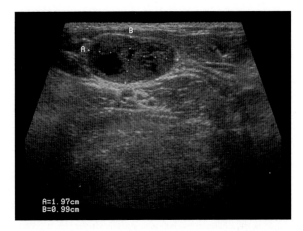

Fɪɢ. 11.30. Anechoic areas within this cervical lymph node are suggestive of necrosis. The FNA cytology confirmed the presence of metastatic squamous cell carcinoma.

[22] (Figs. 11.9 and 11.30). In more than 90% of cases the primary lesion resides as well in the cervical region and the region of location of the metastatic node only suggests the precise location of the primary tumor. It is likely that an ultrasound and FNA for cytology will have already identified the pathology, but the search for the primary will demand endoscopy and other imaging studies which may be an esophagogram, CT, MRI, and PET scan with or without CT linkage.

A cyst pure cyst in level IV without any solid component and abutment with the inferior aspect of the thyroid gland is likely to be of parathyroid origin [23]. Cystic parathyroid adenomas do occur, but these are often intrathyroidal (Fig. 11.31) or may demonstrate a solid component. Pure parathyroid cysts are not associated with hyperparathyroidism (Figs. 11.32, 11.33, and 11.34). The aspirate is crystal clear as water and PTH analysis reveals very high levels in the thousands. In fact, the clear appearance of the fluid and the PTH level is what separates this cyst from a thymic cyst. The histopathology of both cysts may appear to be identical since Hassel's corpuscles can be seen in both.

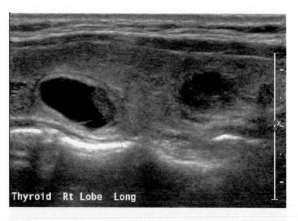

FIG. 11.31. Two hypoechoic masses are noted within the thyroid gland in this patient with primary hyperparathyroidism. The superior lesion (*left*) is a colloid cyst and the inferior lesion (*right*) is the proven intrathyroidal parathyroid adenoma via aspiration for PTH.

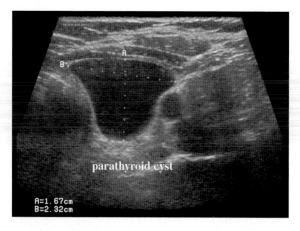

FIG. 11.32. Transverse view of a parathyroid cyst. Note the anechoic internal signal, posterior enhancement, and thin discrete envelope.

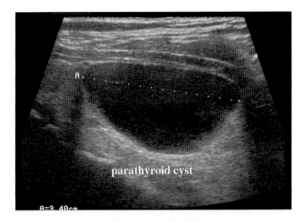

Fig. 11.33. Sagittal view of the same parathyroid cyst.

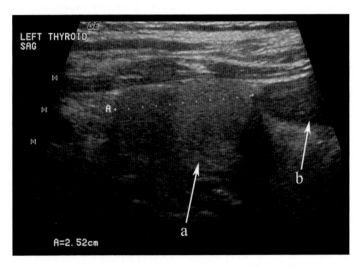

Fig. 11.34. The parathyroid gland (*a*) and parathyroid cyst extending into the anterior mediastinum (*b*) are demonstrated in this sagittal view.

LEVEL V

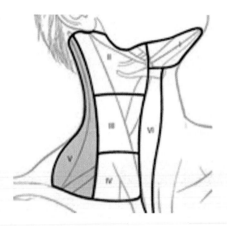

Lymphadenopathy

Lymphomas often present as single or multiple enlarged lymph nodes in level V. Although lymphoma may occur in any of the cervical node basins to include the subcapsular parotid group, they are most often noted in level V as enlarged single or multiple hypoechoic masses [24, 25] (Figs. 11.35 and 11.36). The echoarchitecture is suggestive with an even, homogeneous appearance and loss of the usual hilum. There are no areas of necrosis and the power Doppler pattern may be helpful with peripheral or transnodal vascularity (Fig. 11.37). Of course, multiple and matted adenopathy is a pattern which also frequently defines lymphoma (Fig. 11.38). Although suggestive, these sonographic features are not absolutely diagnostic and demand additional information. When lymphoma is suspected, specimens for cytology are additionally submitted in RPMI solution for flow cytometry.

Inferiorly located nodes in level V with metastatic squamous cell carcinoma are likely to have arisen from a primary of the lung. In addition to an exhaustive search of the head and neck to identify a primary source, A pulmonary CT scan is especially critical when nodes are noted in this area.

Neurofibroma

These may be single or multiple lesions. In patients with von Recklinghausen's disease the diagnosis is relatively straightforward. With ultrasound the mass is noted to be ovoid, homogeneous, and may have a tapered end as noted with a schwannoma.

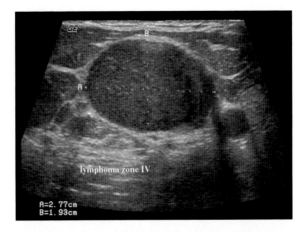

FIG. 11.35. This large lymph node in zone IV fails to demonstrate normal hilar architecture. It is a diffuse non-Hodgkin's lymphoma.

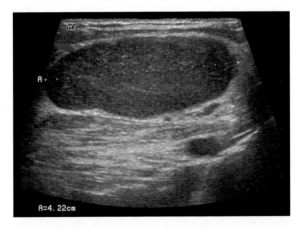

FIG. 11.36. The sagittal view of this same lymphomatous node demonstrates its large size and suspicious homogeneous echoarchitecture.

There is no internal vascularity or hilar architecture. Cytology may be non-diagnostic. One may suspect that this lesion is of neurogenic origin when a painful dysesthesia occurs at the time of needle sampling. Often the clinician assumes that this is an accidental penetration of an adjacent nerve, but if the same painful scenario occurs with a subsequent pass attempts at FNAC should

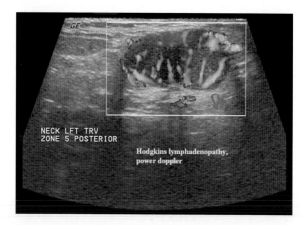

FIG. 11.37. This gray scale Doppler image of a zone V lymph node replaced with Hodgkin's disease demonstrates pathologic transnodal vascularity. This vascular pattern is highly suggestive of malignancy.

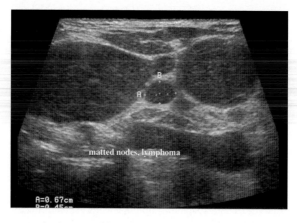

FIG. 11.38. Multiple matted lymph nodes from Hodgkin's disease are demonstrated in this transverse view.

be abandoned in favor of other imaging methods. A traumatic neuroma may resemble a mass lesion (Fig. 11.39). When a linear neural structure enters the mass and FNA is painful, there is little doubt of the diagnosis (Fig. 11.40).

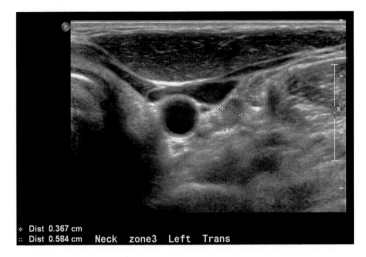

Dist 0.367 cm
Dist 0.584 cm Neck zone3 Left Trans

FIG. 11.39. This patient with prior papillary carcinoma demonstrates a nodule in zone III on transverse ultrasound. This is suspicious for recurrence.

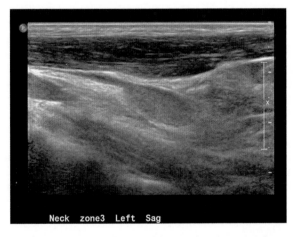

Neck zone3 Left Sag

FIG. 11.40. The sagittal view of the nodule noted in Fig. 11.39 demonstrates a configuration suggesting its association with a nerve. This is the typical appearance of a post operative neuroma and not recurrent carcinoma.

LEVEL VI

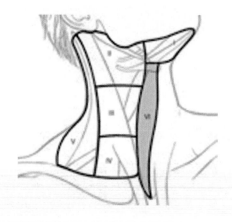

Thyroglossal Duct Cyst

These cysts can occur anywhere from the central suprahyoid region to the thyroid isthmus. Although they share the same sonographic characteristics as cysts elsewhere, there are some special anatomical peculiarities [26]. To begin, the cyst may be multidimensional with an extension posterior to the hyoid bone best seen on the sagittal view (Figs. 11.41 and 11.42) In addition, there may be debris within the cyst which manifests as punctate echogenic lesions throughout the cyst (Fig. 11.43). In the circumstance where a solid component is noted in the cyst, the possibility of a papillary carcinoma must be entertained and appropriate mural samples obtained [27].

Delphian Lymph Node

A midline lymph node in the same distribution as a thyroglossal duct cyst or below even to the cricothyroid membrane may be a marker for a carcinoma within the larynx. Once again, suspicious characteristics of this lesion will require FNA for cytology.

Lingual Thyroid

The key to suspicion of lingual thyroid requires a comprehensive examination of the neck. Lingual thyroid represents an undescended thyroid gland from its origin at the foramen cecum of the midline tongue base. It is an amber submucosal mass and is usually identified through mirror examination of the hypopharynx on routine inspection. However, it may be identified in reverse, i.e., at the time of routine inspection of the neck. If the thyroid gland appears atrophic or absent from its usual orthotopic

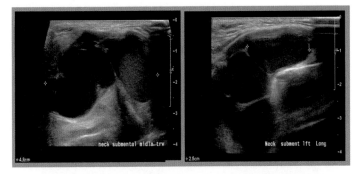

FIG. 11.41. This is a composite transverse and sagittal image of a large thyroglossal duct cyst. Note in the *right* that the superior aspect of the cyst extends deep to the hyoid bone.

FIG. 11.42. This is an intra-operative view of the large thyroglossal duct cyst demonstrated in Fig. 11.41. The *arrow* designates the anterior keel of the thyroid cartilage framework.

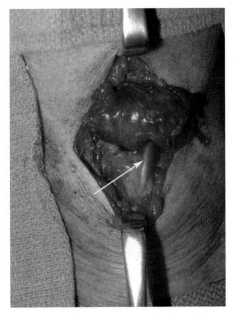

location (Fig. 11.44), then a routine endoscopic and/or nuclear scan will provide the information necessary to establish the diagnosis (Fig. 11.45). Lingual thyroid is not a condition which generally requires any clinical management and is usually simply an embryologic curiosity.

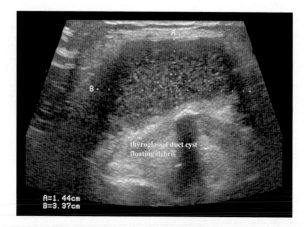

FIG. 11.43. This transverse view of a thyroglossal duct cyst demonstrates the central hyoid bone, a discrete hyperechoic structure with posterior shadowing artifact. Note the multiple punctate hyperlucencies within the cyst which represents debris.

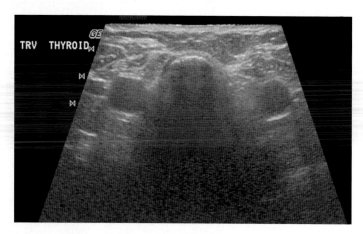

FIG. 11.44. This patient with a tongue base mass demonstrates absence of the normal cervical thyroid gland. Undescended lingual thyroid was diagnosed on initial clinic visit as a result of this ultrasound and demonstration of a typical submucosal tongue base lesion.

Thymus

The thymus gland is usually recognizable in children but generally recedes into adulthood. Its sonographic characteristics are bilateral hypoechoic areas inferior to the lower poles of the thyroid gland with multiple punctate hyperlucencies [28, 29] (Fig. 11.46).

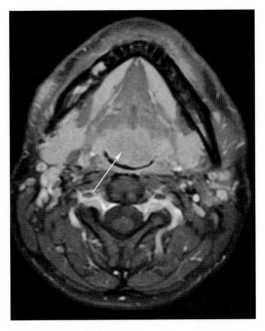

Fig. 11.45. Transverse MRI shows a tongue base mass denoted by the arrow. This is lingual thyroid which has not descended into its normal orthotopic location in the lower neck.

These may be misinterpreted as microcalcifications but are actually Hassel's corpuscles usually found in thymus tissue. The area inferior to the thyroid gland is usually void of this type of lesion and when it is seen by the unwary clinician performing ultrasound the aforementioned characteristics may vaguely simulate papillary carcinoma. The features which suggest benign thymus are its bilateral symmetry and the lack of a confined nodular appearance.

Metastatic Thyroid Carcinoma

Although cervical metastasis from thyroid carcinoma (most often papillary or medullary) is covered elsewhere in this text, it is important to discuss these nodal issues relative to level VI. This is a particularly difficult area to evaluate with ultrasound, but it is important to understand how to optimize this inspection both at the time of initial assessment and during surveillance. The obstacles to proper ultrasound are principally based on anatomy. The clavicle and manubrium are obstacles to ideal positioning

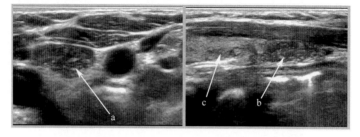

Fig. 11.46. Composite ultrasound image of thymus tissue (*a, b*). The *left* is a transverse image of the left upper mediastinum and the *right* a longitudinal view of the left lobe of thyroid (*c*).

of the transducer and these difficulties can be magnified by body habitus. In very slender patients the depression between the distal sternocleidomastoid muscle and trachea may prevent the transducer from resting evenly on the skin and subcutaneous tissues. Conversely, an obese patient or one with a low-lying larynx may pose a different set of anatomical obstacles. The size of the footprint of the transducer may be a factor, as some narrow probes are easier to manipulate with these anatomical variables in mind. A system which allows manual manipulation to a lower probe frequency may allow better imaging of this deep region. Finally, using a greater depth setting may be assistive in imaging the lower aspect of level VI. Any cystic lesion in the mid or lower neck should be considered to be metastatic papillary thyroid carcinoma until proven otherwise [30] (Fig. 11.47).

Parotid Gland

A portion of the parotid gland may reside in level II and upper level V, but this organ is generally thought of as autonomous along with its subcapsular lymph nodes. Although lesions of the parotid gland would not be related to problems of thyroid origin, it is instructive to give the reader an understanding of what common entities are encountered in an ultrasound survey of the head and neck.

Infection—Acute and chronic parotitis demonstrate many of the same characteristics on ultrasound [31]. Ill-defined areas of hypo or anechoic signal are noted and there may be broad areas of loss of the usual parenchymal architecture (Fig. 11.48). Doppler may show hypervascularity. Hyperplastic lymphadenopathy is usually identified in the upper neck and subcapsular parotid. Confluent anechoic areas would suggest abscess formation.

Cysts—A single parotid cyst may either be due to obstruction of a terminal duct or more commonly a first branchial pouch anomaly.

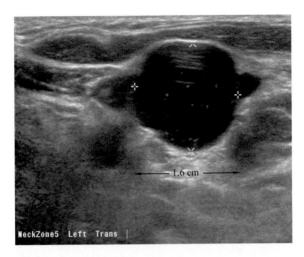

FIG. 11.47. This round, nearly anechoic lymph node in zone V demonstrates posterior enhancement and scattered microcalcifications. It represents metastatic papillary carcinoma.

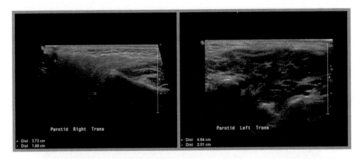

FIG. 11.48. This comparison ultrasound demonstrates the normal parotid parenchyma in the *left* and a heterogeneous pattern in the *right* in a patient with acute parotitis.

These bear the same sonographic characteristics of cysts elsewhere in the neck and body. Multiple cysts are more important to identify and characterize as they are frequently associated with HIV [32]. In fact they are often bilateral and contain debris (Figs. 11.49 and 11.50).

Tumor—The most common tumor of the parotid gland is a pleomorphic adenoma [33, 34] (Fig. 11.51). It has peculiar characteristics which are similar to those of a cyst and may be the only mass lesion which shares the sonographic characteristics of a cystic lesion. The tumor capsule is discrete and the lesion does not extend into the

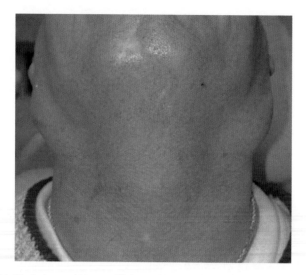

FIG. 11.49. Submental view of bilateral parotid enlargement from a patient with AIDS.

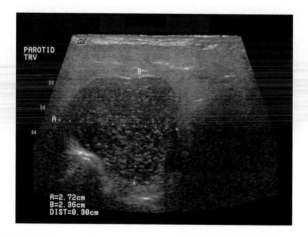

FIG. 11.50. This parotid cyst contains debris which is actually set in motion by the ultrasound waves when visualized in real time. Although a single cyst, it nevertheless is secondary to the patient's HIV status.

surrounding parotid tissues. There are irregular projections from the general perimeter of the mass but these are contained within the same envelope. The most interesting and telling feature is posterior enhancement artifact usually only seen in cysts. This finding is likely

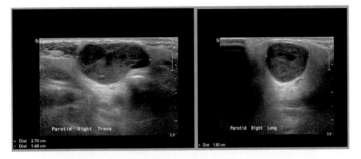

FIG. 11.51. This gray scale ultrasound is typical of a pleomorphic adenoma. The margins are discrete, irregular, and there is posterior enhancement. Posterior enhancement is usually identified in cysts, and this lesion is unique in demonstrating enhancement from a mass.

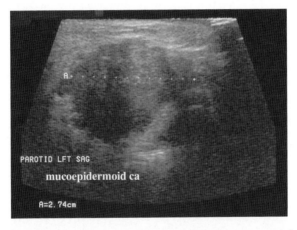

FIG. 11.52. This mass within the parotid gland demonstrates irregularity of its borders which suggests invasion of the surrounding parenchyma. The lesion proved to be a mucoepidermoid carcinoma.

due to the homogeneous nature of the parenchyma. No other parotid tumors demonstrate this finding. Other tumors which are malignant demonstrate irregular margins (Fig. 11.52) and occasionally penetration of their capsule [35]. Often there is no actual separation between the tumor and surrounding parotid tissue. Lesions such as adenoid cystic and mucoepidermoid carcinomas are the most commonly encountered malignancies. In addition to the previously identified malignant features, these tumors often demonstrate adjacent lymphadenopathy.

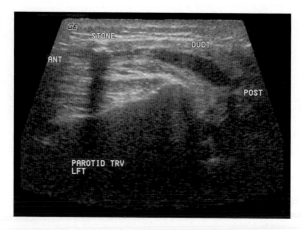

FIG. 11.53. This is a classic image of an obstructing parotid duct calculus. It demonstrates posterior shadowing artifact behind the stone and there is enlargement of the obstructed duct.

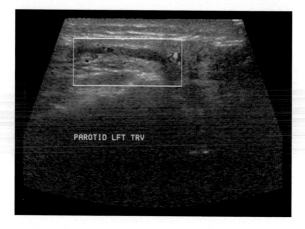

FIG. 11.54. The dilated elongated structure within the parotid gland is proven to be an ectatic duct with color Doppler.

Calculus [36]—The main parotid duct (Stensen's duct) is usually collapsed and does not demonstrate with gray scale ultrasound. Only when the duct is ectatic or enlarged from distal obstruction is it possible to be identified with ultrasound. The duct has the appearance of a tubular structure and without Doppler could be misconstrued as a vessel (Fig. 11.53). The characteristics which identify the actual pathology are as follows: (1) discrete

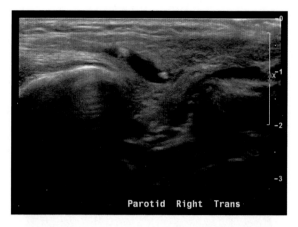

FIG. 11.55. An enlarged obstructed parotid duct demonstrates two internal calculi.

hyperechoic punctate mass in the position of the obstructing lesion (2) tubular anechoic structure at and distal to the calculus (3) absence of vascularity of the duct structure (Fig. 11.54). Occasionally, multiple stones can be noted within the duct (Fig. 11.55). Autoimmune disorder—Sjogren's syndrome is usually noted in patients with recurrent parotid swelling and rheumatoid arthritis [37] (Figs. 11.56 and 11.57). This is condition which affects minor and major salivary glands and produces symptoms of atrophy of the lacrimal glands as well. Thus, these patients experience xerostomia and xerophthalmia (dry mouth and eyes) in addition to the parotid symptoms. The histopathology demonstrates a lymphoproliferative process which is remarkably similar to Hashimoto's thyroiditis. With ultrasound, the homogeneous parenchyma of the parotid gland is replaced with an even small nodular change which has a "Swiss cheese" pattern (Fig. 11.58). This condition is bilateral and usually can be noted by similar ulrasonographic changes in the submandibular glands as well.

MISCELLANEOUS CONDITIONS

Lipoma

This is a mass lesion which on physical examination is often difficult to differentiate from lymphadenopathy or other cervical conditions. These are benign, focal lesions which are located in the subcutaneous domain but can also be seen in other structures

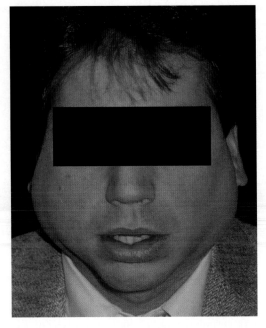

FIG. 11.56. Bilateral parotid swelling is noted in a patient with Sjogren's syndrome.

which contain lipocytes, such as the parotid gland. The mass is ovoid in shape and is traversed with striations along its long axis [38] (Fig. 11.59). It is discrete, avascular with Doppler, and seems separate from its surrounding adipoid tissues.

Vascular Lesions

Lymphangioma and hemangioma have already been discussed as important lesions to identify and differentiate in level I. Other conditions can involve the vascular system in random areas of the neck. For example, it is common for patients who undergo carotid ultrasound to demonstrate unsuspected thyroid lesions and these become a source of referral to endocrinologists and surgeons. Similarly, when performing ultrasound of the thyroid and parathyroid glands it is imperative to survey the neck to identify pathologic lymphadenopathy and any other process which may not be evident with physical examination alone. Atherosclerosis of the carotid artery is often identified as rim or nodular calcification at the carotid bulb (Figs. 11.60 and 11.61). It is not critical to

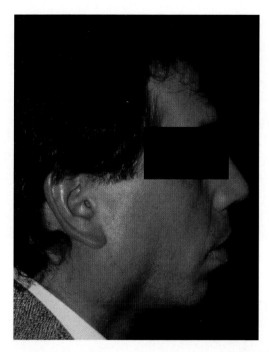

FIG. 11.57. Lateral view of the patient with Sjogren's syndrome. The diffuse swelling demonstrates the full extent of the parotid gland anterior, inferior, and posterior to the auricle.

demonstrate impaired flow distal to the calcification at the bifurcation, as referral for carotid Duplex sonography in an appropriate vascular laboratory will eventually be warranted. Patients who receive or have been administered chemotherapy via a central line may develop IJV thrombosis. This may not have any clinical implications, but some patients may have a progressive thrombophlebitis, neck pain, and serious consequences. The hallmark of identification is the use of Doppler and failure to demonstrate venous flow (Figs. 11.62 and 11.63). Occasionally, patients with invasive thyroid carcinoma may demonstrate thrombosis of the middle thyroid and adjacent jugular veins with Doppler and this important recognition has important implications regarding the extent of surgical planning (Figs. 11.64, 11.65, and 11.66).

In summary, the endocrinologist and clinician who understand thyroid and parathyroid conditions may perform ultrasound with all of its understood advantages for the patient and efficiency of

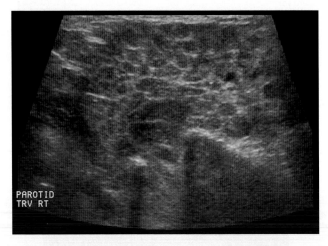

Fɪɢ. 11.58. The normal ground-glass appearance of the parotid gland is replaced by a "Swiss cheese" pattern in the patient with Sjogren's syndrome.

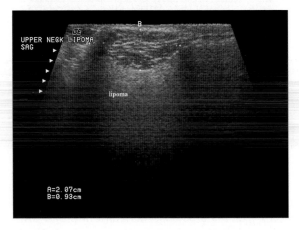

Fɪɢ. 11.59. This discrete, ovoid hypoechoic lesion in the subcutaneous location demonstrates horizontal parallel hyperechoic striations. These findings are typical of a lipoma.

management. Along with this focal interest, it is imperative for these same clinicians to understand how to assess lymph nodes and the ultrasonographic characteristics of metastatic malignancy. This survey process covers the entire neck. Other potential conditions may be identified and this chapter is an effort to cover some

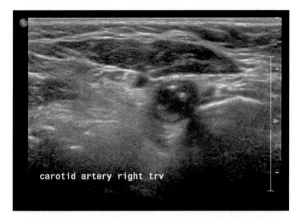

FIG. 11.60. Atherosclerosis of the carotid system is commonly localized to the bulb region (carotid bifurcation). This transverse gray scale ultrasound image demonstrates typical hyperechoic calcifications.

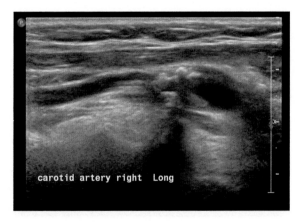

FIG. 11.61. This sagittal ultrasound demonstrates calcifications at the carotid bulb, characteristic of atherosclerosis.

of the more common entities which might be encountered. The reader who performs his or her own ultrasound examination is encouraged to become familiar with normal head and neck anatomy with each examination. Before long, abnormalities will reveal themselves and even if the exact pathology cannot be cataloged

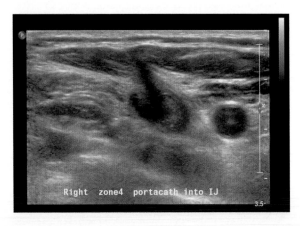

Fig. 11.62. This sagittal gray scale ultrasound demonstrates thrombosis of the internal jugular vein (IJV) in a patient with post central line placement for administration of chemotherapy.

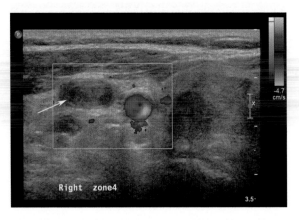

Fig. 11.63. Color Doppler of the thrombosed IJV (designated by the *arrow*) of the patient in Fig. 11.61.

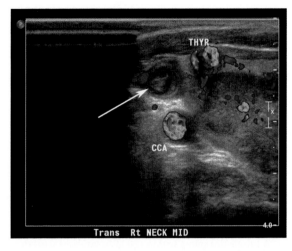

FIG. 11.64. This is a color Doppler image of a thrombosed IJV as designated by the *arrow*. This preoperative ultrasound was performed in a patient with ipsilateral poorly differentiated thyroid carcinoma.

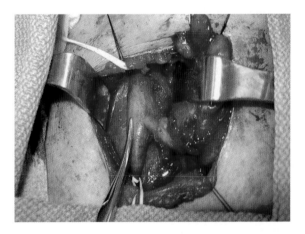

FIG. 11.65. Intraoperative view of the enlarged middle thyroid vein entering the IJV demonstrated with a hemostat in the patient from Fig. 11.63.

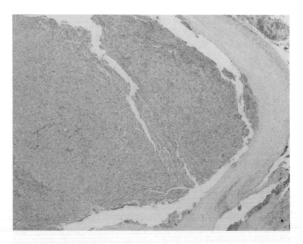

FIG. 11.66. A tumor thrombus within the IJV correlates with the previous ultrasound and intraoperative view.

these changes may be identified as unusual. The decision to invite additional consultation with an appropriate resource may be an additional consideration.

References

1. Ahuja A, Ying M. Sonography of neck lymph nodes: part II. Abnormal lymph nodes. Clin Radiol. 2003;58:359–66.
2. Dumitriu D, Dudea SM, Botor-Jid C, Baciut G. Ultrasonographic and sonoelastographic features of pleomorphic adenomas of the salivary glands. Med Ultrason. 2010;12(3):175–83.
3. Jain P, Jain R, Morton RP, Ahmad Z. Plunging ranulas: high resolution ultrasound for diagnosis and surgical management. Eur Radiol. 2010;20(6):1442–9.
4. Vazquez E, Euriquez G, Castellote A, et al. US, CT, and MR imaging of neck lesions in children. Radiographics. 1995;15:105–22.
5. Milliken JB, Glowacki J. Hemangiomas and vascular malformations in infants and children: a classification based on endothelial characteristics. Plast Reconstr Surg. 1982;69(3):412–22.
6. Benson MT, Dalen K, Mancuso AA, Kerr HH, Caccicarelli AA, Mafee MF. Congenital anomalies of the branchial apparatus: embryology and pathologic anatomy. Radiographics. 1992;12:942–60.
7. Telander R, Filston H. Review of head and neck lesions in infancy and childhood. Surg Clin North Am. 1992;72:1429–47.
8. Haddick WK, Callen PW, Filly RA, Mahoney BS, Edwards MB. Ultrasound evaluation of benign sciatic nerve sheath tumors. J Ultrasound Med. 1984;3:505–7.

9. Fornage BD. Sonography of the peripheral nerves of the extremities. Radiol Med. 1993;5:162–7.
10. Das Gupta TK, et al. Benign solitary schwannomas (neurilemomas). Cancer. 1969;24:355–66.
11. Dickinson PH. Carotid body tumour: 30 years experience. Br J Surg. 1986;73:14–6.
12. Netterville JL, Reely KM, Robertson D, Reiber ME, Armstrong WB, Childs P. Carotid body tumors: a review of 30 patients with 46 tumors. Laryngoscope. 1995;105:115.
13. Arslan H, Unal O, Kutluhan A, Sakarya ME. Power Doppler scanning in the diagnosis of carotid body tumors. J Ultrasound Med. 2000;19(6):367–70.
14. Huang TS, Chen HY. Dual thyroid ectopia with a normally located pretracheal thyroid gland: case report and literature review. Head Neck. 2007;29:885–8.
15. Delozier H, Sofferman RA. Pyriform sinus fistula: an unusual cause of recurrent retropharyngeal abscess and cellulitis. Ann Otol Rhinol Laryngol. 1986;95:377–82.
16. Park NH, Park HJ, Park CS, Kim MS, Park SL. The emerging echogenic tract sign of pyriform sinus fistula: an early indicator in the recovery stage of acute suppurative thyroiditis. AJNR Am J Neuroradiol. 2011;32(3):44–6.
17. Mali VP, Prabhakaran K. Recurrent acute thyroid swellings because of pyriform sinus fistula. J Pediatr Surg. 2008;43(4):27–30.
18. Killian G. La boudre de l'oesophage. Ann Mal Orelle Larynx. 1907;34:1.
19. Westrin KM, Ergun S, Carlsoo B. Zenker's diverticulum—a historical review and trends in therapy. Acta Otolaryngol. 1996;116:351–60.
20. Chang C, Payyapilli R, Scher RL. Endoscopic staple diverticulectomy for Zenker's diverticulum: review of literature and experience in 159 consecutive patients. Laryngoscope. 2003;113:957–65.
21. Mazzeo S, et al. Usefulness of echo color Doppler in differentiating parathyroid lesions from other cervical masses. Eur Radiol. 1997;7(1):90–5.
22. King AD, Tse GM, Ahuja AT, Yuen EH, Vlantis AC, To EW, et al. Necrosis in metastatic neck nodes: diagnostic accuracy of CT, MR imaging, and US. Radiology. 2004;230:720–6.
23. Ihm P, Dray T, Sofferman RA, Nathan M, Hardin NJ. Parathyroid cyst diagnosis and management. Laryngoscope. 2001;111:1576–8.
24. Ahuja A, Ying M, Yang WT, Evans R, King W, Metreweli C. The use of sonography in differentiating cervical lymphomatous lymph nodes from cervical metastatic lymph nodes. Clin Radiol. 1996;51:186–90.
25. Tsang RW, Gospodarowicz MK. Non-Hodgkin's lymphoma. In: Gunderson LL, Tepper JE, editors. Clinical radiation oncology. Philadelphia: Churchill Livingstone; 2000. p. 1158–88.
26. Ahuja AT, King AD, Metreweli C. Thyroglossal duct cysts: sonographic appearance in adults. AJNR Am J Neuroradiol. 1999;20:579–82.
27. VanVuuren PA, Bolin AJ, Gregor RT, et al. Carcinoma arising in thyroglossal remnants. Clin Otolaryngol. 1994;19:509.

28. Fausto CSCV, et al. Thymus: ultrasound characterization. Radiol Bras. 2004;7(3):207–10.

29. Han BK, Suh YL, Yoon HK. Thymic ultrasound II. Pediatr Radiol. 2001;31(7):480–7.

30. Landry CS, Grubbs EG, Busaidy NL, Staerkel GA, Perrier ND, Edeiken-Monroe BS. Cystic lymph nodes in the lateral neck are an indicator of metastatic papillary thyroid cancer. Endocr Pract. 2010;16:1–16.

31. Gritzmann N, et al. Sonography of soft tissue masses in the neck. J Clin Ultrasound. 2002;30:356–73.

32. Shugar J, et al. Multicentric parotid cysts and cervical adenopathy in AIDS patients. A newly recognized entity: CT and MR manifestations. J Laryngol Otolaryngol. 1988;28:272.

33. Webb AJ, Eveson JW. Pleomorphic adenomas of the major salivary glands: a study of the capsular form in relation to surgical management. Clin Otolaryngol Allied Sci. 2001;26:134–42.

34. Stennert E, et al. Histopathology of pleomorphic adenoma in the parotid gland: a prospective unselected series of 100 cases. Laryngoscope. 2001;111:2195–200.

35. Lamont JP, McCarty TM, Fisher TL, et al. Prospective evaluation of office-based parotid ultrasound. Ann Surg Oncol. 2001;8:720.

36. Williams MF. Sialolithiasis. Otolaryngol Clin North Am. 1999;32:819.

37. Mannoussakis M, Mountsopoulos M. Sjogren's syndrome. Otolaryngol Clin North Am. 1999;32:843.

38. Ahuja AT, et al. Head and neck lipomas: sonographic appearance. AJNR Am J Neuroradiol. 1998;19(3):505–8.

CHAPTER 12
Ultrasound-Guided Fine-Needle: Aspiration of Thyroid Nodules

Daniel S. Duick

INTRODUCTION

There are multiple benefits in performing a diagnostic ultrasound examination prior to a thyroid nodule fine-needle aspiration (FNA). These benefits include determining the size and position of a nodule, which allows better selection of needle length and needle size. In patients with a multinodular goiter, ultrasound assures biopsy of the dominant nodule or the nodules most likely to be malignant—those having microcalcifications, increased vascularity, marked hypoechogenicity, blurred irregular borders, or other characteristics associated with malignancy. Finally, ultrasound may redirect the FNA to other areas of suspicion, such as an enlarged, suspicious lymph node or an incidental parathyroid adenoma.

Once a physician acquires the skill to perform thyroid ultrasonography, it is a simple progression to combine the two procedures into an ultrasound-guided FNA (UGFNA). Indeed, this technique is essential to biopsy non-palpable nodules and most nodules less than 1.5 cm in size. UGFNA is also necessary in many obese, muscular, or large frame patients or when a nodule is palpated in the upright position, but cannot be accurately relocated when the patient is supine. UGFNA is indicated for the biopsy of complex or cystic nodules in order to obtain material from the mural or solid component of the nodule and assure adequate cytology. In solid nodules, the best cytology material is usually obtained from the entire nodule. However, many nodules undergo changes

H.J. Baskin et al. (eds.), *Thyroid Ultrasound and Ultrasound-Guided FNA*, **267**
DOI 10.1007/978-1-4614-4785-6_12,
© Springer Science+Business Media, LLC 2013

centrally as they grow and this chapter will describe a number of UGFNA techniques utilized to diagnose problematic nodules. In heterogeneous nodules, the biopsy should be taken from the hypoechoic area of the nodule and any area with any additional suspicious findings (e.g., regions of intranodular Doppler blood flow, microcalcifications, etc.). UGFNA allows for this more precise placement of the needle tip within the nodule.

Multiple investigators have revealed that combining ultrasound and FNA into a single procedure, UGFNA, leads to a three to fivefold increase in satisfactory cellular yields for cytology interpretation compared to conventional FNA [1, 2]. Others have demonstrated an increase in both FNA specificity and sensitivity when UGFNA was performed [3, 4]. UGFNA assures the needle tip is in the nodule (avoiding false negatives) and allows the operator to avoid the trachea and great vessels in the neck. The technique will usually allow the operator to avoid passing the needle through the sternocleidomastoid muscle and thus significantly decreases the discomfort of the procedure. Because UGFNA maximizes the quality and quantity of the cytology, it has become the single best tool with which to evaluate and manage thyroid nodules.

MICRONODULES

The question of whether to biopsy nodules less than 1–1.5 cm (micronodules or "incidentalomas") is controversial. Many argue that nodules of this size seldom present a threat and are so common in the population that routine biopsy of all such nodules is not cost-effective. However, several investigators have shown that the incidence of malignancy in small non-palpable nodules is the same as in palpable nodules [5, 6]. In addition, others have shown that cancers that present less than 1.5 cm in size are often as aggressive as larger cancers [7]. Clearly some judgment is required in deciding which nodules require FNA. The American Association of Endocrinologists (AACE) recommends performing FNA on nodules over 1 cm in size [8]. Smaller nodules in patients who received external radiation to the head or neck during childhood or in patients with a family history of medullary or papillary thyroid cancer also need UGFNA. Patients who have had a hemithyroidectomy for thyroid cancer are candidates for UGFNA if a micronodule should be found in the remaining lobe. Small nodules that appear taller than wide in the transverse view on ultrasound or have an increased intranodular vascular pattern with Doppler interrogation also have a potentially higher risk of malignancy and should have an UGFNA. Other characteristics such as microcalcifications, an irregular/blurred border, or marked hypoechogenicity which is comparable to strap muscles also indicate micronodules that may require UGFNA [9–13]. Most other nodules between 5 and 10 mm in size can safely be observed over a period of time using ultrasound, and FNA can be avoided if there is no significant increase in size [8].

PREPARATION

Prior to consideration of a thyroid nodule aspiration, a history of relative contraindications and rarely absolute contraindication should be obtained. These are the same as with a conventional FNA and include patients who may not be able to lie recumbent due to physical problems; or, who have difficulty in controlling the rate and depth of respiration; and also patients who are uncooperative because of anxiety. Instead of the recumbent position, UGFNA may be able to be performed at 45–60° elevation of the upper body or in a semi-sitting position. Patients with breathing issues or anxiety may often do well with discussion, reassurance, and directions given during the procedure. Younger children may require anesthesia or sedation while adults can be premedicated with an anxiolytic medication in order to obtain a satisfactory biopsy.

An informed written and signed consent should be obtained after a verbal discussion during which all questions have been answered. The consent form should contain in lay language all details and additional information regarding the reason for the procedure, who will be performing the UGFNA, a description of the procedure and risks, as well as patient and witness signatures.

An UGFNA biopsy is defined as utilizing a 25 or 27G needle. Larger needles, cutting needles, coring needles and spring-loaded, needle projecting devices all have an inherently, greater risk for significant bleeding. Also, there is greater risk for puncture site infection and for structural damage to the thyroid, trachea, esophagus, carotid artery, jugular vein, and recurrent laryngeal nerve [8, 9]. Larger needles do not aid in further defining cytologically benign from malignant (indeterminate) follicular nodules. Core needle biopsy can help in obtaining an adequate sample for cytologic interpretation after two or three, repeated FNA "non-diagnostic" aspirates, Thus, the use of an ultrasound-guided, 25 or 27G FNA biopsy of thyroid nodules has become the standard and the preferred technique for reasons of safety, cost, and efficacy [9].

The presence of a severe, uncorrected bleeding, platelet, or coagulopathy disorder rendering the patient incapable of homeostasis is an absolute contraindication for any type of a thyroid needle biopsy. Increased physician concern for performing a UGFNA (e.g., possible relative contraindications) may be due to the patient's use of injectable heparin products; or warfarin with an above therapeutic range INR; or the use of clopidrogrel (Plavix); or dabigatran etexilate mesylate (PRADAXA); *or* large-dose aspirin therapy. The utilization of any of these medications by a patient may be associated with an increased frequency above the normal, low incidence rates for UGFNA of local puncture site bleeding, ecchymoses or hematoma formation. These situations are managed by manual tamponage, followed by a pressure-taped dressing and an ice pack may be utilized as well. If a hematoma occurs, it should be observed by ultrasound to assure stabilization prior to the patient's departure. The individual physician operator's judgment and experience in performing UGFNA in these situations of a potentially increased risk of minor side effects is most important. Full disclosure of risks to the patient is mandatory prior to proceeding with UGFNA. Occasionally for UGFNA, withholding or reducing anticoagulation or other therapy may be appropriate. If there is a decision to defer the procedure, the referring or treating physician should be contacted regarding any concerns or increased risk and plans for problem resolution.

MATERIALS

The ultrasound laboratory should consist of an ultrasound machine with a probe and linear transducer that has a 3.5–5.0 cm footprint and multiple frequency settings ranging between 7.5 and 14 MHz. The machine should also have Doppler imaging capabilities (e.g., color-flow Doppler and power Doppler also). Larger footprint transducers are cumbersome and may impede aspiration capabilities. An additional or utility probe with a similar or lower frequency range is a 2 cm curvilinear or curved linear array transducer (a linear transducer with a convex-curved footprint that produces an image with an increased field of view in a sector format). The smaller curvilinear transducer footprint is useful for imaging and performing an FNA in difficult locations, especially in the lower neck region at the level of the manubrium, clavicles, and insertions of the sternocleidomastoid muscle (Fig. 12.1).

Additional laboratory items should include a mobile ultrasound machine, setup tray/cart, and mobile imaging table or gurney each of which can be easily moved for optimum positioning, visualization, and utilization during an UGFNA or another procedure. The setup tray should include all materials required for

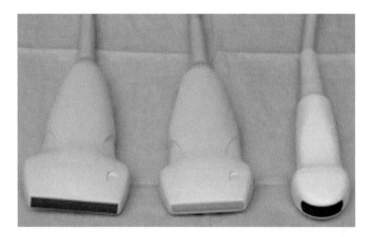

Fɪɢ. 12.1. From *left* to *right* demonstrates different footprint size, linear array transducers with the transducer on the *right* demonstrating a smaller, curvilinear array transducer.

topical cleansing, as well as transducer covers, sterile coupling gel, and an assortment of needles readily assembled and accessible to perform UGFNA. A detachable needle guide adapted for the transducer or transmitted on the monitor screen in a biopsy mode setting on some ultrasound machines may be utilized if desired, but usually is not necessary for routine UGFNA. These devices can be helpful in the FNA of deep or posteriorly located nodules and in performing specialized and prolonged procedures such as drainage of a large cyst followed by percutaneous ethanol injection. Almost any needle will be visible on modern high-resolution ultrasound equipment and this makes use of echogenic needles unnecessary. An assortment of small needles (25–27G) and medium needles (21–23G) and specialty needles (25, 23 or 21G stylet-type needles or spinal needles) of variable lengths and types should be part of the routine setup (Fig. 12.2). The stylet-type needles are used for prolonged fluid aspirations or aspirating structures posterior to the thyroid, which may or may not lie within the thyroid (e.g., exophytic thyroid nodule vs. parathyroid tumor or lymph node). The stylet can be left in while advancing the needle into the lesion of interest and prevents the uploading of thyroid cells into the needle. The stylet also stiffens the needle, making it easier to maneuver prior to withdrawing the stylet when in the nodule and performing an aspirate. Use of commercially available heparinized needles is

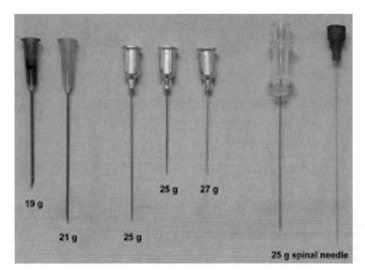

FIG. 12.2. Tray of needles used for ultrasound-guided FNA (UGFNA) (tip viewing of the needle).

not necessary for properly obtained specimens, and heparin may interfere with cytology interpretation.

For aspiration technique, a 10 cc slip-on tip or Luer lock syringe is recommended—preferably with a peripheral or eccentric tip (enhances visibility of the needle hub and bevel).

Pistol grip holders are not recommended since they are cumbersome and often apply excessive negative aspiration pressure, inducing bleeding and poor aspirates. A useful variation of the pistol grip holder is a smaller, spring-loaded aspiration device (e.g., Tao aspirator), which combines both a syringe holder for stabilization and allows for the presetting of the aspiration pressure. This may be especially useful when UGFNA is performed without assistance and when both hands are required for imaging and aspirating. The preset aspiration pressure setting is triggered after needle insertion into the nodule and the other hand continues to hold the transducer and monitor the procedure (Fig. 12.3).

While the use of injectable or topical anesthesia is optional for a 27 or 25G needle procedure, it is the author's practice to routinely use injectable anesthesia. The operator may choose to use one or more of the following for local anesthesia: injectable 1 or 2% lidocaine; or, less commonly, ethyl chloride topical

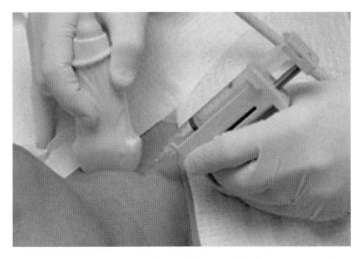

FIG. 12.3. Demonstrates use of a small, spring-loaded aspiration device (Tao) during UGFNA without the use of an assistant for stabilizing the transducer and monitor image during the procedure.

spray or a topical lidocaine gel or patch (applied 1 or 2 h prior to the procedure). Injectable lidocaine should be readily available pending the patient's or physicians preference; or the perceived need of a procedure that is technically difficult (e.g., involve multiple nodules or repetitive aspirations).

TECHNIQUE

The patient should be positioned supine with the neck extended and soft pillow or pad inserted beneath the shoulders to optimize extension of the neck. An additional, small, soft pillow may be placed behind the head for patients who have known neck problems or discomfort with extension of the head and/or rotation of the extended neck. Based on prior knowledge of the planned procedure, the operator should position oneself on either side of the table or at the head of the table for optimal target lesion access during the performance of the aspiration procedure. The monitor should be clearly visible to the operator/physician during the entire procedure. Prior to prepping the neck, an extended field of view should be performed before every needle biopsy. Both lobes of the thyroid, the isthmus, low central region, and the lateral neck should all be observed for any abnormalities or lymphadenopathy not previously detected. Coupling gel is applied to the

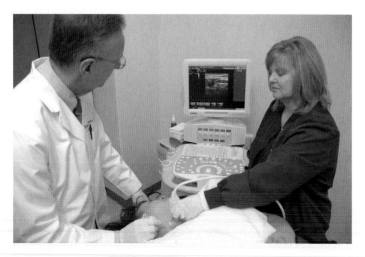

Fig. 12.4. Use of monitor for imaging UGFNA.

transducer face, and the transducer is then enclosed in a sheath or cot to avoid direct contact with any blood products. A low cost alternative transducer cover is Parafilm. The covered transducer is dipped in alcohol, and the neck area is prepped with alcohol swabs. Sterile coupling gel can be applied to the covered transducer face or directly to the prepped neck area (Fig. 12.4).

The key to utilizing ultrasound guidance for performance of the FNA is understanding the orientation of the azimuthal plane, which is the mid-sagittal plane of the transducer face. The transducer sends and receives high frequency ultrasound waves along the azimuthal or mid-sagittal plane of the transducer face. Utilization of the azimuthal plane during UGFNA imaging allows the operator to visualize the needle pathway or approach, adjust the needle insertion angle, and track the entire needle and bevel-up tip by a parallel approach. Alternatively, the needle can be introduced perpendicularly to the sagittal plane, but in this orientation, only the bevel-up tip of the needle will be visible as it crosses the azimuthal plane. Thus, there are basically two approaches for performing the UGFNA based on orientation to the azimuthal plane.

PARALLEL APPROACH

The ultrasound-guided parallel approach tracks the needle from the point of insertion down and along the azimuthal plane to the nodule. The needle is oriented and introduced at either end of the mid portion of the transducer, which is in parallel to the mid-plane of the long axis or sagittal plane. On the monitor screen, the nodule is positioned off-center and closer to the screen's lateral border on the side of planned needle insertion. The needle is best inserted with the bevel tip up towards the transducer since this has angular edges with a flat surface producing greater reflectance and a "brighter" ultrasound image of the tip of the needle. The transducer and needle need to be maintained in the same plane. Upon needle penetration of the skin the needle tip appears at the upper right or upper left corner (depending on orientation of the transducer) of the monitor screen. As the needle is advanced forward and into the nodule, it is carefully guided along and within or adjacent to the azimuthal plane in parallel fashion. This approach allows the operator to observe needle penetration, location, and pathway of the entire needle within the neck, thyroid and nodule, which remain visible on the monitor (Fig. 12.5). If the needle course veers laterally or away from or out of the azimuthal plane even a few degrees, it will be lost from the monitor screen. The parallel technique requires practice and experience to utilize successfully.

PERPENDICULAR APPROACH

In the perpendicular approach, the nodule is imaged and positioned in the mid portion of the screen rather than off center to either lateral side of the monitor. In this way, the point of needle introduction and the nodule beneath for aspiration are both centered in the midpoint of the transducer's side or long axis in order to transversely cross the azimuthal plane at 90° (Fig. 12.6). This again requires experience and skill since the needle itself will not be visualized during the performance of the biopsy. The needle bevel is again introduced with the bevel facing upward toward the transducer to reflect the ultrasound waves and detect its bright image as it crosses the azimuthal plane during needle penetrance of the nodule (Fig. 12.7). Understanding and visualizing the various angles of needle descent is most important and are needed to match the depth of the nodule in the neck when performing UGFNA in the perpendicular approach. The angle of descent dictates whether the needle bevel will be visualized within the nodule (necessary to perform FNA) or above the nodule (descent angle too shallow) or below the nodule (descent angle too steep) as the bevel crosses the narrow beam of the azimuthal plane. Repetitive practice and utilization of both the parallel approach and the perpendicular approach will result in optimizing the orientation and skills of the operator to enhance the performance of UGFNA.

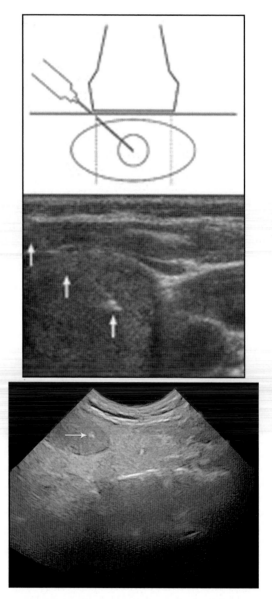

FIG. 12.5. The *upper panel* graphically depicts parallel approach with needle and tip visualization during UGFNA. The two *lower panel* demonstrates ultrasound image of needle and tip (*arrows*) during parallel approach for UGFNA.

FIG. 12.6. Transverse orientation of transducer at 90° to alignment of needle and syringe during perpendicular approach for UGFNA.

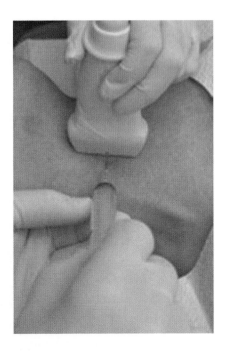

ASPIRATION AND NON-ASPIRATION TECHNIQUES

In general, the use of ultrasound at the time of planned FNA allows the operator to assess for solid, partially cystic, and multicompartmental cystic (complex) nodules. Based on this assessment and the initial pass of an UGFNA, different approaches may be required to obtain adequate sampling and aspirated material for cytologic interpretation. UGFNA can localize tissue areas with vascularity by Doppler interrogation in partially or mostly cystic nodules and enhance acquisition of material for cytology interpretation. There are two basic techniques for needle aspiration of cellular material which are with section or without section.

The closed section, "free hand," technique is performed with a 27 or 25G needle attached to a 10 cc syringe. This needle is introduced into the nodule, under ultrasound guidance, and the plunger is withdrawn for 1–2 cc of negative pressure to induce aspiration. The needle is moved back and forth within diameter of a solid nodule at 3 cycles/s over 3–6 s, the aspiration pressure is released and the needle withdrawn. When liquid or low viscosity diluted material is encountered, this technique may be modified to perform the aspiration in the 2–5 mm subcapsular region (peripherally

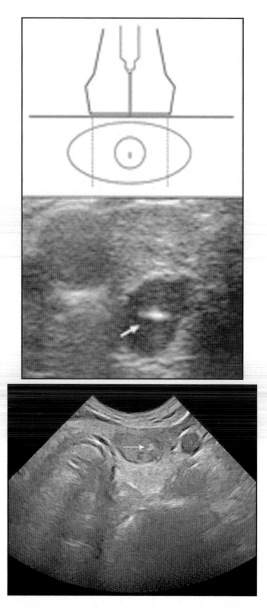

FIG. 12.7. The *upper panel* graphically depicts perpendicular approach with needle tip *only* visualization as it crosses azimuthal plane in a nodule during UGFNA. The two *lower panel* shows ultrasound images of the needle tip *only* as it crosses azimuthal plane (*arrow*) within a nodule during perpendicular approach for UGFNA (*top*, image with a linear transducer; *bottom*, image with a curvilinear transducer).

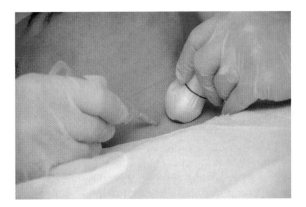

Fɪɢ. 12.8. "Needle only" or Zajdela technique where no aspiration or negative pressure is utilized. Note the stylus of the syringe has been removed from the body of the syringe during the procedure. Also demonstrate is a small footprint, curvilinear transducer.

located tissue is less likely to undergo degenerative changes or dilute the aspirate specimen from complex nodules). The syringe is then detached from the needle, the plunger withdrawn (allowing 2 or 3 cc of air into the syringe), the needle reattached, and the plunger moved slowly forward to extrude aspirated material onto a glass slide for smear and fixation preparation. Many times, however, the nodule is composed of loosely formed microcystic and degenerating tissue and fluid, or the nodule is highly vascularized internally. In these situations a more dilute material rapidly appears in the syringe above the level of the needle hub. If this continues after repeated aspiration attempts with less negative pressure, switching to a non-suction, "needle only" (Zajdela) technique usually improves acquisition of optimum cellular material for slide preparation [11] (Fig. 12.8).

The "needle only" or Zajdela technique utilizes a 27 or 25G needle and the principles of needle bevel nodule penetration and capillary action uploading of cellular material into the needle without aspiration [14]. The needle is grasped at the hub between the thumb and index finger and introduced into the nodule with one to three quick up and down motions over 3–6 s. The index fingertip is then placed over the hub to close the system and the needle is withdrawn, reattached to a syringe with the plunger retracted approximately 2–3 cc, and the material is extruded onto a slide for smear preparation and fixation. Usually two to four separate needle passes are made. A modification of this approach is to remove the plunger from a 10 cc syringe, attach the needle to the syringe (for enhanced control of the needle), and perform an open-system aspirate. The thumb pad is placed over the end of the syringe at the time of needle withdrawal. The needle is detached and reattached to a syringe with a partially withdrawn plunger, and material is extruded onto a slide for smear and fixation. Another modification is to leave the plunger in the syringe and draw up 2–3 cc of air in the syringe prior to aspiration. Cellular material enters the needle via capillary action during the procedure, and the aspirate can then be extruded directly onto a slide.

If the material obtained is frank blood or a watery mixture of interstitial, cystic, and degenerative or bloody fluid, a modification of the "needle only" technique is often helpful. Again, two to four individual needle passes are performed, but an exceedingly rapid, cyclic penetration motion approximating 5–6 cycles/s for a few seconds is utilized rather than a 3 Hz motion. This allows for maximum needle bevel cutting and cellular acquisition with only minimal capillary action time to avoid fluid uploading into the needle.

Air-dried or spray fixation of smears on glass slides are usually preferred for cytologic interpretation. Less commonly, a transport solution containing multiple FNA aspirates for liquid-based cytology (LBC) may be utilized as a primary approach. LBC can also be used as a secondary approach, especially if there is uncertainty of adequacy of material on slides for interpretation and especially if the operator has a high non-diagnostic/insufficient cellularity for interpretation rate. These latter issues can be overcome by utilizing smears and staining one or two slides immediately for assessment of cellular adequacy with a microscope in the laboratory. A written laboratory protocol for the performance of UGFNA and all laboratory associated procedures should be available for reference.

The essence and desired outcome of UGFNA is the acquisition of cellular material and the production of smears on glass slides for fixation and optimal cytologic interpretation. The capability to produce interpretable slides of aspirated material cannot be overemphasized. A high non-diagnostic rate due to inadequate cellularity of smears or the need to solely depend on LBC is usually due to poor training in FNA technique, or smearing techniques, or both. The reader who is poorly trained or repeatedly has non-interpretable slides should either enroll in a slide-making cytology course or attend a training course to learn this and all skills associated with UGFNA.

SUMMARY

There are different methods of performing UGFNA, but there is no single *best method*. The techniques described are those widely utilized; they are not meant to be prescriptive but to provide a starting point for those who desire to start learning this procedure. You will discover many adaptations that can be customized to individual situations. It is important that the physician develop expertise in UGFNA in order to optimize patient care, safety, and outcomes.

References

1. Takashima S, Fukuda H, Kobayashi T. Thyroid nodules: clinical effect of ultrasound-guided fine needle aspiration biopsy. J Clin Ultrasound. 1994;22:536–42.

2. Danese D, Sciacchitano S, Farsetti A, Andreoli M, Pontecorvi A. Diagnostic accuracy of conventional versus sonography-guided fine needle aspiration biopsy of thyroid nodules. Thyroid. 1998;8:15–21.

3. Carmeci C, Jeffery RB, McDougall IR, Noweis KW, Weigel RJ. Ultrasound-guided fine-needle aspiration biopsy of thyroid masses. Thyroid. 1998;8:283–9.

4. Yang GCH, Liebeskind D, Messina AV. Ultrasound-guided fine-needle aspiration of the thyroid assessed by ultrafast papanicolaou stain: data from 1,135 biopsies with a two to six year follow-up. Thyroid. 2001;11:581–9.

5. Hagag P, Strauss S, Weiss M. Role of ultrasound-guided fine-needle aspiration biopsy in evaluation of nonpalpable nodules. Thyroid. 1998;8:989–95.

6. Leenhardt L, Hejblum G, Franc B, Fediaevsky LD, Delbot T, Le Guillozic D, et al. Indications and limits of ultrasound-guided cytology in the management of nonpalpable thyroid nodules. J Clin Endocrinol Metab. 1999;84:24–8.

7. Rosen I, Azadian A, Walfish P, Salem S, Lansdown E, Bedard Y. Ultrasound-guided fine-needle aspiration biopsy in the management of thyroid disease. Am J Surg. 1995;166:346–9.

8. Khoo TK, Baker CH, Hallanger-Johnson J, Tom AM, Grant CS, Reading CC, et al. Comparison of ultrasound-guided fine-needle aspiration biopsy with core-needle biopsy in the evaluation of thyroid nodules. Endocr Pract. 2008;14(4):426–31.

9. Gharib H, Papini E, Paschke R, Duick DS, Valcavi R, Hegedüs L, et al.; AACE/AME/ETA Task Force on Thyroid Nodules. American Association of Clinical Endocrinologists, Associazione Medici Endocrinologi, and European Thyroid Association medical guidelines for clinical practice for the diagnosis and management of thyroid nodules: executive summary of recommendations. Endocr Pract. 2010;16(3):468–75.

10. Papini E, Guglielmi R, Bianchini A, Crescenzi A, Taccogna O, Nardi F, et al. Risk of malignancy in nonpalpable thyroid nodules: predictive value of ultrasound and color-Doppler features. J Clin Endocrinol Metab. 2002;87:1941–6.

11. Baudin E, Travagli JP, Ropers J, et al. Microcarcinoma of the thyroid gland: the Gustave Roussy Institute experience. Cancer. 1998; 83:553–9.
12. Kim E, Park CS, Chung WY, Oh KK, Kim DI, Lee JT, et al. New sonographic criteria for recommending fine-needle aspiration biopsy of nonpalpable solid nodules of the thyroid. AJR Am J Roentgenol. 2002;178:687–91.
13. Marqusee E, Benson CB, Frates MC, et al. Usefulness of ultrasonography in the management of nodular thyroid disease. Ann Intern Med. 2000;133:696–700.
14. Zajdela A, de Maublanc MA, Schlienger P, Haye C. Cytologic diagnosis of orbital and periorbital palpable tumors using fine-needle sampling without aspiration. Diagn Cytopathol. 1986;2:17–20.

CHAPTER 13
Laser and Radiofrequency Ablation Procedures

Roberto Valcavi, Giorgio Stecconi Bortolani,
and Fabrizio Riganti

INTRODUCTION

Percutaneous Laser Ablation (LA) and radiofrequency (RF) are minimally invasive techniques to destroy thyroid nodules and tumors using hyperthermia without surgical removal. The thermal damage caused by heating depends both on the tissue temperature reached and on the duration of heating. For example, heating tissue at 50–55 °C for 4–6 min produces irreversible cellular damage, at temperatures between 60 and 100 °C, near-immediate coagulation of tissue is induced, with irreversible damage to mitochondrial and cytolysic enzymes of the cells, and at over 100–110 °C, tissue vaporizes and carbonizes [1, 2].

The potential advantages of in situ tumor ablation include decreased costs, reduced morbidity, the possibility of performing procedures on outpatients, and the possibility of treating patients who are poor candidates for surgery due to age, comorbidity, or extent of disease. Ablation procedures are performed in the thyroid gland under Ultrasound (US) real time imaging.

LASER ABLATION

LASER is the acronym for Light Amplified Stimulated Emission of Radiation. Laser energy generator is shown in Fig. 13.1. Light energy is applied via optical fibers directly inserted into the tissue [3–7]. Laser technology directs high-level energy to a well-delimited area of tissue in a predictable, precise, and controlled way (Fig. 13.2). A number of laser sources and wavelengths are currently

H.J. Baskin et al. (eds.), *Thyroid Ultrasound and Ultrasound-Guided FNA*, **283**
DOI 10.1007/978-1-4614-4785-6_13,
© Springer Science+Business Media, LLC 2013

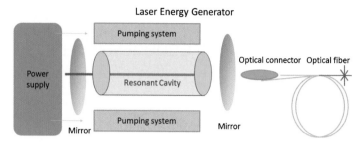

Fig. 13.1. Laser energy generator. The *pumping system* stimulates emission of photons by a *gain medium*. Photons are reflected between two *mirrors* stimulating the emission of other photons as a chain reaction. Laser light escapes from *resonant cavity* through one of the mirrors, which is partially transparent. An *optical connector* conveys *laser beam* into an *optic fiber*.

available and different types of laser fibers, modified tips, and applicators can be used. For example, neodymium:yttrium aluminum garnet (Nd:YAG) or diode (solid state) lasers with a wavelength of 820–1,064 nm are used for percutaneous LA because penetration of light is optimal in the near-infrared spectrum. High power destroys tissue by means of vaporization, charring around the fiber tip surrounded by a coagulation zone, as seen on ultrasound images (Fig. 13.3). Heat deposition is greatest near the thermal source, with a rapid energy decay [8, 9]. Cell death may continue up to 72 h after the procedure due to coagulation of micro vessels and ischemic injury [10]. Microscopically, the coagulation zone is surrounded by a rim of reversible damage that separates necrotic from viable tissue [9, 11]. Figure 13.4 shows gross histology with charring and coagulation zone in a laser nodule resected 1 month after LA. Shrinkage of the nodule will occur because of slow reabsorption of the coagulation zone, eventually resulting in a fibrotic tissue area. We have described microscopic findings after percutaneous LA in benign thyroid nodules [12]. Figures 13.5 and 13.6 exemplify a laser-ablated area, which consisted of a well-defined zone, surrounded by a fibrous capsule filled in by amorphous material. No significant pathologic features were found in the thyroid tissue adjacent to the treated area. Fibrotic changes are seen as hard pattern at elastography (Fig. 13.7).

Charring is the main cause of decreased energy transmission, which in turn limits the coagulation zone. In addition, coagulation necrosis itself reduces optical penetration by about 20% in both normal and tumor tissue [6, 13]. Using a bare tip, almost spherical lesions with a maximum diameter of 12–16 mm can be produced.

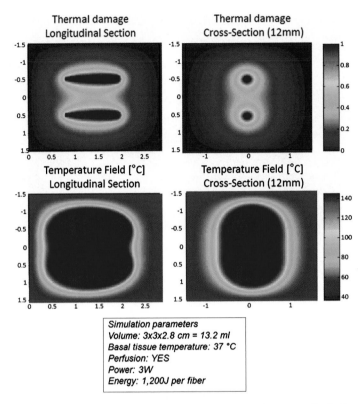

Fig. 13.2. Mathematical model for thermal damage prediction. Multiple-fiber approach: two optical fibers inserted into tissue at 10 mm of distance. Evaluation of thermal damage in terms of percentage of death cells according to Arrhenius model.

Lesion size can be increased by simultaneous use of multiple fibers in an array around the tumor [5], rather than repositioning a single fiber as proposed by some authors.

Laser Ablation in the Thyroid Gland

Outpatient US-guided (US-g) interventional procedures have been proposed to treat benign solid thyroid nodules without open surgery. This new approach is possible thanks to the combined use of ultrasonography (US) and fine-needle aspiration biopsy (FNA), which greatly reduces the need for diagnostic thyroidectomy [14]. The 2009 American Thyroid Association (ATA) management guidelines for patients with thyroid nodules and differentiated thyroid

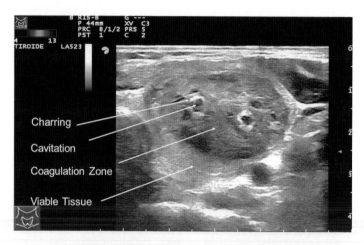

Fig. 13.3. Ultrasound image of a 2-fiber left lobe thyroid nodule laser ablation in a transverse scan. Laser marks are seen as anechoic spots (*cavitation*) surrounded by hyperechoic rims (*charring*) due to tissue vaporization. The *coagulation zone* is hypoechoic parenchyma, clearly cleaved from residual *viable tissue*.

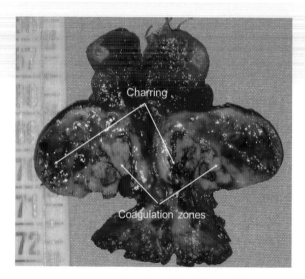

Fig. 13.4. Macroscopic aspect of a benign nodule resected 1 month after LA treatment. *Arrows* show *charring* and *coagulation zones*.

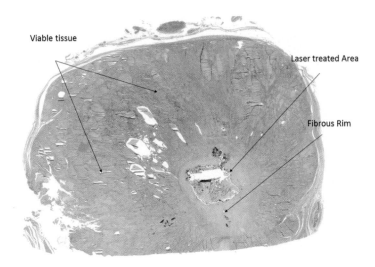

Fig. 13.5. Microscopic changes (×5) occurring in a benign thyroid nodule resected after laser ablation. *Arrows* mark *laser treated area* surrounded by a *fibrous rim*, within hyperplastic thyroid nodular *viable tissue*.

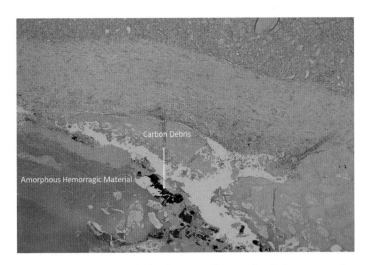

Fig. 13.6. Nodule section at a further magnification (×20) shows *amorphous hemorragic material* with *carbon debris* (*arrows*) due to laser ablation.

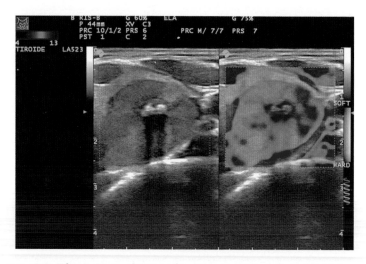

Fɪɢ. 13.7. Fibrotic tissue changes after LA are seen as an hyperechoic zone with posterior shadowing, using standard B-mode imaging (*left*). These changes appear as a *blue colored* hard area using elastography (*right*).

cancer suggest either no treatment or partial/total thyroid surgery for patients with benign solid thyroid nodular disease, depending on nodule size, growth, and symptoms [15], and the 2010 American Association of Clinical Endocrinologists—Associazione Medici Endocrinologi (Italian Association of Clinical Endocrinologists)—European Thyroid Association (AACE-AME-ETA) thyroid nodule guidelines have for the first time introduced US-g interventional approaches as a possible choice for thyroid nodule clinical management [16]. The basic principle of loco-regional treatment is to induce shrinkage of solid thyroid nodules using physical means for tissue destruction. While US-g Percutaneous Ethanol Injection (PEI) is the treatment of choice for cystic nodules, it is no longer recommended for solid nodules [15–17], and HI-FU, successfully experimented in ewes [18, 19], has been used to treat autonomous thyroid nodule in humans in only one case [20]. PLA, the first thermal ablation technique, was introduced by Pacella et al. [21]. Since then several studies have been published on its effects on thyroid cold [22–25], cystic [26], and hot nodules [23, 26–32], including controlled trials [33–36], demonstrating that this new technique is effective and safe (Table 13.1). Indeed, we have been using PLA in patients with benign thyroid cold nodules in Reggio Emilia, Italy since 2002.

Table 13.1 Published papers on the effects of laser ablation procedure on benign thyroid nodules

References	Patients numbers	Nodule type	Initial volume mL: mean±SD	Post-procedure volume mL: mean±SD	Volume reduction (%)	Follow-up (months)
Pacella et al. [21]	2					Feasibility study
Døssing et al. [39]	16	Cold	10±7.9	5.4±5.1	46	6
Spiezia et al. [28]	5	Cold	11.1±4.9	3.7±1.5	74	12
	6	AFTN	3.2±1.3	0.8±0.5	61	12
Døssing et al. [40]	1	AFTN	8.2	4.9	40	9
Pacella et al. [23]	8	Cold	22.7±21.2	10.8±9.2	63	6
	16	AFTN	7.9±6.3	4.1±3.3	62	6
Papini et al. [24]	20	Cold	24.1±15.0	9.6±6.6	64	6
Døssing et al. [33]	15	Cold	8.1±6.1	4.8±3.0	44	6
Amabile et al. [29]	23	Cold	15.0±6.8	9.5±4.2	39/31	3
Cakir et al. [30]	12	Cold	11.9±8.8	2.2±2.3	82	12
Gambelunghe et al. [36]	26	Cold	8.2	4.16	44	7
Døssing et al. [35]	14	AFTN	10.6±2.5	4.6±0.6	44	6
Papini et al. [34]	21	Cold	11.7±5.1	6.6±2.7	43	12
Valcavi et al. [25]	119	Cold	24.8±21.1	12.1±14.9	55	12
Valcavi et al. [37]	122	Cold	23.1±21.3	12.5±18.8	48	36
Rotondi et al. [32]	1	AFTN	55.0	5.0	91	10
Døssing et al. [41]	78	Cold	8.2	4.1	51	38
Amabile et al. [42]	51	Cold	53.5±10.4	//	81	36
(three LA cycles)	26	AFTN	55.3±10.8	//	82	36

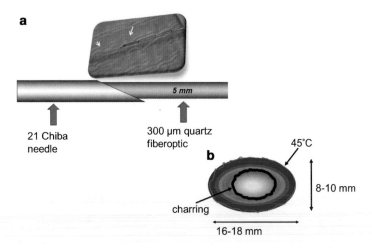

FIG. 13.8. Percutaneous LA flat tip technique. (**a**) A 300 μm plane-cut optic fiber is inserted through the sheath of a 21G Chiba needle, exposing the bare fiber in direct contact with thyroid tissue for a length of 5 mm. (**b**) A single optic fiber, maintained in a still position, destroys only a small amount of tissue (16–18 mm in length, 8–10 mm in width, 8–10 mm in thickness, i.e., about 1 mL volume) when an energy of 1,600–1,800 J with an output power of 2–4 W is delivered.

Technique

LA is an outpatient procedure carried out on fasting subjects. The flat tip technique, proposed and developed by Pacella et al. [21], is based on the insertion of a 300 μm plane-cut optic fiber through the sheath of a 21G Chiba needle, exposing the bare fiber in direct contact with thyroid tissue for a length of 5 mm (Fig. 13.8). In the thyroid gland, multiple fibers are inserted cranio-caudally one at a side of the other at 10 mm distance, in order to obtain an ellipsoid ablation that matches the ellipsoid shape of most thyroid nodules (Fig. 13.9) [25]. At variance with the square multiple fiber technique used for the liver, in the thyroid gland optimal geometrical configuration may be achieved inserting simultaneously the fibers in a triangle or in a line array depending on the nodule shape and size. With four fibers inserted simultaneously, combined with pull-backs, volume ablations up to 30 mL may be attained in a single session (Fig. 13.10).

Procedure

The goal of our procedure is to achieve the maximum ablation volume in a single LA outpatient session. The patient is placed on

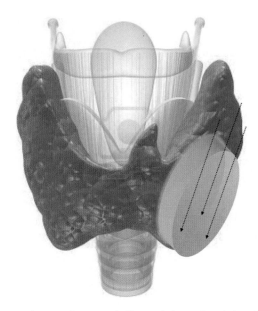

FIG. 13.9. Rendering of a typical ellipsoid thyroid nodule. The greater, intermediate, and smaller diameters are length, width, and thickness, respectively. Multiple fiber ellipsoid configuration is aimed to match this shape. *Arrows* represent three needles inserted in a cranio-caudal direction. Laser firing is started from the bottom part of the nodule, then needles and fibers are pulled back step by step, in accordance to the extent of the lesion.

an operating table in the supine position with hyperextended neck. The operator, seated behind patient's head, watches real time US images on an auxiliary monitor placed on a tower at the patient's feet. US equipment is used by an assistant sitting to the right of the patient. A nurse helps in maneuvers. Procedure is carried out in the dark; a scialytic lamp is used only for needle placement (Fig. 13.11). Real time imaging is the key support and it is used throughout all procedure steps. In Reggio Emilia, Italy in the years 2002–2008 we used an Nd:YAG laser with 1,064 nm near-infrared wavelength emission, equipped with a 4-source beam splitter (DEKA M.E.L.A., Florence, Italy). In 2009, we substituted this with new equipment composed of an ultrasound device and a laser unit (EcholaserX4®, Elesta, Florence, Italy). The EcholaserX4® permits the operator to use up to four laser sources, each with its own

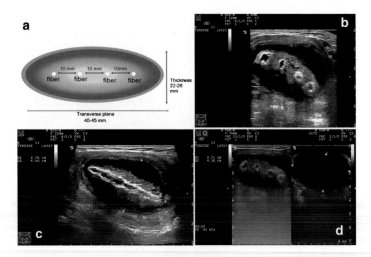

Fig. 13.10. Four-fiber in-line configuration for a large ellipsoid nodule ablation. (**a**) Cartoon of a transverse scan, showing needles inserted one at a side of the other at a distance of 10 mm in order to match ellipsoid nodule shape. With up to four parallel fibers, a coagulation zone up to 40–45 mm wide and 22–26 mm thick may be obtained. (**b**) Ultrasound transverse scan of a left lobe thyroid nodule ablated with four parallel optic fibers. The four laser marks are clearly visible as well the ablation zone. (**c**) Ultrasound longitudinal scan of the same lobe showing laser mark and the hypoechoic ablation zone. (**d**) The ablation area (volume 27.3 mL) is shown by contrast enhancement ultrasound (CEUS). This is extended to almost whole nodule.

energy emission setting and independent activation. This helps matching the ablation zone to nodule size and shape (Fig. 13.12). Contrast enhancement ultrasound (CEUS) study is performed before and after LA in order to estimate ablation volume. Contrast media (Sonovue®, sulfur exafluoride microbubbles) is rapidly injected i.v. (Fig. 13.13). CEUS side effects are very rare; however, contrast media is contraindicated in acute heart ischemia. Light conscious sedation is obtained with i.v. midazolam (2–5 mg) in fractionated boli. Emergency care drugs and equipment, including a defibrillator, are in the interventional suite. Although an anesthesiologist is not present during LA sessions, we recommend performing LA in a healthcare facility where an anesthesiologist and ENT surgery are available. Local anesthesia with 2% ropivacaine HCl subcutaneous and subcapsular infiltration (2–5 mL) is performed under US assistance with a thin (G27)

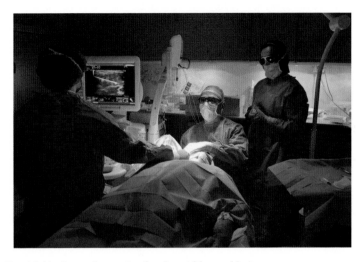

FIG. 13.11. Operative setting for thyroid laser ablation.

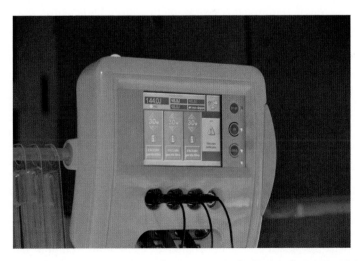

FIG. 13.12. The touch screen of the EcholaserX4® (Elesta, Florence, Italy) display permits the operator to use up to four sources each with its own activation and energy emission setting.

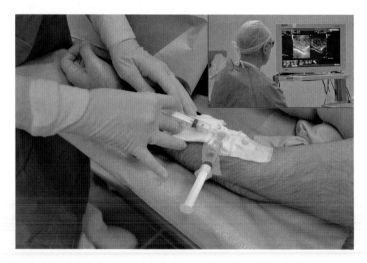

FIG. 13.13. CEUS. Contrast media is rapidly injected through a three-way tap connected to an intravenous catheter. The vein catheter is maintained throughout the procedure and for a couple of hours until patient's discharge.

needle (Fig. 13.14). Chiba 21G needles (1–4) are placed manually along the longitudinal, cranio-caudal, major nodule axis at a distance of 10 mm, matching the anatomy of nodules as closely as possible (Fig. 13.15). Fibers are inserted and laser is immediately turned on. An initial energy of 1,200–1,800 J/fiber with a mean output power of 3 W (range 2–4 W) is delivered starting 10 mm from the bottom of the lesion. A highly echogenic area due to tissue heating and vaporization gradually increases over time until coalescence between fibers is observed (Fig. 13.16). Multiplanar US images on axial and longitudinal scans are performed by the assistant/sonographer throughout laser illumination, allowing real time visual control of each source. By upwards needle/fiber pullbacks of 10 mm, additional doses of laser energy are administered at each step until a distance of 5 mm from the cranial portion of the nodule is reached (Fig. 13.17). While nodules as small as 5 mm may be ablated using a single optic fiber, nodules up to 40–50 mm in width, 30–35 mm in thickness, and 50–70 mm in length (i.e., up to 30–60 mL) may be treated by combining multiple fiber placement, needle/fiber pullback, and high energies. The number of fibers, number of pullbacks, and total energy delivered are tailored to nodule volume. The duration of laser illuminations ranges

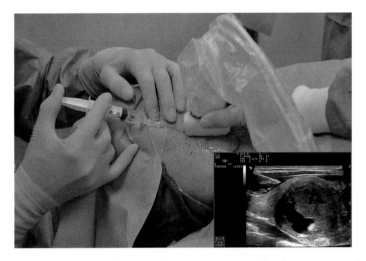

FIG. 13.14. Local anesthesia with 2% ropivacaine HCl subcutaneous and subcapsular infiltration (2–5 mL). External maneuver and US image (*bottom*) showing thyroid subcapsular infiltration.

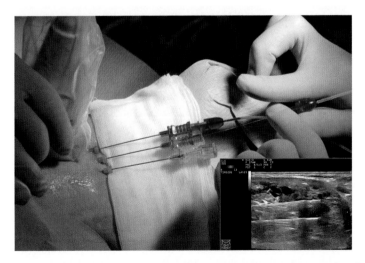

FIG. 13.15. LA procedure with three fibers. Chiba 21G needles are placed manually along the longitudinal, cranio-caudal, major nodule axis, at a distance of 10 mm. Then optic fibers are inserted through the sheath of needles. Real time US images permit to check precise needle/fiber placement (*bottom*).

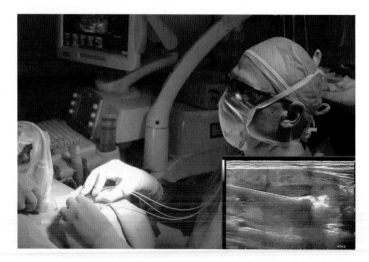

FIG. 13.16. Laser firing. The *bottom* shows longitudinal US images of a needle typically placed within the thyroid nodule. *Left side* of US image is cranial. The needle is parallel to the longitudinal nodule axis. A highly echogenic area due to tissue heating and vaporization is observed during laser firing.

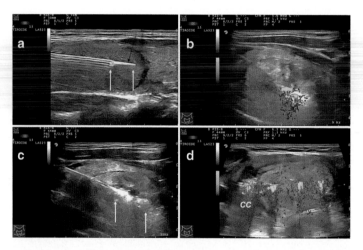

FIG. 13.17. Multiplanar ultrasound imaging of an LA procedure with three fibers in a thyroid nodule. (**a**) Fiber exposed out of the tip of the needle (*arrows*). (**b**) Laser firing, Color-Doppler imaging, longitudinal scan. (**c**) Laser firing, B-mode, longitudinal scan, first pull-back. *Arrows* indicate the pull-back area. (**d**) Laser firing: transverse scan: Color-Doppler images during laser illumination showing the three needles at the same time. *CC* common carotid artery.

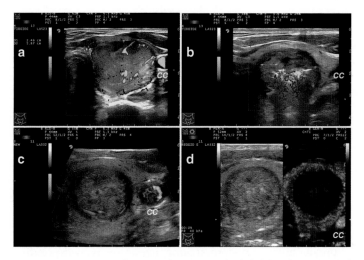

FIG. 13.18. US images of a typical LA case of a left lobe thyroid nodule. Transverse scans. *CC* common carotid artery. (**a**) Nodule Color-Doppler scan before LA. (**b**) Nodule Color-Doppler scan during LA procedure, showing fiber firing. (**c**) Nodule Color-Doppler changes immediately after LA procedure. The nodule is hypoechoic, without internal vascularization. (**d**) CEUS demonstrates complete ablation of the nodule.

from 6 to 30 min, depending on nodule size. Light irradiation is continuous; it is shortly suspended for fiber repositioning only in the event of pain, cough, or other side effects. Figure 13.18 shows US images of a typical LA case before, during, and after LA. CEUS demonstrates complete ablation of the nodule.

PLA Post-procedure Care
Immediately after PLA procedure, all patients receive prednisone 20 mg i.v. bolus. An ice pack with mild pressure is applied on the neck. Patients are then taken to the recovery room, where they receive ketoprofene 100 mg or paracetamol 1 g infusion for 30 min and are kept under observation for about 2 h. Before leaving hospital, all patients undergo US examination. The day after PLA procedure, patients are started on a tapering oral prednisone therapy of 25 mg for 3 days, 12.5 mg for 3 days, and 5 mg for 4 days. Oral pump inhibitors are simultaneously administered (lansoprazole 30 mg) for the 10 days of oral prednisone therapy.

Side Effects

Few complications and side effects have been reported in the published data [22–30, 32–37]. In our own large clinical experience no patient has ever required emergency care or emergency surgery. Intra-operatory pain is usually absent or minimal. Should it occur, laser should be turned off and fibers repositioned in a more central area of the nodule. Post-operatory pain may occur in 8–40% of patients, requiring additional medication [22–25, 33–35, 37]. Intranodular bleeding during needle placement is controlled by rapid fiber insertion and laser illumination and should not prevent regular ablation procedure from being completed. In our hands, infrequent (less than 2.5%) complications were thyroid pericapsular bleeding; vagal symptoms with bradycardia; cough; reversible voice change (complete recovery in 1–2 months after an additional corticosteroid course); tumor rupture with subfascial effusion, disappeared in 3–4 months, with no permanent consequences; cutaneous burn; transient stridor; hyper- or hypo-thyroidism. It should be noted that the list of side effects refers to the series of patients treated with the Nd:YAG laser, including patients at the beginning of the learning curve [37]. With the updated procedure and the introduction of the EcholaserX4®, side effects have been even milder (personal data).

A single case of tracheal laceration 50 days after LA has been reported in the literature. The patient underwent total thyroidectomy and tracheal repair [38].

Clinical Results in Benign Cold Nodules

Nodule shrinkage in the available literature ranges from 36 to 82% of initial volume [20, 23–25, 28–30, 32–37, 39–42]. In our center, we reported safety and effects of Nd:YAG LA treatment in patients with benign nonfunctioning thyroid nodules in a 3-year follow-up [37]. We have now preliminary data on 5-year follow-up in 65 patients (42 females, 23 males, age 52.2 ± 12.3 years). Energy delivered was (mean $\pm$ SD) $8,522 \pm 5,365$ J with an output power of 3.1 ± 0.5 W. Five years after LA, mean $\pm$ SD nodule volume decreased from 28.1 ± 29.3 to 14.5 ± 17.6 mL, with a percent reduction of -49.6% (Fig. 13.19). Volume reduction was related with good clinical response, i.e., cosmetic improvement and compressive symptoms reduction.

According to internal content, nodules were classified as follows: (a) Compact: solid, iso/hypoechoic, homogeneous; (b) Spongiform: aggregation of multiple microcystic components in more than 50% of the nodule. Cystic nodules (fluid content $\geq 50\%$) were excluded from this series. In 44 spongiform nodules, volume

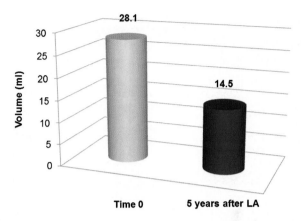

FIG. 13.19. Effects of LA treatment on benign cold thyroid nodules in 65 patients. Mean nodule volume before treatment and 5 years after LA procedure.

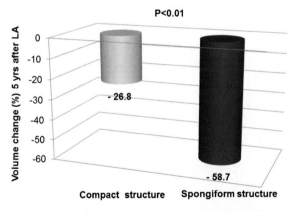

FIG. 13.20. Mean volume changes (%) according to US structure in 65 patients with benign cold thyroid nodules treated with LA in a 5-year follow-up study. LA was more effective in patients with spongiform nodules.

decreased from 24.8 ± 25.9 to 7.7 ± 7.5 mL, with a percent reduction of –58.7%. In 21 compact nodules, volume decreased from 26.4 ± 24.5 to 17.9 ± 22.0 mL, with a reduction of –26.8%. Mean volume shrinkage was significantly greater in spongiform nodules as compared to compact nodules ($P \leq 0.01$) (Fig. 13.20). Our data demonstrate that LA procedure was more effective and durable in patients with

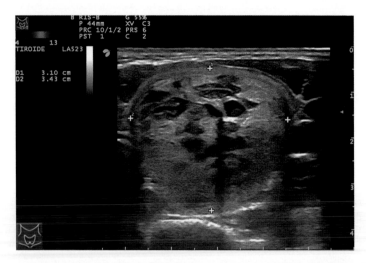

FIG. 13.21. A typical 23.5 mL left lobe spongiform nodule with multiple microcystic elements before LA procedure.

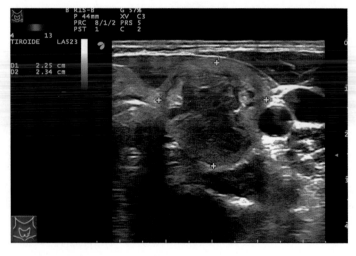

FIG. 13.22. US changes 1 year after LA in the same nodule, with a volume shrinkage to 9.2 mL (–60%).

spongiform nodules. Figure 13.21 shows a typical left lobe spongiform nodule with multiple microcystic elements. Figure 13.22 depicts US changes after LA, with a volume change from 23.5 to

9.2 mL after 1 year. The patients with spongiform nodules are therefore the best candidates for percutaneous LA procedure.

RADIOFREQUENCY ABLATION

The goal of Radiofrequency (RF) is to induce thermal injury to the tissue through electro-magnetic energy deposition. Passage of alternating high-frequency current, between 200 and 1,200 kHz through tissue, leads to a rise in temperature, without muscle contraction or pain [43]. The alternating electric field created in the tissue displaces molecules first in one direction, then in the opposite direction. Such agitation creates frictional heath (Fig. 13.23). In the monopolar mode, which is the one most commonly used, the patient is part of a closed-loop circuit that includes a radiofrequency generator, an electrode needle, and a large dispersive electrode (ground pads). The discrepancy between the small surface area of the needle electrode and the large area of the ground pads causes the heat generated to be concentrated around the needle electrode inserted into target area (Fig. 13.24). A typical treatment produces temperatures of 100 °C or more, resulting in coagulation necrosis within a few minutes, tissue desiccation, and consequent rise in impedance. Small vessels are completely destroyed and large vessels up to 3 mm in diameter are thrombosed [44, 45]. The diameter of the roughly spherical coagulative necrosis is 10–15 mm when using monopolar needle electrode [44, 46]. As for the laser, overheating with carbonization would limit heat transmission and tissue destruction. Internally cooled tip needles maintain probe tip temperatures at around 90 °C without tissue charring. This improves the ability of the radiofrequency applicator to cause ablation (Fig. 13.25). Tissue saline infusion, either in single tip or multitined electrode needles, reduces tissue desiccation with further ablation expansion (Fig. 13.26).

Radiofrequency Ablation in the Thyroid Gland

Current systems used for the thyroid gland are low-perfusion-rate single or expandable multitined needle electrodes [47, 48] (Table 13.2). RF needle thickness ranges from 14G to 18G; the latter thickness, being less invasive, is more used for the thyroid gland.

Technique and Procedure

In contrast with LA technique, where multiple optical fibers are inserted through 21G needles by a cranio-caudal approach

Table 13.2 Effects of radiofrequency ablation procedure on benign thyroid nodules

	Kim et al. [50]	Jeong et al. [51]	Deandrea et al. [49]	Spiezia et al. [52]	Baek et al. [48]	Baek et al. [53]
Number of patients	30	236	31	94	9	15
Number of nodules	35	302	33	94	9	15
Nodule type	Cold	Cold	Cold + AFTN	Cold + AFTN	AFTN	Cold
Solid component (%)	0–100	0–100	>30	>30	60–100	>50
Follow-up period (months)	1–18	1–41	6	12–24	6–17	6–8
V initial (mL)	6.3	6.13	27.7	24.5	15.0	7.5
Volume reduction (%)	64	84	51	79	75	80
Session (mean)	1	1–6 (1.4)	1	1–3 (1.4)	1–4 (2.2)	1
Electrode type	Internally cooled	Internally cooled	Multitined expandable	Multitined expandable	Internally cooled	Internally cooled

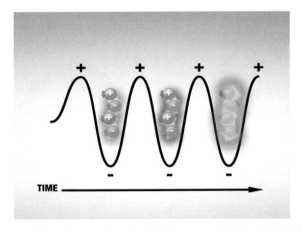

FIG. 13.23. Physical principles of radiofrequency ablation (RFA). Passage of alternating high-frequency current through tissue increases molecular speed, leading to a rise in temperature.

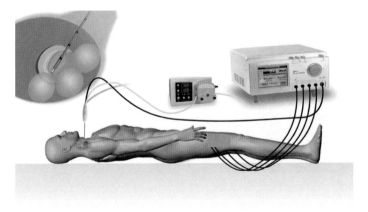

FIG. 13.24. RFA system. The patient is part of a closed-loop circuit that includes a radiofrequency generator, an electrode needle, and a large dispersive electrode (ground pads). *Upper left*: the heat generated by needle electrode is concentrated into target area.

[22, 23, 26–36], RF electrode needle is inserted under US assistance into the thyroid nodule through a transverse approach from the isthmus towards the common carotid artery [47–53]. Different techniques are due to different heat expansion: at the tip of the needle for the laser, at the sides of the needle for RF. The "moving shot" technique uses 7-cm 18G internally cooled needle electrode,

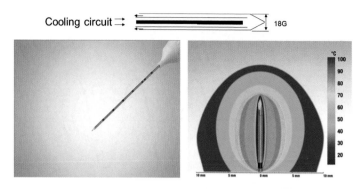

FIG. 13.25. Cooled tip electrode needle (*left*). Cold saline solution is pumped internally in a close circuit at the tip (*top*). Cooling maintains probe tip temperatures at around 90 °C without tissue charring. This improves heat conduction through tissue in a spherical pattern (*right*).

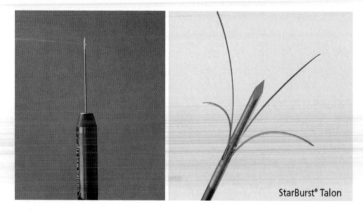

FIG. 13.26. Single tip (*left*) and multitined RF (*right*) electrode needles with tissue saline infusion reduce tissue desiccation with further ablation expansion.

with a 10 mm active tip, inserted through the isthmus without skin incision (Fig. 13.27). CEUS studies before RF helps in visualizing nodule vascularity and viable tissue with greater sensitivity than Color-Doppler (Fig. 13.28).

The thyroid nodule is divided into multiple imaginary ablation units and RF is performed unit by unit. The needle is moved within the thyroid mass by tilting it upwards and backwards from deep to superficial layers of the nodule ("moving shot technique") (Fig. 13.29). Large ablations are obtained without any damage of vital structures (Figs. 13.30 and 13.31).

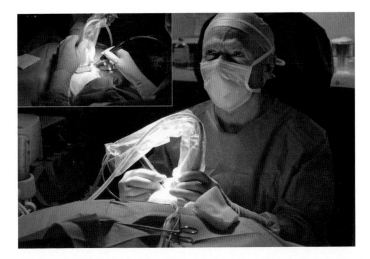

Fɪɢ. 13.27. RF ablation with 18G cool-tip electrode needle, inserted under ultrasound guidance into the thyroid nodule through a transverse approach from the isthmus, using the "moving shot" technique.

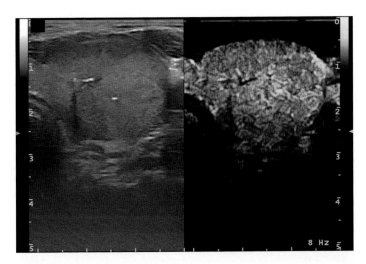

Fɪɢ. 13.28. B-mode and CEUS transverse imaging of a left thyroid nodule. CEUS shows nodule viable tissue with greater sensitivity than Color-Doppler.

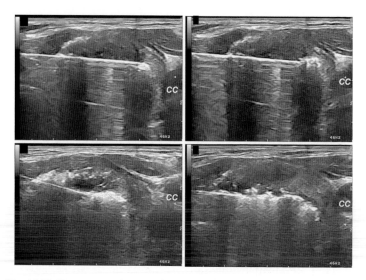

Fig. 13.29. Transverse ultrasound images of the "moving shot" RF ablation technique. (**a**) Insertion of the electrode needle towards the common carotid (*CC*) artery. (**b–d**) The needle is moved within the thyroid mass by pulling it back and tilting it upwards from deep to superficial layers of the nodule.

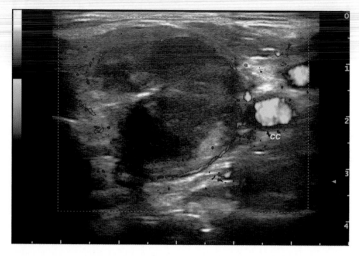

Fig. 13.30. Final ablation, axial ultrasound image, Color-Doppler. Nodular tissue is avascular, markedly hypoechoic with a preexisting central calcification.

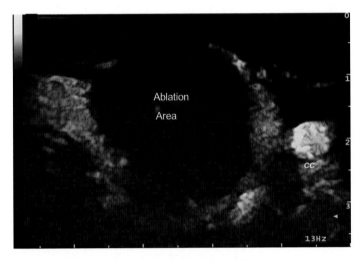

FIG. 13.31. CEUS study demonstrates large ablation of the nodule with minimal residual viable tissue left above vital neck structures.

Side Effects

Our direct experience with RF "moving shot" technique on thyroid nodules matches the available published data reporting minimal side effects [49, 52, 53]. A study carried out on 236 patients treated with the 17G cool tip single electrode needle with the "moving shot" technique reports varying degrees of pain that was managed with oral analgesics [51]. For RF procedure, we used the same protocol as for LA intervention (see before), with minimal, if any, pain. So far we did not encounter any side effect. Complications encountered in a large Korean multicentric study on 1,459 patients who underwent RF ablation of 1,543 benign thyroid nodules were in total 48 (3.3%), 20 major and 28 minor. Details are shown in Table 13.3. A learning curve with comprehension of technical tips is required to prevent complications or properly manage those that occur [54].

Clinical Results in Benign Thyroid Nodules

In a recent study involving 96 elderly patients with benign cold nodules with a mean ± SEM volume of 24.5 ± 2.1 mL, RFA achieved an overall 78.6 and 79.4% mean reduction of initial volume 1 and 2 years after procedure, respectively [52]. Another study with RF reported a mean ± SD change in volume of 46.3 ± 17.1% 6 months after ablation [49]. In a prospective controlled study carried out on

Table 13.3 Complications of thyroid nodule RF ablation in a multicentric Korean study on 1,459 patients [54]

Complication	Number	Incidence (%)	Follow-up results	Detection (days)	Recovery (days)
Voice change	15	0.97	Recovered (13) Follow-up loss (2)	1–2	1–90
Hematoma	15	1.04	Recovered	1	<30
Vomiting	9	0.62	Recovered	1–2	1–2
Skin burn	4	0.28	Recovered	1	<7
Brachial plexus injury	1	0.07	Recovered	1	60
Tumor rupture	2	0.14	Recovered	22–30	<30
Abscess formation with tumor rupture	1	0.07	Surgery	50	–
Hypothyroidism	1	0.07	Medication	180	–

30 patients with cystic or small (mean ± SD volume 7.5 ± 4.9 mL) nodules [51, 53], a mean reduction of 79.7–84.8% of initial volume after 6 months was reported. PEI may obtain similar results in cystic thyroid nodules [17]. PLA vs. RF controlled studies are needed to compare clinical results obtained with these two thermal techniques.

THERMAL ABLATION PROCEDURES IN AUTONOMOUSLY FUNCTIONING THYROID NODULES

The use of thermal ablation techniques for Autonomously Functioning Thyroid Nodule (AFTN), either toxic or pretoxic, was initially proposed as a way to avoid surgery and radioiodine therapy [23, 28, 31, 32, 35, 42, 48, 49, 51, 52]. Also in our experience, early (6–12 months after thermal ablation) follow-up scintiscan showed hot nodule disappearance, with restoration of normal thyroid uptake (Fig. 13.32) and function (personal data). However, as reported with PEI [55], patients with AFTN may have nodule regrowth and recurrent hyperthyroidism. Repeat thermal ablation procedures could stabilize thyroid function.

FOLLOW-UP EVALUATION AFTER THYROID THERMAL ABLATION PROCEDURES

Our thermal ablation follow-up protocol include US evaluation with Color-Doppler and/or CEUS in order to measure nodule volume changes as well as coagulation zone, taken as the avascular, hypoechoic area [56–58]. Laboratory tests (TSH, free T3, free T4, Thyroglobulin, TgAb, TPOAb, and TSH-Receptor Antibodies), side effects, compressive symptoms, and cosmetic signs are also recorded.

INDICATIONS OF THERMAL ABLATION PROCEDURES IN THE ENDOCRINE NECK

Benign Cold Thyroid Nodules

At present, the most important indication for thermal ablation procedures in the thyroid gland [16] is to reduce benign cold thyroid nodules in patients with local pressure symptoms or cosmetic complaints who refuse surgery or who are poor candidates for surgery. There are numerous studies of percutaneous LA in these patients, including controlled trials, homogeneous groups of patients, and investigations of dose–response relationships. The evidence of the effectiveness of LA is thus scientifically more robust than that for radiofrequency thermal ablation [14]. Our data demonstrate that spongiform nodules are the best candidates for laser ablation.

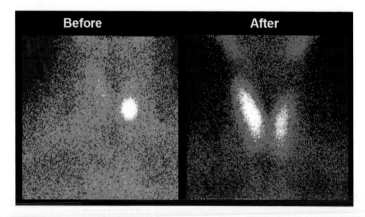

Fig. 13.32. Scintiscan showing an autonomously functioning thyroid nodule (AFTN) before and 6 months after laser ablation.

Other Indications

On the basis of our experience [25, 37] and in accordance with published data [21, 59, 60], thermal ablation is also appropriate in the following cases:

1. Debulking of large AFTNs to bring thyrotoxicosis swiftly under control before radioiodine treatment and to enhance the effectiveness of radioiodine-induced tissue ablation.
2. Palliative treatment of medullary, poorly differentiated thyroid carcinoma and recurrences of malignancies not suited to surgery or radioiodine.
3. LA could be considered as a potential first-line therapy in selected low-risk small papillary cancers (PTC). These patients might be candidates for conservative approaches as they have cause-specific mortality rate at 30 postoperative years of only 1% [61].

CONCLUSIONS

Thermal ablation procedures are a promising, minimally invasive alternative to surgery in specific thyroid pathologies. Before the routine use of these procedures can be recommended, prospective randomized studies are being conducted in order to confirm eligibility criteria and long-term efficacy, assess safety, cost-benefit, and quality-of-life.

References

1. Christophi C, Winkworth A, Muralihdaran V, et al. The treatment of malignancy by hyperthermia. Surg Oncol. 1998;7:83–90.
2. Wheatley DN, Kerr C, Gregory DW. Heat-induced damage to HeLa-S3 cells: correlation of viability, permeability, osmosensitivity, phase-contrast light-, scanning electron- and transmission electron-microscopical findings. Int J Hyperthermia. 1989;5:145–62.
3. Bown SG. Phototherapy in tumors. World J Surg. 1983;7:700–9.
4. Nolsoe CP, Torp-Pedersen S, Burcharth F, et al. Interstitial hyperthermia of colorectal liver metastases with a US-guided Nd-YAG laser with a diffuser tip: a pilot clinical study. Radiology. 1993;187:333–7.
5. Amin Z, Harries SA, Lees WR, et al. Interstitial tumour photocoagulation. Endosc Surg Allied Technol. 1993;1:224–9.
6. Germer CT, Roggan A, Ritz JP, et al. Optical properties of native and coagulated human liver tissue and liver metastases in the near infrared range. Lasers Surg Med. 1998;23:194–203.
7. Heisterkamp J, van Hillegersberg R, Ijzermans JN. Interstitial laser coagulation for hepatic tumours. Br J Surg. 1999;86:293–304.
8. Dachman AH, Smith MJ, Burris JA, et al. Interstitial laser ablation in experimental models and in clinical use. Semin Intervent Radiol. 1993;10:101–12.
9. Pacella CM, Rossi Z, Bizzarri G, et al. Ultrasound-guided percutaneous laser ablation of liver tissue in a rabbit model. Eur Radiol. 1993;3:26–32.
10. Nikfarjam M, Muralidharan V, Malcontenti-Wilson C, et al. Progressive microvascular injury in liver and colorectal liver metastases following laser induced focal hyperthermia therapy. Lasers Surg Med. 2005;37:64–73.
11. Ritz JP, Lehmann KS, Zurbuchen U, et al. Ex vivo and in vivo evaluation of laser-induced thermotherapy for nodular thyroid disease. Lasers Surg Med. 2009;41:479–86.
12. Piana S, Riganti F, Froio E, Andrioli M, Pacella CM, Valcavi R. Pathological findings of thyroid nodules after percutaneous laser ablation: a series of 22 cases with cyto-histological correlation. Endocr Pathol. 2012;23(2):94–100.
13. Ritz JP, Roggan A, Isbert C, et al. Optical properties of native and coagulated porcine liver tissue between 400 and 2400 nm. Lasers Surg Med. 2001;29:205–12.
14. Hegedus L. Therapy: a new nonsurgical therapy option for benign thyroid nodules? Nat Rev Endocrinol. 2009;5:476–8.
15. Cooper DS, Doherty GM, Haugen BR, et al. Revised American Thyroid Association management guidelines for patients with thyroid nodules and differentiated thyroid cancer. Thyroid. 2009;19:1167–214.
16. Gharib H, Papini E, Paschke R, et al. American Association of Clinical Endocrinologist, Associazione Medici Endocrinologi, and European Thyroid Association medical guidelines for clinical practice for the diagnosis and management of thyroid nodules. Endocr Pract. 2010;16 Suppl 1:1–43.

17. Valcavi R, Frasoldati A. Ultrasound-guided percutaneous ethanol injection therapy in thyroid cystic nodules. Endocr Pract. 2004;10: 269–75.

18. Esnault O, Franc B, Monteil JP, et al. High-intensity focused ultrasound for localized thyroid-tissue ablation: preliminary experimental animal study. Thyroid. 2004;14:1072–6.

19. Esnault O, Franc B, Chapelon JY. Localized ablation of thyroid tissue by high-intensity focused ultrasound: improvement of noninvasive tissue necrosis methods. Thyroid. 2009;19:1085–91.

20. Esnault O, Rouxel A, Le Nestour E, et al. Minimally invasive ablation of a toxic thyroid nodule by high-intensity focused ultrasound. AJNR Am J Neuroradiol. 2010;31(10):1967–8.

21. Pacella CM, Bizzarri G, Guglielmi R, et al. Thyroid tissue: US-guided percutaneous interstitial laser ablation-a feasibility study. Radiology. 2000;217:673–7.

22. Døssing H, Bennedbaek FN, Karstrup S, et al. Benign solitary solid cold thyroid nodules: US-guided interstitial laser photocoagulation—initial experience. Radiology. 2002;225:53–7.

23. Pacella CM, Bizzarri G, Spiezia S, et al. Thyroid tissue: US-guided percutaneous laser thermal ablation. Radiology. 2004;232:272–80.

24. Papini E, Guglielmi R, Bizzarri G, et al. Ultrasound-guided laser thermal ablation for treatment of benign thyroid nodules. Endocr Pract. 2004;10:276–83.

25. Valcavi R, Bertani A, Pesenti M, et al. Laser and radiofrequency ablation procedures. In: Baskin BJ, Duick DS, Levine RA, editors. Thyroid ultrasound and ultrasound-guided FNA. 2nd ed. New York: Springer; 2008. p. 198–218.

26. Dossing H, Bennedbaek FN, Hegedus L. Ultrasound-guided interstitial laser photocoagulation of an autonomous thyroid nodule: the introduction of a novel alternative. Thyroid. 2003;13:885–8.

27. Døssing H, Bennedbaek FN, Hegedus L. Beneficial effect of combined aspiration and interstitial laser therapy in patients with benign cystic thyroid nodules: a pilot study. Br J Radiol. 2006;79:943–7.

28. Spiezia S, Vitale G, Di Somma C, et al. Ultrasound-guided laser thermal ablation in the treatment of autonomous hyperfunctioning thyroid nodules and compressive nontoxic nodular goiter. Thyroid. 2003;13:941–7.

29. Amabile G, Rotondi M, De Chiara G, et al. Low-energy interstitial laser photocoagulation for treatment of nonfunctioning thyroid nodules: therapeutic outcome in relation to pretreatment and treatment parameters. Thyroid. 2006;16:749–55.

30. Cakir B, Topaloglu O, Gul K, et al. Effects of percutaneous laser ablation treatment in benign solitary thyroid nodules on nodule volume, thyroglobulin and anti-thyroglobulin levels, and cytopathology of nodule in 1 yr follow-up. J Endocrinol Invest. 2006;29:876–84.

31. Barbaro D, Orsini P, Lapi P, et al. Percutaneous laser ablation in the treatment of toxic and pretoxic nodular goiter. Endocr Pract. 2007;13:30–6.

32. Rotondi M, Amabile G, Leporati P, et al. Repeated laser thermal ablation of a large functioning thyroid nodule restores euthyroidism

and ameliorates constrictive symptoms. J Clin Endocrinol Metab. 2009;94:382–3.

33. Døssing H, Bennedbaek FN, Hegedus L. Effect of ultrasound-guided interstitial laser photocoagulation on benign solitary solid cold thyroid nodules—a randomised study. Eur J Endocrinol. 2005;152:341–5.

34. Papini E, Guglielmi R, Bizzarri G, et al. Treatment of benign cold thyroid nodules: a randomized clinical trial of percutaneous laser ablation versus levothyroxine therapy or follow-up. Thyroid. 2007;17:229–35.

35. Døssing H, Bennedbaek FN, Bonnema SJ, et al. Randomized prospective study comparing a single radioiodine dose and a single laser therapy session in autonomously functioning thyroid nodules. Eur J Endocrinol. 2007;157:95–100.

36. Gambelunghe G, Fatone C, Ranchelli A, et al. A randomized controlled trial to evaluate the efficacy of ultrasound-guided laser photocoagulation for treatment of benign thyroid nodules. J Endocrinol Invest. 2006;29:RC23–6.

37. Valcavi R, Riganti F, Bertani A, et al. Percutaneous laser ablation of cold benign thyroid nodules. A three-year follow-up in 122 patients. Thyroid. 2010;20(11):1253–61.

38. Di Rienzo G, Surrente C, Lopez C, Quercia R. Tracheal laceration after laser ablation of nodular goitre. Interact Cardiovasc Thorac Surg. 2012;14(1):115–6.

39. Døssing H, Bennedbaek FN, Karstrup S, Hegedüs L. Benign solitary solid cold thyroid nodules: US-guided interstitial laser photocoagulation—initial experience. Radiology. 2002;225(1):53–7.

40. Døssing H, Bennedbaek FN, Hegedüs L. Ultrasound-guided interstitial laser photocoagulation of an autonomous thyroid nodule: the introduction of a novel alternative. Thyroid. 2003;13(9):885–8.

41. Døssing H, Bennedbæk FN, Hegedüs L. Long-term outcome following interstitial laser photocoagulation of benign cold thyroid nodules. Eur J Endocrinol. 2011;165(1):123–8.

42. Amabile G, Rotondi M, Pirali B, Dionisio R, Agozzino L, Lanza M, et al. Interstitial laser photocoagulation for benign thyroid nodules: time to treat large nodules. Lasers Surg Med. 2011;43(8):797–803. doi:10.1002/lsm.21114.

43. Siperstein AE, Gitomirsky A. History and technonological aspects of radiofrequency thermoablation. Cancer J. 2000;6:2293–303.

44. McGahan JP, Browning PD, Brock JM, et al. Hepatic ablation using radiofrequency electrocautery. Invest Radiol. 1990;25:267–70.

45. McGahan JP, Brock JM, Tesluk H, et al. Hepatic ablation with use of radio-frequency electrocautery in the animal model. J Vasc Interv Radiol. 1992;3:291–7.

46. Goldberg SN, Gazelle GS, Dawson SL, et al. Tissue ablation with radiofrequency: effect of probe size, gauge, duration, and temperature on lesion volume. Acad Radiol. 1995;2:399–404.

47. Spiezia S, Garberoglio R, Di Somma C, et al. Efficacy and safety of radiofrequency thermal ablation in the treatment of thyroid nodules with pressure symptoms in elderly patients. J Am Geriatr Soc. 2007;55:1478–9.

48. Baek JH, Moon WJ, Kim YS, et al. Radiofrequency ablation for the treatment of autonomously functioning thyroid nodules. World J Surg. 2009;33:1971–7.

49. Deandrea M, Limone P, Basso E, et al. US-guided percutaneous radiofrequency thermal ablation for the treatment of solid benign hyperfunctioning or compressive thyroid nodules. Ultrasound Med Biol. 2008;34:784–91.

50. Kim YS, Rhim H, Tae K, et al. Radiofrequency ablation of benign cold thyroid nodules: initial clinical experience. Thyroid. 2006;16:361–7.

51. Jeong WK, Baek JH, Rhim H, et al. Radiofrequency ablation of benign thyroid nodules: safety and imaging follow-up in 236 patients. Eur Radiol. 2008;18:1244–50.

52. Spiezia S, Garberoglio R, Milone F, et al. Thyroid nodules and related symptoms are stably controlled two years after radiofrequency thermal ablation. Thyroid. 2009;19:219–25.

53. Baek JH, Kim YS, Lee D, et al. Benign predominantly solid thyroid nodules: prospective study of efficacy of sonographically guided radiofrequency ablation versus control condition. AJR Am J Roentgenol. 2010;194:1137–42.

54. Baek JH, Lee JH, Sung JY, Bae JI, Kim KT, Sim J, et al. Complications encountered in the treatment of benign thyroid nodules with US-guided radiofrequency ablation: a multicenter study. Radiology. 2012;262(1):335–42.

55. Guglielmi R, Pacella CM, Bianchini A, et al. Percutaneous ethanol injection treatment in benign thyroid lesions: role and efficacy. Thyroid. 2004;14:125–31.

56. Burns PN, Wilson SR. Microbubble contrast for radiological imaging: 1. Principles. Ultrasound Q. 2006;22:5–13.

57. Wilson SR, Burns PN. Microbubble contrast for radiological imaging: 2. Applications. Ultrasound Q. 2006;22:15–8.

58. Papini E, Bizzarri G, Bianchini A, et al. Contrast-enhanced ultrasound in the management of thyroid nodules. In: Baskin BJ, Duick DS, Levine RA, editors. Thyroid ultrasound and ultrasound-guided FNA. 2nd ed. New York: Springer; 2008. p. 151–71.

59. Monchik JM, Donatini G, Iannuccilli J, et al. Radiofrequency ablation and percutaneous ethanol injection treatment for recurrent local and distant well-differentiated thyroid carcinoma. Ann Surg. 2006;244:296–304.

60. Papini E, Bizzarri G, Pacella CM. Percutaneous laser ablation of benign and malignant thyroid nodules. Curr Opin Endocrinol Diabetes Obes. 2008;15:434–9.

61. Hay ID. Management of patients with low-risk papillary thyroid carcinoma. Endocr Pract. 2007;13:521–33.

CHAPTER 14
Percutaneous Ethanol Injection (PEI) in the Treatment of Thyroid Cysts, Nodules, and Other Neck Lesions

Andrea Frasoldati and Roberto Valcavi

INTRODUCTION

Percutaneous ethanol injection (PEI) was first proposed about 30 years ago for sclerotherapy of different kind of lesions, such as hepatocellular carcinoma, hepatic and renal cysts, adrenal adenoma, and parathyroid hyperplasia [1–5]. Ethanol exerts its sclerosing properties through cellular dehydration and protein denaturation, which lead to coagulative necrosis and small vessel thrombosis. As a consequence, hemorrhagic infarcts and reactive fibrosis are the prevailing histological changes described in tissues exposed to ethanol [6, 7]. In the thyroid gland, the first documented use of PEI for treating thyroid cysts dates to 1989 [8]; shortly after, this technique was also suggested as an alternative therapeutic option to surgery and radioiodine for the treatment of autonomous functioning nodules (AFTN) [9–12]. Since then, PEI sclerotherapy of thyroid cysts has gained a world-wide diffusion, whereas the fortunes of PEI as a candidate first-line therapy for toxic and pre-toxic solid nodules have gradually faded. PEI treatment of thyroid cysts will therefore constitute the heart of the present chapter. PEI has also proved to be quite effective in treating other neck lesions, like thyroglossal duct cysts (TDC), enlarged parathyroid glands, and metastatic lymph nodes. These applications of PEI will also be briefly discussed.

H.J. Baskin et al. (eds.), *Thyroid Ultrasound and Ultrasound-Guided FNA*, **315**
DOI 10.1007/978-1-4614-4785-6_14,
© Springer Science+Business Media, LLC 2013

THYROID CYSTS

PEI has been recognized as the first-line treatment for thyroid cystic lesions [13–15]. Whereas "pure" thyroid cysts are a rare finding (<1% of all thyroid nodules), pseudocystic lesions featuring a major fluid component are quite frequently encountered, accounting for 25–30% of all thyroid nodules detected by US [16, 17]. The fluid content may be quite inhomogeneous, an aggregation of colloidal fluid, blood, and melting necrotic tissue. In the clinical setting, thyroid hemorrhagic cysts typically present as a suddenly occurring visible neck lump, which causes transient tenderness, pain, and pressure symptoms, occasionally associated with hoarseness and dysphagia. Stable regression of the lesion may occur either spontaneously or after fine-needle aspiration; however, thyroid cyst recurrence is the rule [18–20].

In all, results of most studies published over two decades are substantially similar, irrespective of minor technical dissimilarities in the PEI procedure [19–31] (Table 14.1). Ethanol sclerotherapy of thyroid cysts results in a mean volume reduction ranging from 64.0 to 93%, with a 69–95% rate of successful treatments, defined in terms of a ≥50% reduction of thyroid cyst volume (Table 14.1) (Figs. 14.1 and 14.2). Other sclerotherapic agents (e.g., tetracycline and OK-432) have been shown to be as effective as ethanol [21]; yet ethanol instillation has been established world-wide as the standard technique because it is safe, inexpensive, and easily repeatable. As expected, relief from local compressive discomfort and resolution of cosmetic complains tends to parallel the achievement of a significant volume decrease, occurring in about 75–95% of patients treated with PEI. Pressure and/or cosmetic symptoms may be variably recorded and measured. In a recently published series, patients were specifically interviewed and asked to rate symptoms on a 10-cm visual analog scale, while a 1–4 cosmetic score, based on palpation and inspection, was recorded by the physician [31]. After PEI treatment, symptom and cosmetic scores decreased from 3.92 ± 1.54 to 0.39 ± 0.69 and from 3.31 ± 0.90 to 1.17 ± 0.56, respectively [31]. The chance of a stable clinical improvement is 2.5–3-fold higher after PEI as compared to simple evacuation alone [25, 27]. In a well designed, randomized prospective study on 66 consecutive patients followed up for a 6-month period, thyroid cysts were randomly assigned either to ethanol or to isotonic saline flushing, followed in both cases by complete fluid aspiration. After one treatment session, the cure rate was 64% in the ethanol group compared with 18% in the saline group, while at the end of the study results of PEI vs. saline showed a 82% vs. 48% cure rate [25]. These results replicated those obtained in

Table 14.1 Overview of PEI sclerotherapy results in thyroid cystic nodules

	Patients	Mean follow-up (months)	Mean volume at baseline (mL)	Number of PEI sessions	Amount of EtOH injected (% of the extracted fluid)	Mean volume reduction (%)	Success rate (%)[a]	Major side effects
Yasuda et al. [10]	61	6	n.r.	1–3	10	n.r.	72.1	0
Monzani et al. [19]	20	12	~12.0	1–2	~30	n.r.	95	0
Verde et al. [21]	32	12	14.5 (1.5–65.8)	n.r.	n.r. (1–10 mL)	71	75	0
Antonelli et al. [20]	26	12	16.8 ± 9.9	1–5 (mean 2.5)	10–33	n.r.	77	0
Zingrillo et al. [22]	43	37.0 ± 14.0	38.4 (4.8–166)	1–4 (mean 1.5)	10–15	91.9	93	0
Cho et al. [23]	22 (13/9)	3.5 (1–10)	13.0 (3.5–42.0)	1–6	40–100	64.0	68.1	0
Del Prete et al. [24]	98	120 ± 14	35.2 ± 20	1–4 (mean 1.8)	70–150	59.9	93.8	Dysphonia (1)
Kim et al. [26]	20	4.4 (1–6)	15.7 (12.0–48.6)	1–3 (mean 1.8)	40–68	64.0	65.0	0

(continued)

Table 14.1 (continued)

	Patients	Mean follow-up (months)	Mean volume at baseline (mL)	Number of PEI sessions	Amount of EtOH injected (% of the extracted fluid)	Mean volume reduction (%)	Success rate (%)[a]	Major side effects
Bennedbaek et al. [25]	33 (26/7)	6	8.0 (5.0–14.0)	1–3	25–50	100[b]	82.0	Dysphonia (1)
Valcavi et al. [27]	135	12	19.0 ± 19.0	1–3	50–70	85.6[b]	n.r.	Dysphonia (1)
Guglielmi et al. [28]	58	82	13.7 ± 14.0	2.2 ± 1.3	25	86.6	86.2	0
Lee and Ahn [29]	432	36.5 ± 12.9	15.6 ± 12.6	1–7 (mean 2.3)	40–100	66.1	79.4	Dysphonia (3)[c]
Kanotra et al. [30]	40 (24/16)	13.8 ± 5	12.2 (5.8–18.5)	1–3 (mean 1.5)	50	70.0	85.0	0
Sung et al. [31]	36	17.0 ± 7.46	13.8 ± 11.9	1–2 (mean 1.2)	50	93.0	94.4	0

[a]Success rate was defined in most studies a ³50% volume reduction; however, in some studies [25, 28], different criteria were adopted

[b]Median volume reduction

[c]The study reports the effects of PEI treatment in a mixed series of complex cysts (n = 432), solid cold nodules (n = 198), and hot nodules; three patients out of the whole study population developed dysphonia after PEI treatment

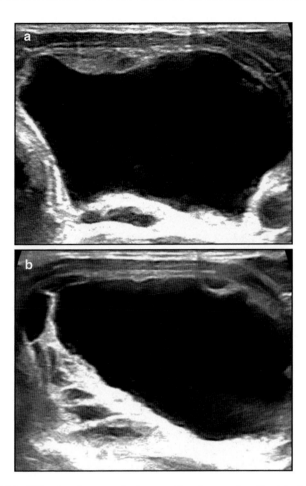

FIG. 14.1. PEI sclerotherapy of a large unilocular cyst localized in the left thyroid lobe ((**a**) longitudinal scan; (**b**) transverse scan). After 1 month, the volume of the lesion was markedly reduced (from 31.3 to 5.9 mL) ((**c**) longitudinal scan; (**d**) transverse scan).

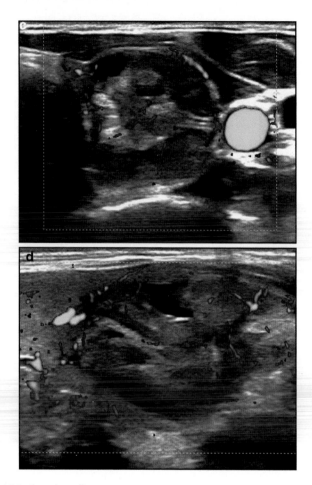

Fig. 14.1. (continued)

a previous open, non-randomized study [20], also confirming a <20% recurrence rate of thyroid cysts after ethanol sclerotherapy. PEI efficacy is durable, with a 3.4% and 6.5% recurrence rate over 5 and 10 years, respectively [24, 28]. PEI feasibility may be to some extent questioned in the treatment of larger (e.g., >40–50 mL) cysts [25, 29], although a negative impact of the initial volume on the final results has not been conclusively demonstrated [22–24, 28, 30]. Instead, the rate of treatment failures recorded by different authors is most likely due to the percentage of "complex" or "mixed" lesions included in their series. In facts, PEI results

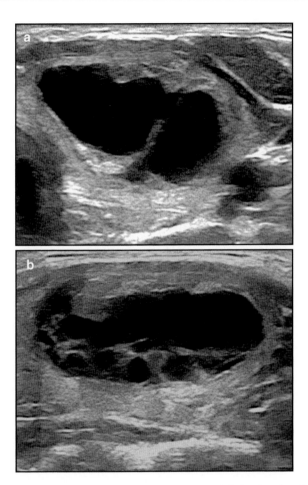

FIG. 14.2. PEI sclerotherapy of a mixed thyroid nodule localized in the left thyroid lobe ((**a**) longitudinal scan; (**b**) transverse scan). After 1 month, the lesion volume decreased from 6.5 to 2.1 mL (**c**, **d**).

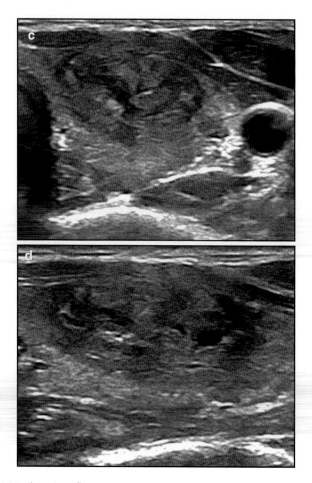

FIG. 14.2. (continued)

are influenced by the lesion structure, with a 60–65% median volume reduction obtained in case of complex cysts featuring a solid component and mixed nodules. This result is significantly worse as compared to the 90–95% reduction expected in "empty body" or "pure" cystic nodules [26, 29, 30]. Multilocular, complex cysts may also require a higher number of treatment sessions [28, 29]. Accordingly, PEI is more effective in cystic vs. "solid" thyroid nodules: in a prospective study on 42 patients, thyroid cysts had a greater volume reduction rate as compared to benign "solid" nodules (64.0% vs. 35.3%, $p < 0.01$) [26]. The resistance exerted by solid thyroid nodules to the action of ethanol is probably linked to their compact cell architecture and to the efficient drainage of ethanol favored by their usually rich vascularization [26, 32]. The relationship between PEI outcome and the structure of the treated nodules may also explain the observation, shared by some, but not all, studies, that the final volume reduction rate is correlated to the volume of the fluid extracted and to the amount of the instilled ethanol [23, 26]. In other words, the larger the fluid content, the more the expected final result. Of course, this rule is likely to be applicable to pure cysts; in series with a prevalence of complex lesions, the smaller the lesion undergoing PEI treatment, the better the results [28, 29]. Another, less predictable, obstacle to a successful PEI procedure is the finding of a viscous and dense cystic content [23, 26, 31]. This may be reliably anticipated during a previous FNA maneuver performed for diagnostic purposes. Nevertheless, the chemical and physical properties of the fluid content may undergo spontaneous changes: thus the results of previous aspiration are not always replicable in the PEI setting. US imaging may sometimes provide some clues about the density of the cyst fluid: the complete absence of any sluggish fluid or particle movement ("snow globe-like effect") after gently enhancing and relieving the probe pressure on the cyst usually indicates a high viscosity of its content.

PEI OF THYROID CYSTS: TECHNIQUE

The patient is placed in a supine position, usually with a pillow under his/her shoulders in order to have the neck fully hyperextended. The neck skin is carefully disinfected and a sterile blanket is placed over the patient's chest, serving as a protection from external contamination and as a work surface. Adequate sterility is also ensured by the use of sterile devices (e.g., probe cover, US gel, and gloves). The patients should be asked to wear a pair of glasses in order to avoid any accidental contact of ethanol with his/her eyes. Local anesthesia is usually unnecessary, especially when using a 20–22 gauge needle; it can however help to minimize the local discomfort when larger needles (e.g., 16–18 gauge) are required and/or the maneuver is likely to be cumbersome. US guidance is mandatory throughout all the procedure. Needle insertion can be accomplished using a needle pointing device, which can be removed once the needle has been safely inserted, thus allowing the needle to be repositioned into the lesion along a different axis. Alternatively, the needle can be inserted free-hand and cautiously directed into the lesion step by step, while kept in full sight by US imaging, with minor adjustments of the probe orientation and pressure. To our knowledge, no controlled studies are available comparing the results of PEI treatment performed with either of these two different approaches. The "free-hand" approach (Fig. 14.3) offers the advantage of a wider range of options for needle positioning through the maneuver, which could be helpful in the case of large, complex cystic lesion. The extraction of the fluid cyst content may be significantly eased by the use of a syringe holder (e.g., the Cameco pistol). After complete fluid extraction, 95% sterile ethanol, contained in 10 mL syringes, is carefully injected into the cyst. At this time, gentle repositioning of the needle inside the lesion may be required. A 20–25 cm tubing connection line between the syringe and the needle, provided with a T clamp system, may facilitate the whole maneuver, reducing the risk to transmit a brusque movement to the needle (Fig. 14.3e–f). The infused ethanol is usually easily visualized on US as a hyperechoic material which progressively refills the cyst (Figs. 14.4 and 14.5). Should the needle get occluded either during the fluid aspiration or the ethanol instillation phases, effective reaming may be obtained by repeatedly passing a stylet through the needle. At the end of the procedure, a short rinsing with normal saline helps reduce the transient pain associated with needle extraction and consequent minimal ethanol leakage to subcutaneous tissues.

Some critical issues must be accurately dealt with during the procedure: (a) the needle tip should be kept under continuous surveillance, especially during the phase of ethanol infusion; (b) abrupt movements should be avoided in order to prevent damaging the cyst walls; (c) the perception of a major resistance to further ethanol injection is a sign to stop the maneuver, verify the needle position, and then carefully retry ethanol injection. As for the amount of ethanol injected, it usually corresponds to approximately 50–70% of the cystic fluid extracted. The choice of the optimal ethanol amount is neither to be aprioristically decided nor blindly calculated on the basis of mathematical formulas. Rather, it should be individualized and based on the pattern of ethanol diffusion as depicted by real-time US imaging, the degree of resistance applied to the tubing connection and the syringe, and the subjective feed-back from the patient.

Basically, PEI may be accomplished according to two alternative strategies: (a) completely evacuate the injected ethanol after a short-time (several minutes) interval, thus limiting the risk of ethanol leakage into the surrounding tissues; (b) leave the infused ethanol inside the cyst in order to prolong its sclerotic effect. As a matter of fact, the comparison of the two treatment modalities did not show any significant difference in terms of sclerotherapy

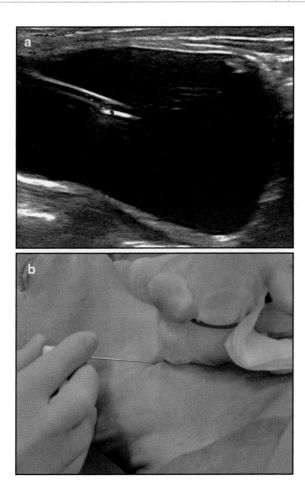

FIG. 14.3. PEI procedure in a unilocular "pure" thyroid cyst (**a**). Needle is inserted under US guidance (**b**); the needle stylet is subsequently gently removed, while the US-probe is temporarily put aside (**c**). The blood content of the cyst spontaneously spills out of the needle hub (**d**); this indicates that the cyst content is quite fluid and that the aspiration phase will be easily carried out. The content of the cyst is then completely aspirated using a 20 mL syringe (**e**). US imaging allows real-time monitoring of the procedure. In case of large cysts, up to 3–4 syringes may be required to complete the drainage of the cyst. At the end of the aspiration phase, an ethanol-containing 10 mL syringe is connected and the ethanol is carefully injected into the lesion under US surveillance (**f**). The entire maneuver is safely accomplished by two operators (one physician and one nurse).

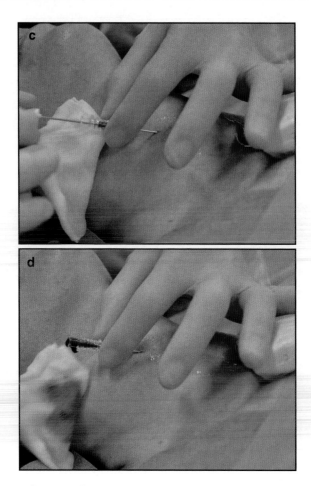

FIG. 14.3. (continued)

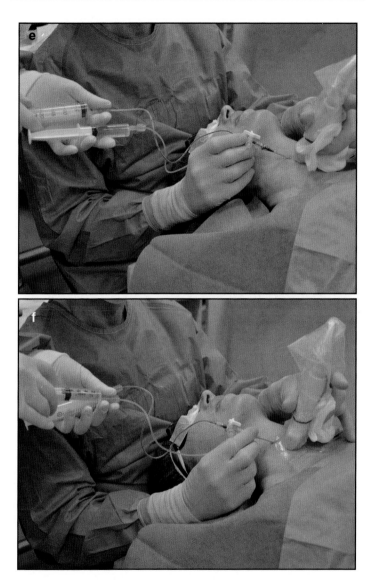

FIG. 14.3. (continued)

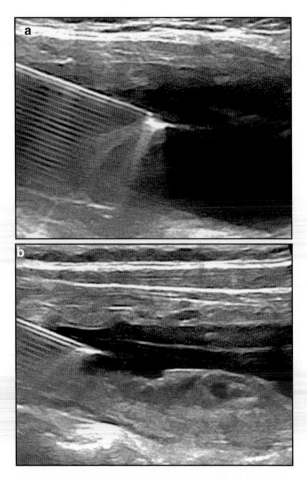

FIG. 14.4. PEI procedure in a large (>50 mL) thyroid cyst (**a**). The fluid is extracted (**b**) and the cyst is refilled with ethanol, visible as a hyperchoic material spilling out of the needle tip (**c**). After ethanol injection, the lesion appears quite inhomogeneous, with ill-defined margins (**d**).

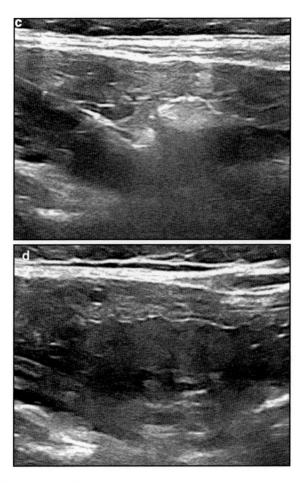

FIG. 14.4. (continued)

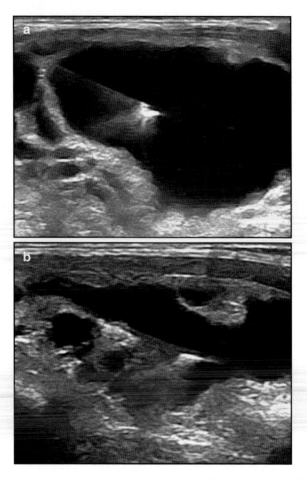

FIG. 14.5. PEI procedure in a large mixed thyroid nodule (**a**). The fluid is thoroughly drained (**b**) and the cyst is then refilled with ethanol (**c**). At the end of the maneuver, the ethanol has partially replaced the fluid content of the lesion (**d**).

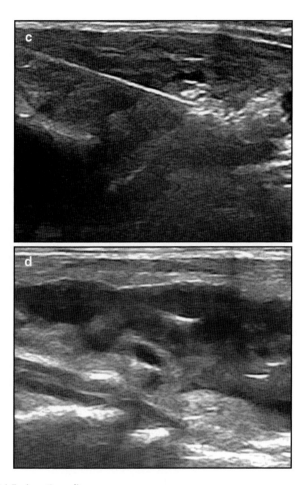

FIG. 14.5. (continued)

results [33]. The latter strategy has probably gained a larger diffusion, notwithstanding ethanol aspiration has been claimed to minimize the risk of ethanol leakage and paraglandular fibrosis [23]. This event is likely to render subsequent surgery on thyroid gland, when needed, more challenging. Therefore, when PEI has previously been performed on posteriorly located thyroid lesions, increased risk of post-surgical hypoparathyroidism or laryngeal nerve palsy should always be considered.

PEI therapy of thyroid cystic lesion is usually devoid of relevant side effects (Table 14.1). As a matter of fact, the fibrous capsule surrounding the cyst acts as a physical barrier to ethanol spreading into the perinodular tissue. Furthermore, the drainage of the fluid content before ethanol injection prevents possible damages to the capsule integrity due to an increased pressure inside the lesion. No substantial differences in safety have been observed in case of complete aspiration of the ethanol-mixed fluid as compared to keeping the ethanol inside the lesion [33]. The limited number (1–2) of sessions usually required by PEI sclerotherapy of thyroid cysts is an additional factor accounting for the low risk of side effects. Nevertheless, reports of recurrent laryngeal nerve (RLN) injury, although extremely rare, still require a high level of alertness throughout the procedure.

AUTONOMOUSLY FUNCTIONING THYROID NODULES

PEI was been proposed two decades ago as an alternative treatment to surgery and radioiodine for AFTNs [9, 11, 12]. Initially welcomed by a large interest, particularly in Europe, ethanol sclerotherapy of "hot" thyroid nodules has lost attraction in the following years due to a number of limitations, like the need for multiple treatment sessions, the uncertain long-term outcome, and the risk of potentially hazardous side effects.

The results published in the first half of the nineties on over 400 patients consistently showed that the vast majority of them (89.6%) were either completely or partially cured by PEI, as indicated by thyroid hormones normalization and reactivation of the extranodular thyroid tissue [9, 11, 12, 32, 34, 35]. At that time, a large multicentric Italian study also demonstrated that PEI success rate was significantly higher in patients with pre-toxic nodules (83.4%) as compared to those with overt hyperthyroidism (66.5%) [36]. Encouraging functional data were paralleled by a significant volume reduction (58.5–90%) of the treated nodules [9, 11, 12, 32, 34, 35, 36]. Apparently, the treatment outcome was influenced by the nodule volume at baseline, with larger nodules being less likely to be effectively cured. Nevertheless, the critical volume cut-off value did not coincide in different studies, ranging from 13 to 40 mL [32, 35, 36]. This issue has been specifically addressed in more recent studies with controversial results [28, 37–39].

The first review articles aiming to draw a balance of PEI treatment in toxic and pre-toxic thyroid nodules correctly underlined that only a few of the available studies reported a over 1-year follow-up time. Therefore, the absence of hyperthyroidism recurrence could not be held as a reliable long-term outcome. Data acquired in a series of 117 patients kept under surveillance for a median follow-up of 2.5 years after PEI treatment indicated a low (13%) rate of treatment failure [40]. Interestingly, only an 11.1% disappearance of hot nodules was recorded, which suggested that full eradication of hyperfunctioning tissue had not been fulfilled. In line with this observation, a 20–35% toxic nodule recurrence has been documented by two long-term studies (mean follow-up 36.7 and 58 months, respectively [29, 41]). Instead, another study on 125 patients (median follow-up 60 months) confirmed a 92.7% PEI success rate with all patients remaining euthyroid throughout the entire study period [39]. As a matter of fact, while it is to be acknowledged that PEI, similarly to radioiodine treatment, is associated with evidence of persisting autonomous tissue at post-treatment scan in at least 30–50% of patients with AFTN, it is still unclear to what extent this finding implies a concrete risk of hyperthyroidism recurrence [13, 42]. Dissimilarities in the number of PEI sessions, the volume of ethanol injected and the follow-up schedule may account for the outcome discrepancies reported above. Moreover, variations in the long-term success rate of PEI may as well depend upon nodule characteristics. In a study on 112 toxic and pre-toxic nodules re-evaluated 5 years after treatment, a fluid component greater than 30% and an initial volume <15 mL were associated with a favorable outcome, irrespective of the functional status (overt or subclinical hyperthyroidism at baseline) [28]. PEI has also been proposed in combination with radioiodine administration as a multi-modal therapeutic strategy for large AFTNs with promising results [13, 42]. This approach may combine the advantages of a limited number of PEI sessions and of a reduced ^{131}I dose [13].

An overall 3.9% frequency of dysphonia, due to RLN palsy, was reported in the first series of patients with AFTN treated with PEII [35]. Although usually transient, this complication has been correctly seen as troublesome, because it is serious and unpredictable. In fact, RLN my suffer either from ethanol spillage beyond the capsule of posteriorly located nodules or from compression due to intra- or extranodular bleeding. Risk of ethanol extranodular seepage cannot be completely prevented; it can however be reduced following two fundamental rules: injecting ethanol at a low pressure, especially in case of already treated, fibrotic nodules, and carefully monitoring the location of the needle tip within the nodule. The sudden onset of intense pain in the course of the maneuver, in the absence of US signs of hemorrhagic swelling inside or around the nodule, may signal extrathyroidal leakage of ethanol. Learning curve of PEI operators as well as improved resolution of US imaging probably account for the lower rate of dysphonia (0.7–0.8%) reported in more recent studies [39, 41]. Other major side effects such as hematoma, ipsilateral facial dysesthesia, jugular vein thrombosis, septic complications, and worsening of thyrotoxicosis have been occasionally described. Two anecdotic cases of injury of cervical sympathetic chain causing transient Horner's syndrome induced by PEI treatment of thyroid nodules have also been reported [43]. Finally, sporadic reports of Graves' disease occurring in patients previously treated with PEI raised concern about a possible relationship between ethanol injection and induction of anti-thyroidal autoimmune response [44].

In conclusion, the available data indicate that in most patients with "hot" thyroid nodules, PEI sclerotherapy restores a normal thyroid function and achieves a significant volume reduction. Nevertheless, these results are usually obtained at the expense of multiple sessions of therapy, each one associated with a concrete risk of relevant side effects. Besides, hyperthyroidism recurrence cannot be completely excluded in the long term. In the everyday clinical practice, these limitations have overwhelmed the possible advantages of PEI approach as compared to radioiodine or surgery. Thus, the role PEI in the treatment of hyperfunctioning thyroid nodules has been confined to a very limited range of indications, namely symptomatic patients for various reasons not susceptible to cure by the traditional first-line treatments. However, other kinds of US-guide interventional techniques introduced in the last decade (e.g., LTA and radiofrequency) are currently threatening PEI to be definitely eclipsed also in this frame.

BENIGN "COLD" NODULES

The use of PEI for sclerotherapy of benign "cold" nodules has been quite limited, mainly because of the higher risk of hazardous side effects as compared to cystic nodules as well as the lower beneficial results as compared to other recently introduced US interventional techniques, namely LTA and RF. Another point of concern is related to the risk of occult cancer: false negative cytological results are possible, and histological evidence of papillary thyroid cancer (PTC) has been occasionally reported in patients previously treated with PEI who finally underwent thyroid surgery [7].

Notwithstanding these premises, the data available from the few published series were not discouraging [26, 29, 45–47]. In a randomized, prospective study on 50 patients with single solid nodules, the reductive effects of PEI in benign cold nodules have been convincingly better than those achieved with L-thyroxine (LT4) administration with a 47% vs. 9% mean volume reduction and a 56% vs. 32% relief of pressure and cosmetic complains [46]. A large retrospective series on 198 solid nodules followed up for about 36 months described even more satisfactory results, with a 75.1% ± 12.3 (mean ± SD) volume reduction [29]. Notably, a ≥50% reduction was recorded in 88.9% of the treated nodules [29]. These results were similar to those obtained in a previous study on 54 patients treated either with PEI alone or with PEI in combination with lT4, showing a ~70% mean volume reduction [45]. On the other hand, the mean rate of volume reduction turned out remarkably lower (~38%) in a study comparing PEI effects in solid vs. cystic nodules [26]. As for PEI treatment of AFTN, the advent of other US-guided interventional techniques will probably make PEI sclerotherapy of benign "cold" solid nodules obsolete in the next few years.

OTHER NECK LESIONS

TDC are a common congenital neck abnormality arising from the embryonic thyroglossal duct structures, located along the midline, between the hyoid bone and the thyroid gland [48, 49]. Ethanol sclerotherapy of TDC have been attempted [50–52] in order to avoid the morbidity and risks associated with surgery, still considered the treatment of choice [49, 53]. Whereas first reports on a very limited number of patients have shown only partially successful results, a recently published series of 11 patients with TDC consecutively treated with PEI indicate an 80% success rate, without any relevant side effects [52]. In this study, the main technical limitation of PEI in TDG, i.e., a too viscous content of the cyst, has been effectively managed by using a large bore needle (14–16 gauge) and irrigating with saline the cyst walls [52]. In line with these data, at our institution, PEI is routinely used for TDC sclerotherapy with durable results (Fig. 14.6). Thus, PEI should be considered as an alternative option to surgery in patients with TDC.

"True" Parathyroid (PT) cysts are nonfunctioning lesion, derived from embryological remnants [53, 54]. They are commonly viewed as rarely occurring lesions, with less than 300

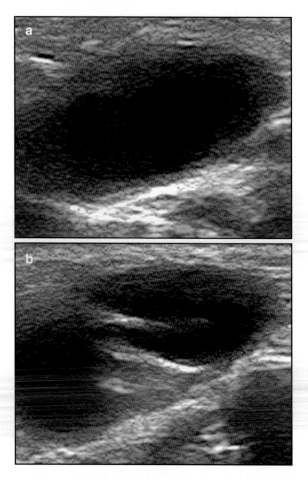

FIG. 14.6. PEI procedure performed in a 21-year girl with a small, yet spontaneously recurring, thyroglossal duct cyst (18×14×10 mm, volume = 1.3 mL) (**a**). As expected, the fluid content was quite viscous and its complete drainage was not possible, notwithstanding a 16 gauge needle was used. Partial fluid aspiration was followed by the injection of a small amount of ethanol and subsequent rinsing of the cyst consent (**b**, **c**). At the end of the maneuver, US texture of the lesion is inhomogenous, with minor anechoic portions (**d**).

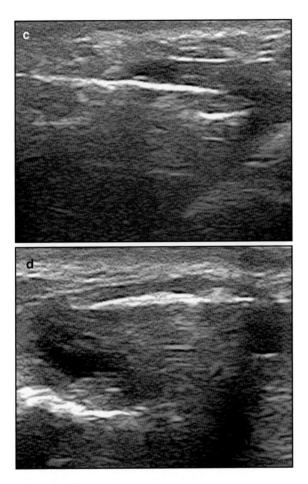

Fɪɢ. 14.6. (continued)

cases reported in the literature; yet, their frequency is likely to be underestimated. Firstly, PT cysts are often deeply located, and not clinically evident at inspection and/or palpation; secondly, they are easily mistaken for thyroid cysts [55]. Interestingly, detection of microcystic changes in otherwise normal parathyroid glands is a frequent finding at autopsy (40–50%), suggesting that the cystic component may be the final outcome of gradual retention of secretions [54]. In line with this observation, a PT cyst may occasionally correspond to a parathyroid adenoma featuring a fluid component [56]. US-guided FNA completed with parathyroid hormone (PTH) assay in the fluid within the cyst is critical for the diagnosis [56–59]. Similarly to thyroid cysts, PT cysts frequently recur after FNA; therefore, ethanol or other sclerosing agents (e.g., tetracycline) have been proposed as an alternative to surgical treatment [60–63]. According to the available evidence, PEI of PT cysts is an effective and safe procedure (Fig. 14.7). PEI has long been used for treating parathyroid hyperplasia in patients with chronic renal failure suffering from secondary or tertiary hyperparathyroidism with excellent results [64–67]. A recent study documented an 89.5 and 95.2% success rate in dialysis patients with recurrent and persistent hyperparathyroidism after subtotal parathyroidectomy, respectively [67]. Parathyroid adenomas in high-surgical risk patients with primary hyperparathyroidism have also been treated with PEI with partial success [68, 69].

PEI treatment of PTC neck recurrences (NR), first attempted at Mayo Clinic in the nineties [70, 71], has recently met a renewed interest, due to a number of reasons. Firstly, second surgery is always a challenging option, and in case the target lesion is located in the surgical bed, the patient is exposed to a higher risk of RLN injury and/or hypoparathyroidism [72]. Collateral damages of surgery need also to be weighted against the chance of treatment failure, as detection of small NR in the surgical field may prove to be difficult and disease eradication may be an elusive task. Secondly, the indolent course of most PTC recurrences tends to discourage the choice of an aggressive and potentially hazard-ous treatment. Unfortunately, radioiodine effectiveness is limited because NR often behave as non-iodine-avid lesions. At least four large series of thyroid cancer NR treated with PEI, all referring to patients with PTC, are currently available in the literature [73–76]. All these studies unanimously report excellent results, with a 16.5–66.0% rate of complete lesion regression and a remarkably low incidence of major side effects (Table 14.2). In the majority, if not the totality (86–100%), of patients, PEI was successful in con-trolling neck disease throughout the study period. Interestingly, efficacy of PEI sclerotherapy in the management of PTC NR does not apparently seem to be influenced by the structure (solid vs. cystic) of the target lesion, at variance with the experience col-lected in thyroid nodules. In conclusion, PEI can be considered a valuable therapeutic option for patients presenting with PTC NR, who are not amenable to second surgery and/or radioiodine therapy. Further studies are needed to balance the pros and cons

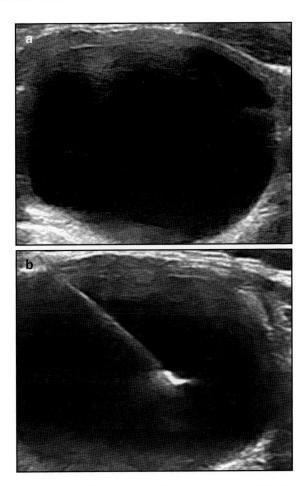

FIG. 14.7. PEI procedure on a left lower parathyroid gland cyst ($43 \times 41 \times 31$ mm, volume = 29.0 mL) (**a**). The watery cyst fluid is complete drained (**b**) and the cyst is filled with ethanol (**c**). One week after the maneuver, the lesion size is frankly reduced ($33 \times 31 \times 13$ mm, volume = 7.0 mL).

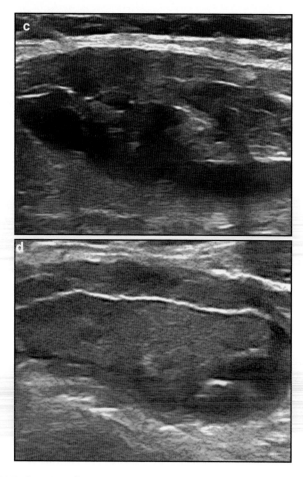

Fig. 14.7. (continued)

Table 14.2 PEI sclerotherapy in neck recurrences of papillary thyroid carcinoma

	NR (pts)	Mean follow-up (months)	Location (central vs. lateral neck compartment)	Basal lesion size	Mean volume decrease (%)	Complete regression (%)	RLN injury
Lewis et al. [71]	29 (14)	18 (2–77)	n.r.	492 mm³	95.9	31.3	0
Lin et al. [73]	24 (16)	24 (13–43)	11 vs. 13	9.9 (5.5–29.0) mm	37.5–43.5	16.5	1
Kim et al. [74]	47 (27)	26 (10–38)	7 vs. 40	678.8 ± 87.4 mm³	93.6 ± 12.6	44.7	1
Heilo et al. [76]	109 (63)	32 (3–72)	49 vs. 60	340 (10–3,560) mm³	n.r.	66.0	0

of ethanol sclerotherapy vs. other kinds of US interventional procedure in this clinical setting [72, 77].

References

1. Bean WJ. Renal cysts: treatment with alcohol. Radiology. 1981;138: 329–31.
2. Bean WJ, Rodan BA. Hepatic cysts: treatment with alcohol. AJR Am J Radiol. 1985;144:237–41.
3. Solbiati L, Giangrande A, DePra L, et al. Percutaneous ethanol injection of parathyroid tumors under US guidance: treatment for secondary hyperparathyroidism. Radiology. 1985;155:607–10.
4. Livraghi T, Giorgio A, Mario G, et al. Hepatocellular carcinoma and cirrhosis in 746 patients: long term results of percutaneous ethanol injection. Radiology. 1985;197:101–8.
5. Rossi R, Savastano S, Tommasselli AP, et al. Percutaneous computer tomography-guided ethanol injection in aldosterone-producing adrenal adrenocortical adenoma. Eur J Endocrinol. 1995;132:302–5.
6. Crescenzi A, Papini E, Pacella CM, et al. Morphological changes in a hyperfunctioning thyroid adenoma after percutaneous ethanol injection: histological, enzymatic and sub-microscopical alterations. J Endocrinol Invest. 1996;19:371–6.
7. Monzani F, Caraccio N, Basolo F, et al. Surgical and pathological changes after percutaneous ethanol injection therapy of thyroid nodules. Thyroid. 2000;10:1087–92.
8. Rozman B, Benze-Zigman Z, Tomic-Brzac H, et al. Sclerosation of thyroid cysts by ethanol. Period Biol. 1989;91:1116–8.
9. Livraghi T, Paracchi A, Ferrari C, et al. Treatment of autonomous thyroid nodule with percutaneous ethanol injection: preliminary results. Radiology. 1990;175:827–9.
10. Yasuda K, Ozaki O, Sugino K, et al. Treatment of cystic lesions of the thyroid by ethanol instillation. World J Surg. 1992;16(5):958–61.
11. Martino E, Murtas MI, Liviselli A, et al. Percutaneous intranodular ethanol injection for treatment of autonomously functioning thyroid nodules. Surgery. 1992;112:1161–5.
12. Papini E, Panunzi C, Pacella CM, et al. Percutaneous ultrasound-guided ethanol injection: a new treatment of toxic autonomously functioning thyroid nodules? J Clin Endocrinol Metab. 1993;76:411–6.
13. Pacini F. Role of percutaneous ethanol injection in management of nodular lesions of the thyroid gland. J Nucl Med. 2003;44:211–2.
14. Cooper DS, Doherty GM, Haugen BR, et al. Revised American Thyroid Association management guidelines for patients with thyroid nodules and differentiated thyroid cancer. Thyroid. 2009;19(11):1167–214.
15. Gharib H, Papini E, Paschke R, et al. American Association of Clinical Endocrinologists, Associazione Medici Endocrinologi, and EuropeanThyroid Association Medical Guidelines for Clinical Practice for the Diagnosis and Management of Thyroid Nodules. Endocr Pract. 2010;16 Suppl 1:1–43.

16. De Los Santos ET, Keyhani-Rofagha S, Cunningham JJ, et al. Cystic thyroid nodules: the dilemma of malignant lesions. Arch Intern Med. 1990;150:422–7.

17. Sheppard MC, Franklyn JA. Management of the single thyroid nodule. Clin Endocrinol. 1994;41:719–24.

18. Jensen F, Rasmussen SN. The treatment of thyroid cysts by ultrasonographically-guided fine needle aspiration. Acta Chir Scand. 1976;142:209–11.

19. Monzani F, Lippi F, Goletti O, et al. Percutaneous aspiration and ethanol sclerotherapy for thyroid cysts. J Clin Endocrinol Metab. 1994;78:800–2.

20. Antonelli A, Campatelli A, Di Vito A, et al. Comparison between ethanol sclerotherapy and emptying with injection of saline in treatment of thyroid cysts. Clin Investig. 1994;72(12):971–4.

21. Verde G, Papini E, Pacella CM, et al. Ultrasound guided percutaneous ethanol injection in the treatment of cystic thyroid nodules. Clin Endocrinol. 1994;41:719–24.

22. Zingrillo M, Torlontano M, Chiarella R, et al. Percutaneous ethanol injection may be a definitive treatment for symptomatic thyroid cystic nodules not treatable by surgery: five-year follow-up study. Thyroid. 1999;9:763–7.

23. Cho YS, Lee HK, Ahn IM, et al. Sonographically guided ethanol sclerotherapy for benign thyroid cysts: results in 22 patients. AJR Am J Roentgenol. 2000;174(1):213–6.

24. Del Prete S, Caraglia M, Russo D, et al. Percutaneous ethanol injection efficacy in the treatment of large symptomatic thyroid cystic nodules: ten-year follow-up of a large series. Thyroid. 2002;12:815–21.

25. Bennedbaek FN, Hegedus L. Treatment of recurrent thyroid cysts with ethanol: a randomized double blind controlled trial. J Clin Endocrinol Metab. 2003;88:5773–7.

26. Kim JH, Lee HK, Lee JH, et al. Efficacy of sonographically guided percutaneous ethanol injection for treatment of thyroid cysts versus solid thyroid nodules. AJR Am J Roentgenol. 2003;180:1623–726.

27. Valcavi R, Frasoldati A. Ultrasound-guided percutaneous ethanol injection therapy in thyroid cystic nodules. Endocr Pract. 2004;10:269–75.

28. Guglielmi R, Pacella CM, Bianchini AP, et al. Percutaneous ethanol injection treatment in benign thyroid lesions: role and efficacy. Thyroid. 2004;14:125–31.

29. Lee SJ, Ahn I-M. Effectiveness of percutaneous ethanol injection therapy in benign nodular and cystic thyroid disease: long-term follow-up experience. Endocr J. 2005;52:455–62.

30. Kanotra SP, Lateef M, Kirmani O. Non-surgical management of benign thyroid cysts: use of ultrasound-guided ethanol ablation. Postgrad Med J. 2008;84(998):639–43.

31. Sung JY, Kim YS, Choi H, et al. Optimum first-line treatment technique for benign cystic thyroid nodules: ethanol ablation or radiofrequency ablation. AJR Am J Roentgenol. 2011;196(2):W210–4.

32. Di Lelio A, Rivolta M, Casati M, et al. Treatment of autonomous thyroid nodules: value of percutaneous ethanol injection. AJR Am J Roentgenol. 1995;164:207–13.
33. Kim DW, Rho MH, Kim HJ, et al. Percutaneous ethanol injection for benign cystic thyroid nodules: is aspiration of ethanol-mixed fluid advantageous? AJNR Am J Neuroradiol. 2005;26(8):2122–7.
34. Livraghi T, Paracchi MA, Ferrari C, et al. Treatment of autonomous thyroid nodules with percutaneous ethanol injection—a 4 year experience. Radiology. 1994;190:529–33.
35. Ferrari C, Reschini E, Paracchi A. Treatment of the autonomous thyroid nodule: a review. Eur J Endocrinol. 1996;135(4):383–90.
36. Lippi F, Ferrari C, Manetti L, et al. Treatment of solitary autonomous thyroid nodules by percutaneous ethanol injection. Results of an Italian multicenter study. J Clin Endocrinol Metab. 1996;81:3261–4.
37. Monzani F, Caraccio N, Goletti O. Five year follow-up of percutaneous ethanol injection for the treatment of hyperfunctioning thyroid nodules: a study of 117 patients. Clin Endocrinol. 1997;46:9–15.
38. Zingrillo M, Torlontano M, Ghiggi MR, et al. Radioiodine and percutaneous ethanol injection in the treatment of large toxic thyroid nodule: a long-term study. Thyroid. 2000;10:985–9.
39. Del Prete S, Russo D, Caraglia M, et al. Percutaneous ethanol injection of autonomous thyroid nodules with a volume larger than 40 ml: three years of follow-up. Clin Radiol. 2001;56(11):895–901.
40. Tarantino L, Francica G, Sordelli I, et al. Percutaneous ethanol injection of hyperfunctioning thyroid nodules: long-term follow-up in 125 patients. AJR Am J Roentgenol. 2008;190:800–8.
41. Yano Y, Sugino K, Akaishi J, et al. Treatment of autonomously functioning thyroid nodules at a single institution: radioiodine therapy, surgery, and ethanol injection therapy. Ann Nucl Med. 2011;25(10): 749–54.
42. Zingrillo M, Modoni S, Conte M, et al. Percutaneous ethanol injection plus radioiodine versus radioiodine alone in the treatment of large toxic thyroid nodules. J Nucl Med. 2003;44:207–10.
43. Pishdad GR, Pishdad P, Pishdad R. Horner's syndrome as a complication of percutaneous ethanol treatment of thyroid nodule. Thyroid. 2001;21:327–8.
44. Regalbuto C, Le Moli R, Muscia V, et al. Severe Graves' ophthalmopathy after percutaneous ethanol injection in a nontoxic thyroid nodule. Thyroid. 2012;22(2):210–3.
45. Caraccio N, Goletti O, Lippolos PV, et al. Is percutaneous ethanol injection a useful alternative for the treatment of the cold benign thyroid nodule? Five years' experience. Thyroid. 1997;7:699–704.
46. Bennedbaek FN, Nielsen LK, Hegedus L. Effect of percutaneous ethanol injection therapy versus suppressive doses of l-thyroxine on benign solitary sold cold nodules: a randomized trial. J Clin Endocrinol Metab. 1998;83:830–5.
47. Bennendbaek FN, Hegedus L. Percutaneous ethanol injection therapy in benign solitary cold thyroid nodules: a randomized trial comparing one injection with three injections. Thyroid. 1999;9:225–33.

48. Mondin V, Ferlito A, Muzzi E, et al. Thyroglossal duct cyst: personal experience and literature review. Auris Nasus Larynx. 2008;35(1): 11–25.

49. Clark OH. Parathyroid cysts. Am J Surg. 1978;35:395–402.

50. Fukumoto K, Kojima T, Tomonari H, et al. Ethanol injection sclerotherapy for Baker's cysts, thyroglossal duct cysts, and branchial cleft cysts. Ann Plast Surg. 1994;33:615–9.

51. Baskin HJ. Percutaneous ethanol injection of thyroglossal duct cysts. Endocr Pract. 2006;12:355–7.

52. Kim SM, Baek JH, Kim YS, et al. Efficacy and safety of ethanol ablation for thyroglossal duct cysts. AJNR Am J Neuroradiol. 2011;32:306–9.

53. Clark OH, Okerlund MD, Cavalieri RR, et al. Diagnosis and treatment of thyroid parathyroid and thyroglossal duct cysts. J Clin Endocrinol Metab. 1979;48:983–8.

54. Ippolito G, Fausto Palazzo F, Sebag F, et al. A single institution 25-year review of true parathyroid cysts. Lagenbecks. Arch Surg. 2006;391: 13–8.

55. Ujiki MB, Nayar R, Sturgeon C, et al. Parathyroid cyst: often mistaken for a thyroid cyst. World J Surg. 2007;31:60–4.

56. Frasoldati A, Valcavi R. Challenges in neck ultrasonography: lymphadenopathy and parathyroid glands. Endocr Pract. 2004;10(3):261–8.

57. Pacini F, Antonelli A, Lari R, et al. Unsuspected parathyroid cysts diagnosed by measurement of thyroglobulin and parathyroid hormone concentration in fluid aspirates. Ann Intern Med. 1985;102:793–4.

58. Silverman JF, Khazanie PG, Norris HT, et al. Parathyroid hormone (PTH) assay of parathyroid cysts examined by fine-needle aspiration biopsy. Am J Clin Pathol. 1986;86:776–80.

59. Prinz RA, Peters JR, Kane JM, et al. Needle aspiration of nonfunctioning parathyroid cysts. Am Surg. 1990;56(7):420–2.

60. Okamura K, Ikenoue H, Sato K, et al. Sclerotherapy for benign parathyroid cysts. Am J Surg. 1992;163:344–5.

61. Sanchez A, Carretto H. Treatment of a nonfunctioning parathyroid cysts with tetracycline injection. Head Neck. 1993;15:263–5.

62. Akel M, Salti I, Azar ST. Successful treatment of parathyroid cyst using ethanol sclerotherapy. Am J Med Sci. 1999;317:50–2.

63. Baskin HJ. New applications of thyroid and parathyroid ultrasound. Minerva Endocrinol. 2004;29:195–206.

64. Solbiati L, Giangrande A, Pra LD, et al. Ultrasound-guided percutaneous fine-needle ethanol injection into parathyroid glands in secondary hyperparathyroidism. Radiology. 1985;155:607–10.

65. Fugakawa M, Kitaoga M, Tominaka Y, et al. Guidelines for percutaneous ethanol injection therapy of the parathyroid glands in chronic dialysis patients. Nephrol Dial Transplant. 2003;18 Suppl 3:31–3.

66. Douthat WG, Cardozo G, Garay G, et al. Use of percutaneous ethanol injection therapy for recurrent secondary hyperparathyroidism after subtotal parathyroidectomy. Int J Nephrol. 2011;2011:246734.

67. Chen HH, Lin CJ, Wu CJ, et al. Chemical ablation of recurrent and persistent secondary hyperparathyroidism after subtotal parathyroidectomy. Ann Surg. 2011;253(4):786–90.

68. Cercueil JP, Jacob D, Verges B, et al. Percutaneous ethanol injection into parathyroid adenomas: mid- and long-term results. Eur Radiol. 1998;8:1565–9.
69. Harman CR, Grant CS, Hay ID, et al. Indications, technique and efficacy of alcohol injection of enlarged parathyroid glands in patients with primary hyperparathyroidism. Surgery. 1998;124:1011–20.
70. Hay ID, Charboneau JW. The coming of age of ultrasound-guided percutaneous ethanol ablation of selected neck nodal metastases in well-differentiated thyroid carcinoma. J Clin Endocrinol Metab. 2011;96:2717–20.
71. Lewis BD, Hay ID, Charboneau JW, et al. Percutaneous ethanol injection for treatment of cervical lymph node metastases in patients with papillary thyroid carcinoma. AJR Am J Roentgenol. 2002;178:699–704.
72. Monchik JM, Donatini G, Iannuccilli J, et al. Radiofrequency ablation and percutaneous ethanol injection treatment for recurrent local and distant well-differentiated thyroid carcinoma. Ann Surg. 2006;244:296–304.
73. Lim CY, Yum JS, Lee J, et al. Percutaneous ethanol injection therapy for locally recurrent papillary thyroid carcinoma. Thyroid. 2007;17:347–50.
74. Kim BM, Kim MJ, Kim EK, et al. Controlling recurrent papillary thyroid carcinoma in the neck by ultrasonography-guided percutaneous ethanol injection. Eur Radiol. 2008;18:835–42.
75. Sohn YM, Hong SW, Kim EK, et al. Complete eradication of metastatic lymph node after percutaneous ethanol injection therapy: pathologic correlation. Thyroid. 2009;19:317–9.
76. Heilo A, Sigstad E, Fagerlid KH, et al. Efficacy of ultrasound-guided percutaneous ethanol injection treatment in patients with a limited number of metastatic cervical lymph nodes from papillary thyroid carcinoma. J Clin Endocrinol Metab. 2011;96(9):2750–5.
77. Baek JH, Kim YS, Sung JY, Choi H, Lee JH. Locoregional control of metastatic well-differentiated thyroid cancer by ultrasound-guided radiofrequency ablation. AJR Am J Roentgenol. 2011;197:W331–6.

CHAPTER 15

Ultrasound-Guided FNA and Molecular Markers for Optimization of Thyroid Nodule Management

Daniel S. Duick

Thyroid nodules are a common clinical problem. The prevalence range by palpation is 3–7%. Imaging with thyroid ultrasonography detects numerous additional nodules with prevalence rate ranging from 20 to 76% of the general adult population [1]. The prevalence risk for malignancy in a thyroid nodule is less than 5% [2]. A risk-based strategy has been developed to evaluate thyroid nodules and includes: clinical history and physical examination; serum TSH assay; and high-resolution, diagnostic ultrasonography. High-resolution ultrasonography enhances thyroid nodule selection and the need for fine needle aspiration (FNA) selection by sonographically defining size, consistency, and features suggestive of malignancy. [1].

Thyroid nodule FNA, especially with ultrasound guidance (UGFNA), enhances the yield of interpretable, nodular-aspirated material for cytologic interpretation by 3–5-fold over simple FNA without ultrasound guidance. UGFNA results in about 70–75% of nodules being classified as cytologically benign and approximately 4–5% as malignant [1]. This leaves a large pool of 20–25% of FNA samples, which are characterized as "indeterminate" by cytopathologic interpretation. Based on the Bethesda System For Reporting Thyroid Cytopathology, these indeterminate FNAs are cytologically categorized and risk-ranked (% risk of malignancy) as: atypical cells or follicular lesion of undetermined significance (FLUS) 5–10%; follicular neoplasm (FN) or suspicious for FN

H.J. Baskin et al. (eds.), *Thyroid Ultrasound and Ultrasound-Guided FNA*, **347**
DOI 10.1007/978-1-4614-4785-6_15,
© Springer Science+Business Media, LLC 2013

15–30% and Hurthle cell neoplasm (HCN) or suspicious for HCN 15–45%; and suspicious for malignancy 60–75% [3]. In an updated, multicenter meta-review of 8,937 resected thyroid nodules, cytology and histopathology revealed that two thirds of indeterminate nodules were benign with an average yield for malignancy of 34% [4]. Therefore, the FNA indeterminate group presents a challenging problem from a diagnostic standpoint and a great need to better characterize nodule status preoperatively in order to enhance management strategy and avoid unnecessary surgery.

Many centers have reported their experience with immunohistological studies in an attempt to differentiate a benign vs. malignant diagnosis from indeterminate FNA specimens [5, 6]. The major problem with immunohistological markers including, but not limited to, galectin-3, fibronectin-1, HBME-1, cytokeratin-19, and CITED-1, either individually or as panels is a lack of sensitivity and specifically to differentially characterize the FNA indeterminate cytopathologic subgroups of atypia/FLUS from FN/HCN or from suspicious for malignancy categories. Additionally, there is significant overlap of immunohistologic markers between cytopathologically indeterminate nodules and differentiated thyroid cancer [7, 8].

In the past decade, there has been a progressive interest in the characterization of malignancies by mutation detection. Somatic mutations are present in approximately 42% of papillary thyroid cancer (PTC) and 65% of follicular thyroid cancer. Additionally, technologies have advanced in the ability to acquire, transport, store, retrieve, and detect somatic mutations from thyroid nodule FNA-derived cells [9]. Initial studies centered mostly around one mutation detection, BRAF, which approaches 100% predictability for PTC and a few studies for the gene rearrangements, RET/PTC and PAX8/PPARg. More recent studies have analyzed various combinations or a panel of mutations (e.g., 2–6 or more somatic mutations) including BRAF, RAS, RET/PTC, and PAX8/PPARg and other markers [9].

In a retrospective review of 20 previous publications on FNA of thyroid nodules and molecular markers, the authors selected four larger studies with data derived from panels of somatic mutations performed on thyroid nodules with cytologically indeterminate diagnoses. Additionally, these studies correlated FNA diagnoses, mutation detection rates, and the final surgical histopathologic diagnoses [10].

Noteworthy was the "suspicious for malignancy" subgroup (2 of the 4 studies reported in the indeterminate category) that was excluded from the analysis. In virtually all studies, the "suspicious for malignancy" has a much higher risk for malignancy and therefore enhances sensitivity and specificity reporting. The authors then combined and recalculated the false positive, false negative, sensitivity, and specificity from these four studies to primarily produce a larger analysis of mutation panels in the atypica/FLUS and FN/HCN subgroups.

There were 243 operated, indeterminate nodules with histologic correlation and the rate for malignancy was 27.6% ($N = 67$) with 63/67 representing PTC or follicular variant of papillary thyroid cancer (FVPTC). The combined means and (ranges) were: false positive/FP = 0.25, (0–4); false negative/FN = 9 [1–21]; sensitivity = 63.7% (38–85.7%); and specificity = 98% (95–100%) for the reanalyzed four studies [10].

More recently, a large, multi-institutional experience was reported on 1,056 consecutive thyroid FNA samples with indeterminate cytology [11]. There were 967 (92%) samples adequate for determination of BRAF, RAS, RET/PTC, and PAX8-PPARg [11]. FNA cytology subgroups included: atypia/FLUS; FN; suspicious for FN or HCN; and suspicious for malignancy. There were 497 patients (531 nodule samples) who underwent thyroidectomy and data was analyzed and correlated for cytology, histologic diagnosis, and molecular mutation studies. Results of this data are as follows:

1. Atypia/FLUS: 247 samples (malignant/benign = 35/212; mutation +/− =22/13; sensitivity/specificity was 63% and 99% with a NPV of 94%, respectively.
2. FN/HCN or suspicious FN/HCN: 214 samples (malignant/benign = 58/156; mutations +/− = 33/25; and sensitivity/specificity was 57% and 97% with a NPV of 86%, respectively.
3. Suspicious for malignancy: 52 samples (malignant/benign = 28/24; mutations +/− = 19/9; and sensitivity/specificity was 68% and 96% with a NPV of 72%, respectively.

There were 121 malignancies diagnosed from the 513 specimens. Seventy-four mutation positive and 47 mutation negative cancers were represented in all three subgroups. The risk for a cancer mutation negative status was 6%, 14%, and 28% for the indeterminate subgroups of atypia/FLUS, FN/HCN, and suspicious for malignancy, respectively.

RAS determination was most prevalent in the malignancy group, but there was low-level detection of RAS in each of the benign subgroups as well and this has been previously reported [12, 13]. The presence of BRAF confirmed the presence of papillary cancer with 100% predictability. Of the 74 mutation positive malignancies, three were PAX8/PPARg and 1 RET/PPC.

A surgical management approach was recommended based on testing of the mutations as follows; a mutation positive patient should undergo total thyroidectomy based on the cancer risk of 88%, 87%, and 95% in each indeterminate subgroup, respectively. For mutation negative patients, lobectomy was recommended as the first procedure in the suspicious for FN/HCN and the suspicious for malignancy subgroups. In the atypia/FLUS subgroup, the overall cancer rate for mutation negative status was 6%. In this subgroup, a lobectomy was recommended vs. ultrasound observation with or without a repeat FNA [11].

A novel, alternative approach for evaluating FNA indeterminate thyroid nodules was the development of a gene expression classifier (GEC) utilizing high-dimensionality genomic data to molecularly categorize thyroid nodules [14]. The GEC was based on assessment for genomic wide expression levels of more than 247,000 mRNA transcripts and FNA samples from 315 thyroid nodules subsequently proven to be histopathologically benign or malignant. An algorithm was developed and tested on more than 400 samples and tested again on two independent sample sets to assess its performance. The GEC is comprised of mRNA transcripts from 142 genes representing well known cancer biologic pathways, some additionally not previously implicated in cancer. These GEC genes encode proteins involved in cellular metabolism, apoptosis, tumor growth and inhibition, as well as transcription regulation. Standard testing of the GEC has been observed to have a 96% NPV for malignancy [14].

The GEC was developed to optimize surgical selection and avoid unnecessary surgery by excluding asymptomatic benign nodules, and as a corollary, enhance the surgical pool with malignant nodules.

A theoretical, cost-effectiveness model has been reported utilizing the GEC [15]. In the United States annually, there are approximately 75,000 operations for FNA, cytologically indeterminate nodules resulting in the resection of 25,000 malignancies. The model suggests that utilization of the GEC in the FNA cytologically indeterminate group (17% of 450,000 FNAs that occur annually) could result in a 74% reduction in surgical procedures performed in patients with benign nodules. The ramifications of both the avoidance of unnecessary surgical procedures and the potential for significant cost savings in healthcare dollars by utilizing the GEC will require validation of the theoretical model in clinical trials as well as clinical practice experience [15].

More recently, numerous reports focused on microRNA (miRNA or miR) have proliferated in all forms of cancer including malignant thyroid nodules. MicroRNA are short RNA, noncoding molecules averaging only 22 nucleotides in length. These miRNA function as regulators, usually negative, for the expression of protein-encoding genes and are involved in cell development, apoptosis, growth, immune response, and may act as tumor suppressor genes or oncogenes. Dysregulation of miRNAs, and specifically different miRNAs, has been described in various thyroid cancers including papillary (PTC), follicular (FTC), and anaplastic thyroid cancer (ATC) [16–18]. Also reported are different levels of miRNAs in different types of thyroid cancers, suggesting that these various cancers harbor specific signatures of miRNA expression [19, 20].

Research continues to evolve on the diagnostic utility of miRNAs from FNAs of thyroid nodules. MicroRNAs can characterize aberrantly activated metabolic pathways in malignant thyroid tumors [21, 22]. MicroRNAs can create variations of functionally active, new miRNAs from their native miRNA by changing the structures of precursors and also by modifying sequencing responsible for targeting mRNA [23]. MicroRNAs have complex interactions with SNPs (single nucleotide polymorphisms) that modify the miRNA's precursor mRNA and result in new and different miRNAs with altered functional roles. The latter is also an explanation for the hereditary predisposition to thyroid cancer [22, 24].

In summary, the approach and management of thyroid nodules still remains in the hands of decision-making clinicians. Currently, molecular test panels are available which can aid in the decision-making process for the management of FNA-derived, cytologically indeterminate thyroid nodules. Continuing research, refinement, and validation of these and newer tests in development should help the clinician in the very near future to further hone in on the optimum diagnosis and management of indeterminate thyroid nodules in particular and thyroid cancer in general.

References

1. Gharib H, Papini E, Paschke R, Duick DS, Valcavi R, Hegedüs L, et al. AACE/AME/ETA task force on thyroid nodules. Endocr Pract. 2010;16 Suppl 1:1–43.
2. Hegedüs L. Clinical practice. The thyroid nodule. N Engl J Med. 2004;351(17):1764–71.
3. Cibas ES, Ali SZ. The Bethesda system for reporting thyroid cytopathology. Thyroid. 2009;19(11):1159–65.
4. Wang CC, Friedman L, Kennedy GC, Wang H, Kebebew E, Steward DL, et al. A large multicenter correlation study of thyroid nodule cytopathology and histopathology. Thyroid. 2011;21(3):243–51.
5. de Matos PS, Ferreira AP, de Oliveira Facuri F, Assumpção LV, Metze K, Ward LS. Usefulness of HBME-1, cytokeratin 19 and galectin-3 immunostaining in the diagnosis of thyroid malignancy. Histopathology. 2005;47(4):391–401.

6. Saggiorato E, De Pompa R, Volante M, Cappia S, Arecco F, Dei Tos AP, et al. Characterization of thyroid 'follicular neoplasms' in fine- needle aspiration cytological specimens using a panel of immunohistochemical markers: a proposal for clinical application. Endocr Relat Cancer. 2005;12(2):305–17.

7. Faggiano A, Caillou B, Lacroix L, Talbot M, Filetti S, Bidart JM, et al. Functional characterization of human thyroid tissue with immunohistochemistry. Thyroid. 2007;17(3):203–11.

8. Freitas BC, Cerutti JM. Genetic markers differentiating follicular thyroid carcinoma from benign lesions. Mol Cell Endocrinol. 2010;321(1):77–85.

9. Eszlinger M, Paschke R. Molecular fine-needle aspiration biopsy diagnosis of thyroid nodules by tumor specific mutations and gene expression patterns. Mol Cell Endocrinol. 2010;322(1–2):29–37.

10. Ferraz C, Eszlinger M, Paschke R. Current state and future perspective of molecular diagnosis of fine-needle aspiration biopsy of thyroid nodules. J Clin Endocrinol Metab. 2011;96(7):2016–26.

11. Nikiforov YE, Ohori NP, Hodak SP, Carty SE, LeBeau SO, Ferris RL, et al. Impact of mutational testing on the diagnosis and management of patients with cytologically indeterminate thyroid nodules: a prospective analysis of 1056 FNA samples. J Clin Endocrinol Metab. 2011;96(11):3390–7.

12. Ezzat S, Zheng L, Kolenda J, Safarian A, Freeman JL, Asa SL. Prevalence of activating ras mutations in morphologically characterized thyroid nodules. Thyroid. 1996;6(5):409–16.

13. Vasko VV, Gaudart J, Allasia C, Savchenko V, Di Cristofaro J, Saji M, et al. Thyroid follicular adenomas may display features of follicular carcinoma and follicular variant of papillary carcinoma. Eur J Endocrinol. 2004;151(6):779–86.

14. Chudova D, Wilde JI, Wang ET, Wang H, Rabbee N, Egidio CM, et al. Molecular classification of thyroid nodules using high-dimensionality genomic data. J Clin Endocrinol Metab. 2010;95(12):5296–304.

15. Li H, Robinson KA, Anton B, Saldanha IJ, Ladenson PW. Cost-effectiveness of a novel molecular test for cytologically indeterminate thyroid nodules. J Clin Endocrinol Metab. 2011;96(11):E1719–26.

16. He H, Jazdzewski K, Li W, Liyanarachchi S, Nagy R, Volinia S, et al. The role of microRNA genes in papillary thyroid carcinoma. Proc Natl Acad Sci USA. 2005;102(52):19075–80.

17. Pallante P, Visone R, Ferracin M, Ferraro A, Berlingieri MT, Troncone G, et al. MicroRNA deregulation in human thyroid papillary carcinomas. Endocr Relat Cancer. 2006;13(2):497–508.

18. Visone R, Pallante P, Vecchione A, Cirombella R, Ferracin M, Ferraro A, et al. Specific microRNAs are downregulated in human thyroid anaplastic carcinomas. Oncogene. 2007;26(54):7590–5.

19. Weber F, Teresi RE, Broelsch CE, Frilling A, Eng C. A limited set of human MicroRNA is deregulated in follicular thyroid carcinoma. J Clin Endocrinol Metab. 2006;91(9):3584–91.

20. Sheu SY, Grabellus F, Schwertheim S, Worm K, Broecker-Preuss M, Schmid KW. Differential miRNA expression profiles in variants

of papillary thyroid carcinoma and encapsulated follicular thyroid tumours. Br J Cancer. 2010;102(2):376–82.

21. Mazeh H, Mizrahi I, Halle D, Ilyayev N, Stojadinovic A, Trink B, et al. Development of a microRNA-based molecular assay for the detection of papillary thyroid carcinoma in aspiration biopsy samples. Thyroid. 2011;21(2):111–8.

22. de la Chapelle A, Jazdzewski K. MicroRNAs in thyroid cancer. J Clin Endocrinol Metab. 2011;96(11):3326–36.

23. Starega-Roslan J, Krol J, Koscianska E, Kozlowski P, Szlachcic WJ, Sobczak K, et al. Structural basis of microRNA length variety. Nucleic Acids Res. 2011;39:257–68.

24. Jazdzewski K, Liyanarachchi S, Swierniak M, Pachucki J, Ringel MD, Jarzab B, et al. Polymorphic mature microRNAs from passenger strand of pre- miR-146a contribute to thyroid cancer. Proc Natl Acad Sci USA. 2009;106(5):1502–5.

CHAPTER 16
Ultrasound Elastography of the Thyroid

Robert A. Levine

It has long been recognized that palpably hard thyroid nodules are suspicious for cancer [1]. Conventional gray-scale ultrasound provides information regarding characteristics such as shape, echogenicity, edge definition, calcification, and vascular flow, which have been shown to be correlated with risk of cancer. However, it does not provide direct information corresponding to the hardness of a nodule. Elastography is a technique that utilizes ultrasound to analyze the stiffness of a nodule by measuring the amount of compression that occurs when the nodule is subjected to external pressure. The technique was described two decades ago, but the first report of application to thyroid nodules appeared in 2007 [2]. A number of subsequent studies have shown that elastography can provide additional information regarding the probability of malignancy in a nodule [3].

Multiple techniques have been employed to provide external pressure and strain to a nodule. The most common technique is manually applying external pressure using the ultrasound transducer, after placing a linear transducer over the region of interest. An alternative technique uses pulsation from the carotid artery as the compression source [4]. Multiple sites within and around the nodule are analyzed, and the ultrasound software compares the deformation of the nodule to the surrounding tissue.

Presently there are two major techniques for interpretation of elastography data. In the most commonly utilized technique, the relative stiffness is shown on a color display, superimposed on a B-mode image (Fig. 16.1). For statistical analysis, the

H.J. Baskin et al. (eds.), *Thyroid Ultrasound and Ultrasound-Guided FNA*, **355**
DOI 10.1007/978-1-4614-4785-6_16,
© Springer Science+Business Media, LLC 2013

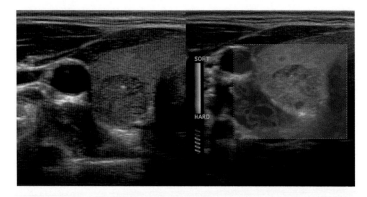

FIG. 16.1. This nodule has a hypoechoic echotexture and a possible microcalcification, but otherwise does not have a highly suspicious grayscale appearance. The elastogram shows it to have hard regions. FNAB and surgical pathology revealed a papillary carcinoma.

qualitative information provided on the color display is then assigned a numerical value (color score) corresponding to a stiffness index. Reproducibility of the numerical value is a limitation of this operator dependent technique. Alternatively, a strain ratio may be calculated by dividing the mean strain within a lesion by the mean strain in the surrounding tissue [5]. This semiquantitative method has better reproducibility than the color score, but still requires operator input in selecting both the boundaries of the lesion and the surrounding tissues, leading to some degree of subjective imprecision [6].

Recently, shear wave elastography has been introduced as a technique that does not require manual compression. Utilizing a separate ultrasonic pulse (the shear wave), the change in wave propagation speed is tracked to obtain an elasticity value. It is operator independent, reproducible, and quantitative [7].

Ultrasound elastography has been used to analyze nodules and predict malignant potential in breast [8, 9], prostate [10], pancreas, and lymph nodes [11]. It has been used to measure liver fibrosis [12], as well as stiffness of cardiac tissue following myocardial infarction. It remains an ancillary technique in these organs with clinical application still predominantly in the research setting.

Early experience with breast nodules demonstrated promise for elastography in predicting malignancy. An early large study looking at breast elastography demonstrated a sensitivity of 86% and a specificity of 90% [8]. A recent study reported a sensitivity of 69.5% and a specificity of 83.1% [9]. The authors demonstrated the specificity to exceed that of conventional B-mode sonography, reducing the false positive rate. However, the false negative rate exceeded 30%, casting doubt as to whether a negative finding would be sufficient to eliminate the need for biopsy of a breast nodule.

In an early study of thyroid elastography, Rago at al. [13] reported results of real-time ultrasound elastography in 96 consecutive patients with a solitary thyroid nodule undergoing surgery for either compressive symptoms or suspicion of malignancy on a prior fine needle aspiration biopsy. Tissue stiffness was scored from 1 to 5 based on subjective analysis of the elastogram color image. They reported that scores of 1 or 2 were found in 49 cases, all benign lesions. A score of 3 was found in 13 cases with one case of carcinoma, and 12 from benign lesions. Thirty cases had scores of 4 or 5 and all were carcinomas. They reported a sensitivity of 97% and a specificity of 100% for a score of 4 or 5 to predict malignancy.

Lyshchik et. al. [14] performed a prospective study involving 52 thyroid nodules in 31 consecutive patients. Of the 52 nodules, 22 were malignant and 30 were benign. Both real-time elastography and off-line processed ultrasound elastograms were utilized. The strain of the nodule was compared to the strain of the surrounding normal thyroid tissue. The results for the off-line strain ratio analysis were far superior to the real-time studies. They reported that the off-line processed elastogram was the strongest independent predictor of thyroid gland malignancy, with 96% specificity and 82% sensitivity. However, they also reported that off-line strain image processing is time consuming and labor intensive.

In a recent meta-analysis, Bojunga [15] compiled data from eight clinical studies (including both of the above studies) analyzing 639 nodules in 530 patients. The overall sensitivity was 92% and specificity was 90%. The false negative rate was 10.4%, misclassifying 16 of 153 cancers, including four of nine follicular carcinomas.

Several recent studies have looked at whether elastography will be useful in patients with a prior indeterminate thyroid biopsy. Rago et al [16] studied 142 nodules with a prior FNAB cytology interpreted as indeterminate and found a sensitivity of 96.8% and specificity of 91.8%. Only one of 31 carcinomas (3.2%) was misclassified in this study. However, in a subsequent report from the same institution, Lippolis [17] reported contradictory results in 102 patients undergoing surgery for a nodule with a prior follicular biopsy. With very few nodules demonstrating high elasticity (low stiffness), they reported a sensitivity of 88.9% but a specificity of only 6%. The false positive rate was 89% (59/66) and the false negative rate was 11% (4/36). The discordant results observed in these two studies remain unexplained, but it emphasizes the fact that real-time elastography is a very subjective and user dependent process. Additional trials are underway to further assess the role of elastography in nodules with indeterminate biopsies and to assess the reproducibility of elastography data.

A number of modifications of technique have been proposed to improve the accuracy and reproducibility of elastography. As noted above, shear wave elastography provides a quantitative value without need for external pressure application by the sonographer and is a very promising technique. Calculation of the percentage of the nodule exhibiting a hard texture (hard area ratio) has been reported to have a greater area under the receiver operating characteristic curve than either the strain ratio or color score [6].

The general applicability of most of the studies reported thus far is limited due to selection bias. In the meta-analysis performed by Bojunga, the incidence of malignancy was 24% [15]. Most analyses report an incidence of malignancy of 2–5% in nodules selected for biopsy, and the incidence of malignancy is much lower in unselected nodules [1]. The predictive value of a test varies with the incidence of malignancy in the population studied and elastography will need to be studied in unselected populations with thyroid nodules in order to determine its true predictive value.

A single study has evaluated the utility of elastography in assessment of cervical lymph nodes suspected of containing metastatic cancer. Lyshchik et. al. [11] examined 141 peripheral lymph nodes in 43 consecutive patients referred for surgical treatment of suspected thyroid or hypopharyngeal cancer. By comparing the strain of lymph nodes and surrounding neck muscles, a strain index was calculated. An index cutoff of 1.5 resulted in a 98% specificity and 85% sensitivity. The results were superior to conventional gray-scale ultrasound criteria utilizing the short to long axis ratio.

Figures 16.1–16.6 illustrate the images provided by elastography. Figure 16.1 shows a papillary carcinoma with a single microcalcification. Figure 16.2 shows a papillary carcinoma of the thyroid with psammomatous calcification. As would be expected, this nodule was very firm on physical examination. The figure shows that areas of the nodule are very hard and very suggestive of a malignant nodule. Note the scale at the right edge of the image indicating a color scale ranging from soft (SF) to hard (HD). Figure 16.3 shows a nodule with soft consistency on

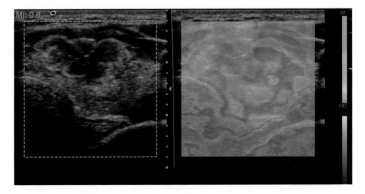

FIG. 16.2. This nodule has several suspicious features including peripheral microcalcifications, scalloped margins, and hypervascularity on power Doppler (not shown). The elastogram shows significant areas indicated as "Hard" (see scale located on the right of the image. HD = Hard, SF = Soft.). Surgical pathology confirmed a papillary carcinoma.

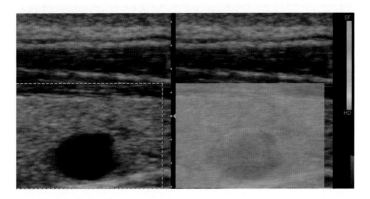

FIG. 16.3. This hypoechoic nodule appears very soft on elastography, suggesting a lower risk of malignancy.

the elastogram. Figures 16.4 and 16.5 are from a single patient. Bilateral nodules were present. The larger left (dominant) nodule had previously demonstrated benign aspiration cytology. It had a soft texture on elastography. The right sided nodule had more suspicious sonographic features (heterogeneous hypoechoic echotexture, irregular margins, and microcalcifications) as well as a hard texture at elastography and proved to be a papillary carcinoma. Figure 16.6 is from a 38-year-old male with diffusely multifocal

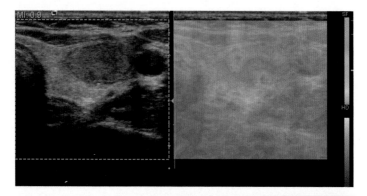

FIG. 16.4. This 34-year-old woman had bilateral nodules. The figure shows the left nodule, which was the larger of the two and was previously biopsied with benign cytology. The elastogram shows the nodule to be predominately soft.

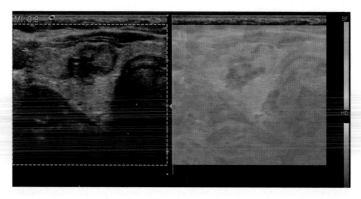

FIG. 16.5. In the same patient as Image 14.3, the right nodule was smaller, but had several suspicious features including a heterogeneous echotexture, irregular margins, and microcalcifications. The elastogram shows the nodule to have a hard composition. Pathology confirmed papillary carcinoma.

infiltrative tall cell variant of papillary carcinoma, stage T3N1BM0. Multiple areas of hard tissue are shown on the elastogram.

Not all nodules are amenable to elastography. Due to an inability of the ultrasound beam to penetrate the nodule, elastography cannot be performed on nodules with peripheral rim calcification. Complex nodules with a large cystic component may provide misleading results because the elasticity is more dependent on the

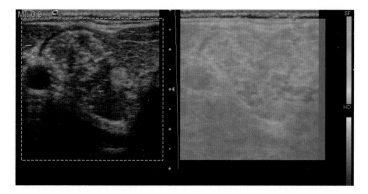

Fig. 16.6. This image is from a 38-year-old male with diffusely multifocal infiltrative tall cell variant of papillary carcinoma, stage T3N1BM0. Multiple areas of hard tissue are shown on the elastogram.

liquid content than the solid portion of the nodule. Small nodules probably can be measured accurately with elastography, but the limits of acceptable size have not been fully tested. Multinodular goiters with multiple confluent nodules without normal intervening thyroid parenchyma cannot be assessed by conventional elastography, but may be amenable to measurement with shear wave elastography. The impact of background Hashimoto's thyroiditis or other abnormalities of the thyroid parenchyma has not been adequately assessed.

There are two potential major roles for elastography in the analysis of thyroid nodules. The first is indicating the need for biopsy in a nodule that otherwise would be considered low suspicion and not undergo biopsy. Current guidelines state that nodules smaller than 1–1.5 cm with no suspicious features (indistinct margins, microcalcifications, taller than wide shape, extreme hypoechogenicity, or strong vascular flow) can be monitored without biopsy [1]. However, if the positive predictive value of elastography is high, an otherwise non-suspicious nodule demonstrated to be hard by elastography would be considered for biopsy. On the other hand, if the negative predictive value of elastography is adequate, it could be used to help determine which nodules can be safely observed without biopsy. Approximately 4% of the population has a palpable thyroid nodule, and over 50% have a small nodule detectable by ultrasound [1]. Clearly all nodules found by physical examination or incidentally during other neck studies cannot undergo fine needle biopsy. Any technique used to determine which nodules can be safely monitored without biopsy needs to have an extremely low false negative rate. Unfortunately, in most of the studies reported to date, the false negative rate is too high.

In summary, while the initial reports of elastography of thyroid lesions are very exciting, additional large studies on unselected populations with thyroid nodules are needed to determine whether the technique has sufficient sensitivity and negative predictive value to obviate the need for biopsy or surgery.

References

1. Cooper D, Doherty G, Haugen B, et al. Revised American Thyroid Association management guidelines for patients with thyroid nodules and differentiated thyroid cancer. Thyroid. 2009;19(11):1167–214.
2. Lyshchik A, Tatsuya H, Ryo A, et.al. (2004) Ultrasound elastography in differential diagnosis of thyroid gland tumors: initial clinical results. RSNA, Abstract.
3. Hegedus L. Can elastography stretch our understanding of thyroid histomorphology? J Clin Endocrinol Metab. 2010;95(12):5213–5.
4. Bae U, Dighe M, Dubinsky T, et al. Ultrasound thyroid elastography using carotid artery pulsation: preliminary study. J Ultrasound Med. 2007;26(6):797–805.
5. Xing P, Wu L, Zhang C, Li S, Liu C, Wu C. Differentiation of benign from malignant thyroid lesions – calculation of the strain ratio on thyroid sonoelastography. J Ultrasound Med. 2011;30:663–9.
6. Ding J, Cheng H, Ning C, Huang J, Zhang Y. Quantitative measurement for thyroid cancer characterization based on elastography. J Ultrasound Med. 2011;30:1259–66.
7. Sebag F, Vaillant-Lombard J, Berbis J, Griset V, Henry JF, Pent P, Oliver C. Shear wave elastography: a new ultrasound imaging mode for the differential diagnosis or benign and malignant thyroid nodules. J Clin Endocrinol Metab. 2010;95(12):5281–8.
8. Itoh A, Venu E, Tohno E, et al. Breast disease: clinical applications of US elastography for diagnosis. Radiology. 2006;239(2):341–50.
9. Navarro B, Ubeda B, Vallespi M, Wolf C, Casas L, Browne JL. Role of elastography in the assessment of breast lesions. J Ultrasound Med. 2011;30:313–21.
10. Pallwein L, Mitterberger M, Struve P, et al. Real-time elastography for detecting prostate cancer: preliminary experience. BJU Int. 2007; 100(1):42–7.
11. Lyshchik A, Higashi T, Asato R, et al. Cervical lymph node metastases: diagnosis at sonoelastography-initial experience. Radiology. 2007;243(1):258–67.
12. Friedrich-Rust M, Ong M, Herrman E, et al. Real-time elastography for noninvasive assessment of liver fibrosis in chronic viral hepatitis. Am J Roentgenol. 2007;188(3):758–64.
13. Rago T, Santini F, Scutari M, et al. Elastography: new developments in ultrasound for predicting malignancy in thyroid nodules. J Clin Endocrinol Metab. 2007;92:29–2922.

14. Lyshchik A, Higashi T, Asato R, et al. Thyroid gland tumor diagnosis at US elastography. Radiology. 2005;237(1):202–11.
15. Bojunga J, Herrmann F, Meyer G, Weber S, Zeuzem S, Freidrich-Rust M. Real time elastography for the differentiation of benign and malignant thyroid nodules. Thyroid. 2010;20:1145–50.
16. Rago T, Scutari M, Santini F, Loiacono V, Piaggi P, Di Coscio G, Basolo F, Berti P, Pinchero A, Vitti P. Real-time elastography: useful tool for refining the presurgical diagnosis in thyroid nodules with indeterminate or nondiagnostic cytology. J Clin Endocrinol Metab. 2010;95(12):5274–80.
17. Lippolis PV, Tognini S, Materazzi G, Polini A, Mancini R, Ambrosini CE, Dardano A, Basolo F, Seccia M, Miccoli P, Monzani F. Is elastography actually useful in the presurgical selection of thyroid nodules with indeterminate cytology? J Clin Endocrinol Metab. 2011; 96(11):e1826–30.

CHAPTER 17
Authoring Quality Ultrasound Reports

J. Woody Sistrunk and H. Jack Baskin, Sr

"What to leave out and what to leave in".....Bob Seger (Against the Wind)

FOREWORD

In the past decade since endocrinologist-performed thyroid ultrasound became mainstream, consider the impact this has meant to patients with thyroid and parathyroid disorders. The physician-performed ultrasound evaluation, ultrasound-guided FNA, and ultrasound thyroid cancer surveillance have changed thyroid and parathyroid disease management forever.

From the initial 14-page American Association of Clinical Endocrinologists Thyroid Ultrasound Course Syllabus that presented virtually all there was to know about thyroid ultrasound, to this present volume, much has changed with the concerned endocrinologist performing their own procedures.

With this relatively new science, inherent responsibilities exist. Quality measures such as American College of Endocrinology's Certification in Neck Ultrasound (ECNU) and American Institute of Ultrasound Medicine (AIUM) Practice Accreditation have been put in place. But keep in mind *neither certification nor accreditation will ever take the place of quality work*.

As endocrinologists performing thyroid ultrasound, one of the most difficult steps in the learning process is writing reports. A critical factor in generating a quality report is to have a desire and direction to create a meaningful and worthwhile report. It is a skill that requires practice in order to be clear and concise and yet not overwrite. Taking advantage of reviewing every report, yours

H.J. Baskin et al. (eds.), *Thyroid Ultrasound and Ultrasound-Guided FNA*, **365**
DOI 10.1007/978-1-4614-4785-6_17,
© Springer Science+Business Media, LLC 2013

as well as others, will help define the end result. Thyroid ultrasound reporting should yield a consistent product that shows the quality of the work done. Throughout this chapter, we hope to give an idea of what it takes to author a quality ultrasound report.

EXAMPLES OF WHAT TO AVOID

We have all seen poor reports that left unanswered questions that are unfortunately answered with a surgeon's knife. Below are actual ultrasound reports as examples of what to avoid. Hopefully, this will incite interest in the need to author quality reports. One must take responsibility for quality work.

- "There are multiple nonspecific hypodensities and small cystic nodules in the thyroid gland. Their appearance is nonspecific."How much more nonspecific can one be?
- "This solitary PULMONARY nodule has a differential diagnosis of carcinoma, adenoma, thyroiditis or hemorrhage." Close, but wrong organ.
- "Multiple bilateral solid nodules. None distinguishes itself as being different than any of the others and there is no dominant nodule. I recommend correlation with a nuclear medicine thyroid scan as most thyroid cancers are cold by nuclear medicine. If any cold nodule is determined to be present on the nuclear medicine study, then we will direct biopsy to that area." Money doesn't talk, it swears.....*Bob Dylan (It's Alright, Ma).*
- "Heterogeneous thyroid echotexture suggests thyroid cellular disease."Perhaps suggesting that not all thyroid glands are made of cells.
- "Multinodular thyroid gland likely related to a multinodular goiter"Rocket science!
- "Multiple small benign adenomatous nodulations are present in the gland, more on the left. No suspicious focus seen."

In order to write good reports one should read and critique every report they see. Learn from others good aspects of reporting, and then take that extra step to be even better. Consider your audience: the referring doctor—an ultrasound report is a demonstration of the quality of your work and dedication to the practice of thyroidology; the subsequent surgeon whose appropriate decision will depend upon your report; and yourself when you are performing serial follow-up. Table 17.1 outlines the elements of a diagnostic ultrasound report. Let us review each of these in detail.

1. *Identification Data.* Although not required for reports submitted for ECNU because of HIPPA regulations, it is

Table 17.1 Components of a thyroid ultrasound report [3]

		ECNU Requirement
1.	Identification data	No
2.	Indication for performing procedure	Yes
3.	Explanation of procedure	No
4.	Thyroid size (measurements)	Yes
5.	Thyroid description	Yes
6.	Description of pathology	Yes
7.	Impression	Yes
8.	Recommendations	Yes
9.	Cartoon	No

essential for those done in the course of practice. At a minimum it should include patient name, date of birth, ID number (social security or patient/clinic number), facility name, and date of procedure.

2. *Indication*. Aside from being necessary for third party payment, the indication guides the report. Consider the clinical question to be answered by ultrasound. Be succinct in giving the indication, but keep it brief. Examples are:

- "multinodular goiter"
- "diffuse thyroid enlargement"
- "hyperthyroidism"
- "right thyroid nodule found on CT"
- "history of papillary thyroid cancer in sister"

Occasionally, a more complicated indication is necessary such as "1.9 cm right tall cell papillary cancer, s/p total thyroidectomy and subsequent I^{131} therapy. T1b, N0, M0 (Stage I)," but always keep the indication brief and to the point.

3. *Explanation of Procedure*. This should be a simple overview of how the procedure is carried out. Examples would be:

- "Using physician-performed, real-time ultrasound limited to the thyroid gland and anterior neck, longitudinal and transverse images were obtained of both lobes and isthmus."
- "Using physician-performed, real-time ultrasound limited to the thyroid bed and neck including nodes (Levels I, II, III, IV, V, VI) longitudinal and transverse images were obtained."

There is no set number of ultrasound images required [1–3]. The number would be more for a sonographer taking images for the physician to read than it would be if the physician were performing the ultrasound in real-time. It would be even less if a video of the study were made. As a minimum one should have images of both lobes in the transverse and longitudinal views plus documentation of all pathology in three dimensions. Always ask yourself if enough images were obtained to answer the clinical question at hand for performing the procedure. NOTE: No one cares about the brand of ultrasound machine or the MHz of the probe. While details like these may have their place in NASCAR, they have no place in ultrasound reporting.

4. *Thyroid Size.* Clearly, thyroid size matters; however, no gold standard thyroid in a felt lined box exists in Helsinki, Finland, with which to compare. The size of a normal thyroid gland correlates with the amount of iodine in the diet. The United States is replete with dietary iodine, and the normal thyroid has anterior-posterior and transverse dimensions of 2 cm or less with a longitudinal dimension of 4.5–5.5 cm and weighs approximately15–20 g. In Europe which has less dietary iodine, the normal gland may be up to 40 g. Therefore, we measure each thyroid lobe in three planes (longitudinal, anterior-posterior and transverse) and the anterior–posterior of the isthmus. It is best to avoid words such as length, depth, width, etc. since these do not refer to a definite plane of measurement, and a limited vocabulary will yield more consistency in reporting. While you may calculate the volume of the thyroid, this has no routine role in clinical thyroidology and is considered optional. Measurements can be given in centimeters or millimeters, but be consistent throughout your report. A statement at the beginning of a report stating: "All measurements are in millimeters in the Longitudinal X Anterior-Posterior X Transverse planes" avoids having to do this after each measurement.

5. *Thyroid Description.* While we are often compelled to go directly to pathology, at this point it is prudent to make a concerted effort to pause and describe the thyroid parenchyma, including a check for increase in Doppler flow. This allows one to look at the "Big Picture" prior to focusing on pathology and leads to a more consistent reporting style. Additionally, other considerations of underlying disease states such as Hashimoto's thyroiditis, thyroid lymphoma or Graves' disease may be discovered that without thoughtful consideration would be lost in the search to find a thyroid

nodule. Begin your statement with "Overall" to make certain that the reader understands this is a summation statement of the gland. Examples would be:

- "Overall, the thyroid is symmetric with a homogeneous echotexture."
- "Overall, the thyroid gland is symmetrically enlarged, diffusely heterogeneous and hypervascular."
- "Overall, the thyroid gland is enlarged and asymmetric with a prominent right lobe; echotexture is homogeneous."

6. *Description of Pathology*. What did you see and where did you see it? Location is critical; the more descriptive the report is, the more reproducible your exam will be. No absolute convention exists, but we strongly recommend starting on the right and then move to the left. Nothing is more confusing in an ultrasound report than to describe nodules in an inconsistent pattern. Consistency equals quality. As a minimum divide the thyroid into upper, mid, and lower lobes as well as into lateral and medial to describe the location of a nodule. The isthmus is usually omitted unless it is enlarged or contains a nodule.

Nodules

In describing a nodule: Is it solid or cystic? Is it hypoechoic, hyperechoic, or isoechoic? Is it homogeneous or heterogeneous? By considering these three questions, an on-going process begins that will help identify suspicious or benign nodules while performing the study. Measure nodules in three dimensions and *do* calculate the volume because it is a more accurate measure to monitor the size of a nodule over time. Nodules that are taller than they are wide (Anterior-posterior > transverse) should be noted. Keep in mind that both benign and malignant nodules are still nodules. They are not lesions, masses, growths, hypodensities, polyps, goiters, areas, nodularities, geographic hypoechogenicities, or nodulations. They are just nodules! This actual example, "Impression—A 3.4 mm complex mass is seen in the right lobe" seems to be designed to create anxiety if read by the patient and could easily become an invitation for unnecessary surgery. Also do not confuse your reader with newly coined meaningless terms like inhomogeneous, nonhomogeneous, etc. Cysts can be subdivided into *simple cyst* (only cystic content), *complex cyst* (more cystic than solid material) and *complex nodule* (more solid than cystic material). As referenced in the 2009 American Thyroid Association guidelines, a *spongiform nodule* is defined as an "aggregation of multiple microcystic components in more than 50 % of the nodule volume is 99.7 % specific for identification of a benign thyroid nodule" [4]. If a nodule is seen that has this typical appearance, describing it as a spongiform nodule is helpful. It can be of critical importance in reassurance of the clinician and the patient.

Other nodule characteristics must also be noted when present. Calcifications can be broadly classified into eggshell calcifications, dense calcifications with posterior acoustic shadowing, or microcalcifications without shadowing. The borders of a nodule may be smooth with or without a halo, irregular, or infiltrative. Vascularity can be described as central or peripheral or one can use the Grades 1 through 4 described by Fukunari et al. [5] that has become a standard for description of Doppler flow in nodules. Finally, the presence of a comet tail artifact in a colloid nodule should always be mentioned. Like the spongiform nodule, it reduces the likelihood of malignancy to less than 1 %.

Lymph Nodes

An assumption is made with every neck ultrasound that an attempt was made to look at the lymph nodes. This is a cursory look, not lymph node mapping. Your report should reference it for completeness sake. If no nodes with a Short/Long Axis Ratio > 0.5 are seen, a summation statement in the impression can be: "No significant cervical adenopathy is seen." Any lymph node with an anterior–posterior dimension >0.5 cm and a Short/Long Axis Ratio >0.5 should be reported along with a note about the presence or absence of a hilar line, cystic necrosis (often revealed by posterior acoustic enhancement), and calcifications. Doppler flow is described as central along the hilar line or peripheral; the Grades used in evaluating nodules do not apply with lymph nodes. If a single node is seen of doubtful clinical significance, document that node in the body of the report. It may have importance later, particularly after the confirmation of malignancy with an FNA.

Lymph Node Mapping

Preoperative or postoperative node evaluation in thyroid cancer patients is much more comprehensive and a consistent protocol is of critical importance. Place a map (Fig. 2 on page 1,178 (2009) of the American Thyroid Association Guidelines) above your ultrasound machine, and refer to it with every description you make. Nodes are located in Levels, not zones. Although no absolute convention exists, mapping and reporting nodes are easier to interpret when a consistent pattern is followed. Start with the central neck (Level VI), then Level IA and IB of both sides of the neck. Continue to Right Levels IIA, IIB, III, IV, VA, and VB. Then examine Left IIA, IIB, III, IV, VA, and VB. The criteria mentioned above are used to identify suspicious nodes that may be malignant. The cartoon (Fig. 17.1) can be copied and used to diagram the size and location of suspicious lymph nodes for the surgeon.

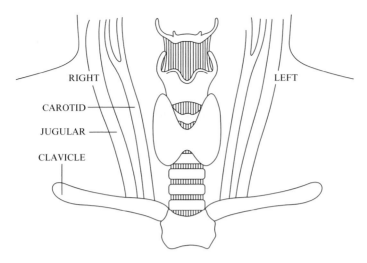

FIG. 17.1. AACE ECNU cartoon.

Parathyroid glands

Because normal parathyroid glands are seldom or never seen with ultrasound, those that are seen are enlarged and represent adenoma, hyperplasia, cyst, or carcinoma. They should be measured in three dimensions, lateralized right or left, and their location noted (i.e., posterior to thyroid, intrathyroidal, in thyro-thymic ligament, etc). State the echogenicity (almost always Hypoechoic) and describe the vascularity, especially the presence or absence of a polar artery.

7. *Impression.* One should not consider the impression as a chance to restate the entire body of your report; it is an *impression*, keep it brief. Some examples would be:

- "Prominent thyroid gland with a 2 cm solid, hypoechoic, heterogeneous nodule in the right lateral mid lobe."
- "The thyroid gland is surgically absent compatible with the clinical history of thyroidectomy and subsequent I131 therapy for papillary cancer."
- "Symmetrically enlarged diffusely heterogeneous goiter, compatible with the clinical history of Hashimoto's thyroiditis."

8. *Recommendations.* As part of the ECNU certification, recommendations should be included in the report e.g., "Recommend follow-up in one year" or "Correlation with thyroperoxidase antibody is recommended," The impression

and specific recommendations may be combined e.g., "A suspicious dominant nodule with microcalcifications is present in the left lobe; an UGFNA is recommended to confirm or rule out malignancy." This type of statement will benefit the referring physician and explains to the third party payer why the UGFNA is necessary.

9. *Cartoon.* While not required by ECNU or AIUM, a drawing demonstrating pathology may be of great help to the referring physician, the surgeon or the patient. Sketching the findings in the presence of the patient solidifies in the mind of the patient an overview of the pathology and its relevance. Using copies of Fig. 17.1 facilitates this.

WHAT NOT TO DO

Do not overwrite; avoid the use of *qualifiers*, words that are unnecessary, inappropriate and only serve to confuse or muddy the report. A nodule is not *rather* hypoechoic, it is hypoechoic. A lymph node is not *very* flat, it is flat with a Short/Long Axis Ratio <0.5. Avoid incriminating statements such as these actual examples:

- "A follow-up ultrasound is recommended every 3 months to ensure stability."
- "With Hashimoto's thyroiditis, development of lymphoma is possible; therefore follow-up on a regular basis, for instance annually"
- "Low density asymmetric nodule in the right lobe. The differential diagnosis for this would be adenoma, thyroiditis, carcinoma, or hemorrhage. Follow-up diagnostic scan may be of some further diagnostic benefit"

SUMMARY

An excellent ultrasound examination may come to naught if the ultrasound report is deficient. Extracting all the useful information from an ultrasound study and presenting it in a cohesive, concise manner is a skill that one develops with practice over time. As the science advances to include elastography, incorporating data from biometric material obtained by UGFNA to formulate decision making, and ultrasound-guided PEI and other ablative procedures; ultrasound reports will need to be expanded. Developing a firm foundation in writing reports is essential.

In this chapter we have attempted to outline our approach to writing an informative, constructive, and practical report. We urge that you critique other's reports as well as your own, constantly striving to improve; remember the *perfect* ultrasound report has yet to be written. Writing better ultrasound reports will improve your ultrasound examination techniques that, in turn, will improve your future reports. Consistency, quality and reproducibility are the hallmarks of a good report. Keep the vocabulary simple and remember the T-shirt that says "Help stamp out and eradicate superfluous redundancy."

References

1. Endocrine Certification in Neck Ultrasound (ECNU) Handbook. https://www.aace.com/files/CandidateHandbook.pdf
2. American Institute of Ultrasound in Medicine (AIUM) Practice guidelines for performance of a thyroid and parathyroid ultrasound examination. http://www.aium.org/ publications/guidelines/thyroid.pdf
3. American College of Radiology (ARC)—American Institute of Ultrasound in Medicine (AIUM) Practice guideline for the performance of a thyroid and parathyroid ultrasound examination. http://www.arc.org/SecondaryMainMenueCategories/qualitysafty/guidelines/us/usthyroidparathyroid.aspx
4. Cooper DS, et al. Revised American Thyroid Association management guidelines for patients with thyroid nodules and differentiated thyroid cancer. Thyroid. 2009;19:1167–214.
5. Fukunari N, et al. Clinical evaluation of color Doppler imaging for the differential diagnosis of thyroid follicular lesions. World J Surg. 2004;28(12):1261–5.

Index

H.J. Baskin et al. (eds.), *Thyroid Ultrasound and Ultrasound-Guided FNA*, **375**
DOI 10.1007/978-1-4614-4785-6,
© Springer Science+Business Media, LLC 2013

Printed in the United States of America